THERAPEUTIC COMMUNICATION
Knowing What to Say When

Other Books by PAUL L. WACHTEL

Psychoanalysis and Behavior Therapy: Toward an Integration

Resistance: Psychodynamic and Behavioral Approaches
(*Editor*)

The Poverty of Affluence: A Psychological Portrait
of the American Way of Life

Family Dynamics in Individual Psychotherapy:
A Guide to Clinical Strategies (*with Ellen F. Wachtel*)

Action and Insight

THERAPEUTIC COMMUNICATION
Knowing What to Say When

PAUL L. WACHTEL, Ph.D.
CUNY Distinguished Professor
City University of New York

With a Postscript by Ellen F. Wachtel, Ph.D.

THE GUILFORD PRESS
New York London

© 1993 Paul L. Wachtel
Published by The Guilford Press
A Division of Guilford Publications, Inc.
72 Spring Street, New York, NY 10012
www.guilford.com

Paperback edition 1998

Printed in the United States of America

This book is printed on acid-free paper.

Last digit is print number: 19   18   17   16   15   14   13   12   11

Library of Congress Cataloging-in-Publication Data

Wachtel, Paul L., 1940–
    Therapeutic communication : knowing what to say when /
Paul L. Wachtel
        p.   cm.
    Includes bibliographical references and index.
    ISBN-10: 0-89862-260-3   ISBN-13: 978-0-89862-260-7 (hc.)
    ISBN-10: 1-57230-416-2   ISBN-13: 978-1-57230-416-1 (pbk.)
    1. Psychotherapist and patient.   2. Psychotherapists—
Language.   3. Communication in psychiatry.
4. Psychotherapy.   I. Title.
    [DNLM: 1. Communication.   2. Professional–Patient
Relations.   3. Psychotherapy—methods.   WM 420 W1145t]
RC480.8.W333   1993
616.89′14—dc20
DNLM/DLC   92-49431
for Library of Congress   CIP

*This book is dedicated to my patients and to
my students, who over many years have shaped
the questions that have occurred to me about the
process of psychotherapy and have stimulated
the answers that have emerged.*

Preface

This is a book about therapeutic technique—about how to move from understanding the patient to putting that understanding into words. It aims to fill a gap in the literature and in many training programs, a gap that can leave the student-therapist (and even the therapist with considerable experience) feeling, "I think I know what's going on with the patient, but what should I actually *say*?" My aim in this book is to examine in great detail precisely what the therapist *can* say that can contribute to the process of healing and change. The goal is to put things in a way that is therapeutic, to confront difficult truths and feared inclinations without damaging the patient's self-esteem or arousing needless distress and resistance.

Although a practical book, this volume is also an exploration of theory. It presents an integrative theory of psychological disorder and psychological change, a theory rooted in the psychodynamic tradition while drawing upon the insights and discoveries of other approaches as well. Throughout the book, the rationales for the clinical interventions recommended are described in detail, and the reader is shown why one way of saying things is preferred to another.

A central focus of the book is on the nuances of phrasing and meaning that I believe can make a crucial difference between comments to patients that are genuinely therapeutic and comments that unwittingly perpetuate the very problems the patient brings for treatment. But as important as this aspect of therapeutic practice is, it is obviously not all there is to skillful clinical work. Although the volume gives unusual prominence to the crafting of comments, to the exact way in which interpretations and other messages to the patient are put into words, its concern is by no means limited to wording or phrasing alone. The theoretical chapters at the beginning of the book provide a comprehensive picture of the methods and processes that must be brought to bear in effective therapeutic work. And throughout this volume as the therapist's options for what to say in any particular clinical situation are

examined, they are considered in the context of the overall set of factors
that create a thrust for change.

A book about the implications of the language we use must be particularly concerned about the problems created by the longstanding tendency of our language to treat the human race as if it consisted of just one
gender. The use of "he" and "his" to refer to generic human beings has
been widely recognized as problematic. But I know of no effort to solve
this linguistic challenge that is fully satisfactory. Sentences full of "he or
she" and "his or her" are extremely awkward, and restricting oneself to
plurals can lose the immediacy and vitality that comes with inviting the
reader to imagine a concrete, singular human being. What I have chosen to do to address the problem is as follows: whenever the generic human being referred to is the therapist, I will employ the pronouns "she"
and "her"; when it is the patient, I will use "he" or "him."

This convention seems to me to have several advantages. To begin
with, it obviates the need for littering the page with multiple pronouns
or restricting oneself to plurals. But it also addresses more directly the
most common prejudices and stereotypes that make our traditional
language forms problematic. In our stereotypes, it is the professional,
the "doctor," who is male; the patient role, however, is one we often
imagine occupied by women. The convention employed here reverses
that stereotype. It calls attention to the fact that a growing number of
professionals in our field are women and reserves the more conventional use of the male pronoun for references to individuals in treatment or to people caught in one or another of the neurotic dilemmas
that I describe. Moreover, using male and female pronouns in different
but systematically distinguished contexts affords greater clarity for the
reader in those sections in which both therapist's and patient's responses or feelings are discussed.

No solution to the vexing problem that our linguistic "foreparents"
have bequeathed us is perfect. I hope, however, that the convention I
have chosen serves reasonably well the (oft competing) twin goals of, on
the one hand, clarity and felicity of expression and, on the other, attention to the sensitivities of half the human race and to the need to
challenge the preconceptions that have created obstacles to the full
realization of the human potential of both women and men.

On a different linguistic front, I have had to make a decision about
the use of the terms "patient" and "client." Some therapists prefer the
term client to patient, feeling it puts the person one works with on a
more equal footing. In this book, however, I continue to use the term
patient, partly because I was brought up on it, and it simply feels more
comfortable and natural to me, and partly because "client" connotes too

great an emphasis on the business aspect of the relationship. *Accountants* have clients; for therapists to adopt the same word seems to me less than satisfactory.

To be sure, "patient" too is problematic. (Indeed, all words are problematic for describing this most puzzling of human relationships.) But a participant at a workshop I held with my wife at Cape Cod a number of years ago made a point I found reassuring: apparently, the Latin root of the word *patient* is "one who suffers," whereas the root of *client* is "one who depends." Thus, if the aim is to remove the putatively demeaning or condescending implications of patient, client is not a very good choice. Nor, in this context, is patient a bad one to convey what it is that brings the person into therapy and that defines his relationship to the therapist.

Finally, with regard to one more issue of language, it is my strong conviction that obscurity of presentation reflects not profundity but unclarity of thought. To the best of my ability I have foresworn jargon and attempted to put into clear English my view of what goes on in the therapist's office, why it works, and when it goes astray. There is something subtly authoritarian about prose that is intimidatingly dense. It attempts to ward off criticism with the implicit message "You are not smart enough to make a judgment." It is my hope that the reader, whether she agrees or disagrees with what I am saying, will feel that I have been clear enough for her to feel smart enough.

This book draws heavily on my own practice and on my experience in teaching, supervising, and giving workshops to students and practitioners at varying levels of experience. In drawing on the precise particulars of clinical interactions with patients—both my own and those of my students and supervisees—I have been concerned to assure their anonymity. Not only the names of patients but some of the identifying details of patient profiles have been changed to assure that the patients' privacy is protected.

The nature of this book's focus requires it to be rich in clinical detail. Many of the arguments are built inductively around concrete illustrations from clinical practice, and throughout I aim to enable the reader to see precisely how the principles described are used in actual clinical interaction. Particularly in the last few chapters, I present extended excerpts of sessions in order to provide a sense of how the dialogue between patient and therapist is played out and how the process of working through proceeds. But, although it is certainly my intent to be persuasive, and the emphasis on concrete clinical detail is in part designed to further that end, when all is said and done, the material presented is clearly more properly understood as illustration than evidence. Ultimately, it will take systematic research to establish with any degree of certainty how best to achieve the changes patients seek in coming to therapy.

It should be evident to the empirically minded reader, however, that although the book is decidedly clinical in its orientation, there are manifold research implications in the formulations it presents. Many of the principles and assumptions presented here lend themselves quite clearly to empirical testing. One can readily imagine process studies in which the therapist's comments are rated for the degree to which they embody or fail to embody one or another of the principles advocated here, and the immediate in-session consequences of utilizing or failing to utilize them are examined. Similarly, it is not difficult to envisage outcome studies in which samples from treatments are rated for the degree to which they embody one or another of these principles and the impact on therapeutic success or failure is assessed.

Studies demonstrating the importance of conceptualizing psychological difficulties in terms of the kinds of circular patterns described in both the theoretical and clinical sections of this book will be more difficult to conduct. Such studies require a still greater degree of complexity and sophistication, especially if they are to show how the linear formulations that presently predominate are but part of a larger pattern, the full understanding of which gives us considerably greater understanding and therapeutic possibility. Such research is possible, however, and, I believe, presents both a challenge and an opportunity to the methodologically innovative investigator. I will follow closely any efforts to test empirically the ideas presented here, and I look forward to the modifications and further development of these ideas that such research will inevitably require and stimulate.

It is a pleasure to acknowledge the close reading and extremely helpful comments of Sidney Blatt, Kenneth Frank, Stanley Messer, David Wolitzky, and Daniel Wile. Their comments were at once tough minded and supportive, and they greatly enriched my own appreciation of the task I had set myself.

My wife, Ellen, also read every chapter, but she went a step further. She *wrote* one. Sensing strong affinities between the principles described here and the ways she works as a couples therapist (an aspect of clinical practice in which she is particularly expert), she offered to write a chapter on the applications of these principles to couples work. I was delighted, and the Postscript on therapeutic communication with couples that constitutes Chapter 13 was the result. I am grateful to her for a chapter that significantly enhances the value of the book—and even more for the love she has offered over so many years.

Contents

CHAPTER 1

The Talking Cure

Psychotherapy is the talking cure. Yet surprisingly little has been written about what therapists actually say. Whereas the patient's every word is examined for subtle nuances of meaning and inflection, the *therapist's* words go largely unnoticed. Her participation is addressed primarily in terms of listening and understanding. That she also talks is almost an afterthought.

Fortunately, the days are waning when this absence of attention to the therapist's words was paralleled by a relative absence of the words themselves. Where once, based in part on a misunderstanding of the implications of Freud's theories, many therapists tended to view as desirable a rather severe limitation on their participation in the therapeutic process, now most therapists—even psychoanalytically oriented therapists—talk back.

The merciful decline of the caricaturable silent therapist—a loss, perhaps, for the cartoonists of *The New Yorker* but a more than compensating gain for patients in therapy—has not, however, been accompanied by a corresponding increase in the attention therapists pay to what they say. Therapists may now reveal to their supervisors that they talk, but they still are usually not taught to give their own words the kind of careful scrutiny they are taught to give to the words of their patients.

Training programs continue to emphasize primarily the development of therapists' listening skills. They teach therapists (as, of course, they should) to cultivate an empathic capacity to enter into the patient's or client's world. But the question of precisely how to *communicate* that understanding in the therapeutically most effective way tends to get far less attention. Implicitly or explicitly, the assumption is made that if one really understands, what to say will become clear rather readily.

Over the years I have become convinced, both from my work with students learning to do psychotherapy and from observing my own behavior as a therapist, that what to say does *not* follow automatically from one's understanding of the patient. The framing of therapeutically effective comments is a skill, just as achieving proper understanding is a skill; and although the crafting of therapeutic comments is obviously not independent of one's understanding of the patient, it is far from completely determined by that understanding.

I am also persuaded by my experience that creating therapeutically helpful comments is a *teachable* skill. Both beginning students and seasoned practitioners can benefit from paying more attention to just how they phrase what they say to patients. After a time, one begins to get a feel for ways of saying things that are significantly less productive of resistance and significantly more respectful of the patient's self-esteem. And this not because one pulls one's punches or avoids painful realities but because how one gets one's message across is as important as what that message is.[1]

FOCAL MESSAGES AND "META-MESSAGES"

Central to the argument of this book is the idea that every overt message that the therapist intends to convey, every communication of a particular understanding of the patient's experience or dynamics (what I will call the *focal message*), carries with it a second message, a *meta-message* if you will, that conveys an attitude about what is being conveyed in the focal message.[2] It is often in this meta-message—frequently unnoticed or unexamined—that the greatest potential for therapeutic transformation (or therapeutic failure) lies.

It is by now widely recognized that, when listening to a patient, it is at least as important to notice *how* the patient communicates as to hear *what* he says—indeed that very often the "how" is the most important "what" that the astute listener can pick up (see particularly, Reich, 1949; Shapiro, 1965, 1981, 1989). But a corresponding literature on the how of the *therapist's* communications is scarcely to be found.

No doubt, effective therapists develop considerable skill in framing comments whose meta-messages are consistent with their therapeutic aims; but it is likely that even many therapists whose metacommunica-

---

[1]Indeed, the "what" of the message and the "how" of the message are not really separable. To a signifcant degree, how one gets the message across determines what the message really "is." In the terms introduced next, the meta-message is an intrinsic—and crucial—part of the overall message conveyed to the patient.

[2]My use of the term meta-message may call to mind for some readers Bateson's (1972, 1979) discussions of metamessages and metacommunication. His approach, however, has rather different emphases, deriving from his interest in Whorf's (1956) theory of language and Whitehead and Russell's (1910–1913) theory of logical types.

tional skills are quite impressive rarely think about such matters explicitly, and that little emphasis was placed on this dimension of their work in the course of their training. When standard texts approach the topic, it is most often under such rubrics as tact and timing. The focus of this book is considerably broader than what is typically included in the notion of tact, but it does overlap in certain ways with what is commonly conveyed by that concept.

My concern in this volume, however, is with more than just tact. Indeed, there are ways in which some of the recommendations made here can be seen as suggesting an *alternative* to tact—not, I hasten to add, in the sense that I advocate being tactless; but in the sense that in ordinary social intercourse being tactful at times implies a degree of evasion of difficult issues, a skillful avoidance of an uncomfortable truth. What I hope to show are ways *to* address the disagreeable matters whose evasion is often at the heart of the patient's difficulties—but to do so in such a way that the patient will hear what is said and will be inclined to deal with the issue rather than to find new ways to ward it off.

An interpretation whose message is accurate but whose meta-message is poorly wrought can have an effect similar to that of a potentially curative organ transplant that is rejected by the patient's body because it is registered as alien. Such an interpretation is potentially healing in principle but unhelpful in actual effect because it is experienced as a dangerous intrusion of alien material. Like the needed organ, it too is rejected and thereby prevented from exercising its curative potential. "Tissue rejection," one may well say, is an issue in the psychotherapeutic process as well.

For that reason, I will concentrate a good deal on the larger meaning of the therapist's message—on what view of himself it induces in the patient; whether it elicits cooperation or resistance; whether it enhances the patient's self-esteem; whether it leads to conflict-resolving or fear-reducing or skill-enhancing action; what it conveys about the therapist's view of the patient; etc.

It is striking how often in the literature basic details are omitted regarding what the therapist actually says, with the consequence that the full implications of what is said remain unexamined. In the psychoanalytic literature, for example, it is not uncommon to find phrases such as "I interpreted for her the Oedipal origins of her transference to me." Such a description of what transpired can hide a multitude of sins (or, for that matter, of virtues). It could be referring to statements as opposite in their implications as *You are inappropriately feeling sexual toward me as you inappropriately felt sexual toward your mother* or *You are made uncomfortable by healthy loving feelings toward me as you were taught to feel uncomfortable about similar feelings toward your mother.* The therapeutic implications of these two versions of "interpreting the transference" differ enormously.

Even many seemingly concrete and communicative reports, whether in the literature or in supervisory sessions, can be seen on closer inspection to leave a crucial ambiguity about what was actually said and, hence, to be considerably less useful or revealing than they might first appear. When a supervisee reports, for example, "I told the patient that I thought his forgetting was related to his anger at his wife," his actual comment could have varied anywhere from *You were angry at your wife, and you tried to hide it by forgetting* to *You've told me about a number of things your wife did that I would imagine made you angry; perhaps you forgot because you were trying so hard not to be angry at her.* The tone and meaning of these two ways of "telling him his forgetting was related to his anger at his wife," the meta-messages they convey, diverge quite substantially. Unless one examines the actual comments in their concrete detail, one's appreciation of what transpired will be incomplete and potentially quite misleading.

ATTENDING TO THE PATIENT'S EXPERIENCE OF THE THERAPIST'S REMARKS

In considering the implications of the ideas and examples just discussed, it is essential to be clear that the meaning *to the patient* of the therapist's comment is not objectively given in the comment itself. The patient will inevitably experience the comment "in his fashion," filtering it through his past experiences, expectations, needs, fears, and working models of human relationships. Put differently, the ubiquitous phenomenon of transference will make it likely that the patient's experience of the comment will differ in certain respects from what the therapist thinks she is conveying.

The ramifications of this understanding of the communicative process are substantial and will be explored in various ways throughout this book. It is important, however, that appreciation of the crucial role of the patient's subjectivity in determining the meaning of the therapist's remarks not mislead one into downplaying the importance of what the therapist actually says. As discussed in Chapter 4 (see also Wachtel, 1981), transferential reactions, though idiosyncratic, are far from arbitrary. They are significantly shaped by the actuality of the situation, even as they give a particularized meaning to that actuality (cf. Gill, 1982, 1983; Hoffman, 1983). The way the therapist chooses to phrase her communication will not completely determine how the patient experiences it, but it is highly relevant to that experience. Though the vagaries of transference will render the impact of the comment prob-abilistic and partially indeterminate, the *likely* impact—and especially the *range* of likely impacts—can be usefully estimated, especially as the therapist gets to know her patient and the patient's particular way of construing experiences.

It is absolutely central to the point of view presented in this book that the therapist must not simply *assume* how the patient will experi-ence the comment and that she must be constantly alert to the meaning *the patient* gives to the remark. However, the therapy will be much the worse for it if this important truth is used by the therapist to obscure the equally crucial reality that the particular way one says something has a powerful impact, and that, when the therapist has learned to pay atten-tion to the meta-messages embodied in her remarks, the probable im-pact can be estimated with a reasonable degree of accuracy. If the fact of transference becomes a nihilistic cliche, justifying the therapist's lack of attention to how she phrases her comments on the grounds that they will mean something different to the patient than the therapist intended anyway, the therapist's ability to be genuinely therapeutic is notably impoverished. Throughout this book, I intend to weave together the implications of two important realities of the therapeutic process and relationship—that, on the one hand, the meaning of the therapist's comments is ultimately the meaning as experienced by the patient, and on the other, that that experience is significantly determined by the actual shape and tone of the therapist's remarks.

"THERAPIST NOISES"

Critical or countertherapeutic meta-messages are often not easy to de-tect. Psychotherapists have developed a variety of commonly used forms to carry their messages, and these forms are often quite effective (at least initially) in disguising the meta-message that is being conveyed. Indeed, that is in large measure their purpose.

Consider, for example, the following brief interaction between a patient, Linda, and her therapist. The therapist described Linda as someone who frequently put her off balance, who asked questions that she did not know how to respond to. On one occasion, for example, Linda asked her, "You're not Jewish, yet you're married to a Jewish man. How come?"

The therapist, feeling flustered and uncertain, called upon a kind of comment that will probably sound familiar to almost all readers. "It's interesting," she said, "that you ask so many questions."

"Interesting" is one of those words that seem to convey the neutrality that is widely believed to be the proper stance for the therapist to maintain. By commenting that the patient's behavior is interesting, it may seem we are simply calling attention to it, attempting to stir the patient's curiosity about his own mental processes. But is "interesting" in this instance neutral? Most of us are usually pleased when we are told that something we have said or done is interesting. Would the present comment produce the same self-satisfied glow? I doubt it.

It is not difficult to detect that the real message conveyed by this expression of interest is disapproval. Calling the patient's behavior "interesting" in this context puts her in her place, affirms that she is a clinical "case." We all have images of therapists in bad movies saying to the patient, in a heavy Viennese accent, "verrry interrressting," and again we know that this is not meant as a compliment.

Such locutions are what I call "therapist noises." They are the familiar phrasings that we all call upon when uncertain, phrasings that at once convey a bolstering sense of professionalism and serve to protect us from further revelation of our reactions. It is difficult for me to imagine any therapist (myself included) doing entirely without these protective colorations. Doing therapy makes one too vulnerable to give them up completely. Moreover, their close relatives are perfectly legitimate expressions of the stance of participant observation (Sullivan, 1953, 1954), the odd combination of engagement and reflectiveness that characterizes psychotherapy at its best. Indeed, sometimes the very same phrase can be in one instance a therapist noise and in another an expression of the therapist's competent professionalism. That is, after all, why such phrases actually do soothe and protect us. They would not *feel* competently professional if they were not versions of something that on other occasions really was competently professional.

If one is attuned to the idea of therapist noises, however, they are not hard to detect. When one is making therapist noises one has a characteristically hollow feeling, a sense of discomfort, fraudulence, or stiltedness that, subjectively, is painfully obvious, however hard one tries to keep it from being noticed by the patient. One is aware, and not in a positive way, of "sounding like a therapist." When I have introduced this concept to students, they have had little trouble recognizing instantly what I was referring to and have indeed noted that it was an all too common accompaniment of their efforts to take on the therapist's role. One gauge that I have only half jokingly suggested to students as a rough indication of whether they are drifting into making therapist noises is to keep track of their *perhaps-to-maybe ratio*. When one is in the stilted, "therapist noises" stance, one is likely to use rather frequently the word *perhaps* ("perhaps you're feeling such and such") rather than the more informal *maybe*. Such subtleties of tone can be useful in alerting the therapist to what can be a rather important dimension of her interaction with the patient.

Phrases such as *I wonder what you mean by that?* or *I wonder why you're asking me that?* or *What do you think you should do?* or a host of others all can be appropriate and facilitative of the therapeutic process; completely excising them from our therapeutic vocabulary would impoverish our work very substantially. But they can also be stultifying clichés that keep the patient at bay, protect the therapist's fragile sense of expertise, and prevent real life from entering the interaction between patient and therapist. The discussions in this book are designed both to help the therapist become more aware of when her communications take on this quality and to help her build a repertoire of more genuinely therapeutic comments that can obviate the need for "therapist noises" and promote contact rather than uncomfortable self-protection.

EXCEPTIONS TO THE RULE

Although the general paucity of writings on the crucial details of technique addressed in this book is rather striking, a number of writers have seen clearly the importance of the topic and have made valuable contributions. Leston Havens, for example (Havens, 1986), has written on matters of wording and phrasing from a perspective that combines existential and interpersonal points of view. He offers a rather elaborate taxonomy of types of therapeutic statements, which he broadly categorizes into empathic language, interpersonal language, and performative language. Much like the present volume, his book is filled with detailed examinations of particular ways of saying things and their implications for the therapeutic process. I will have occasion in a number of places in this book to draw on his interesting observations.

Ralph Greenson, in his authoritative text on psychoanalytic technique, shows considerable interest in and thought about the wording of comments to patients and discusses his choice of words in some detail. As he puts it,

> My language is simple, clear, concrete, and direct. I use words that cannot be misunderstood, that are not vague or evasive. When I am trying to pin down the particular affect the patient might be struggling with, I try to be as specific and exact as possible. I select the word which seems to portray what is going on in the patient, the word which reflects the patient's situation of the moment. If the patient seems to be experiencing an affect as though he were a child, for example, if the patient seems anxious like a child, I would say: "You seem scared," because that is the childhood word. I would never say, "you seem apprehensive" because that would not

fit, that is a grown-up word. Furthermore, "scared" is evocative, it stirs up pictures and associations, while "apprehensive" is drab. I will use words like bashful, shy, or ashamed, if the patient seems to be struggling with feelings of shame from the past. I would not say humiliation or abasement or meekness.

In addition, I also try to gauge the intensity of the affect as accurately as possible. If the patient is very angry, I don't say, "You seem annoyed," but I would say, "You seem furious." I use the ordinary and vivid word to express the quantity and quality of affect I think is going on. I will say things like: You seem irritable, or edgy, or grouchy, or sulky, or grim, or quarrelsome, or furious, to describe different kinds of hostility. How different are the associations to "grouchy" as compared to "hostile." In trying to uncover and clarify the painful affect and the memories associated to that specific affect, the word one uses should be right in time, quality, quantity, and tone. (1967, pp. 108–109)

Warren Poland, another analyst who has appreciated the importance of what the therapist or analyst actually says, shows as well how certain assumptions of standard psychoanalytic thought can obscure and constrain that appreciation. Poland, pointing in his own way to the dimension I addressed above in terms of the distinction between the focal message and the meta-message, notes that "The analyst's music carries messages as important as those in the manifest words." He alerts the reader to "buried messages," to the fact that "Even simple remarks carry implied messages beyond the manifest" (Poland, 1986, p. 248).

In a more critical vein, Poland notes the "artificial separation of pure messages from hidden forces" that has characterized psychoanalytic thought on clinical language. He cites as an example of the conceptual confusions that can arise the claim by the highly respected analyst Rudolf Loewenstein (1956) that the well-functioning analyst excludes from his speech any appeal or effort to affect the patient, "limiting himself specifically to the cognitive function in relation to facts concerning his present addressee: the patient" (Loewenstein, 1956, p. 462).

"Such tidiness of concept is appealing," says Poland, but "unfortunately" such a model, in which "the patient reports his inner world and like an objective outside observer, the analyst interprets," does not square with experience. The idea of "simply saying," of speech that is not also "an action upon the other," seems to Poland highly questionable, and he states quite explicitly (and correctly, I believe) that

The analyst speaks for effect. No matter the analyst's desire to see his role as that of an impartial researcher helping catalyze the uncovering of buried truth, the analytic work is done for purpose. If the analyst were to have no impact on the patient and the analysis . . . then the analyst and the analysis would be meaningless. (Poland, 1986, p. 264)

Poland provides a number of interesting illustrations of how language may be used, when the therapist or analyst is aware, to enhance the likelihood of getting through to the patient. One of my favorites involves an instance in which a patient presented to him a dream in which "the manifest content repudiates an urge, one the patient would prefer to disown." In speaking about the dream, the patient adds that he "would never do anything so outrageous as the dream suggests." To this Poland replied, "You wouldn't even dream of such a thing" (1986, pp. 246–247).

Poland's way of framing his comment provides a potential opening that a more direct confrontation would likely fail to provide. The paradoxical quality of the comment (both acknowledging the patient's claim that he wouldn't dream of such a thing and pointing out that he just did) provides a gentle nudge, and, as Poland notes, the patient can choose to hear it in whatever way he is ready to. Not only is such a comment less heavy-handed than something like *You say you wouldn't do such a thing yet you went ahead and dreamt it;* it also creates a tone in which analyst and patient are standing side by side rather than facing each other as adversaries. Poland is giving the patient credit for being able to see the humor and paradox in his comment, and they can both appreciate it together.

Poland further notes that the analyst's style of speech can have as significant an impact on the patient as do the words. In a fashion similar to the approach taken in the present book, Poland points to the "how" of the therapist's comment as well as the what, its "official" or manifest focus. With regard to the "never dream of it" comment, he points out that

spoken with regard to the patient in his struggles, the statement is helpful. Spoken with an edge of sarcasm, it ridicules and belittles. Interpretations . . . are undermined if the message itself is not truly respectful and nonprovocative. (Poland, 1986, p. 264)

A somewhat similar strategy of communication is illustrated in another of Poland's descriptions: a woman patient, whom Poland perceived as having considerable conflict and anxiety over sexuality and body damage, described to him her fears of her male supervisor's comments. Poland's comment—"You're afraid of a penetrating remark"— differs quite considerably from a comment such as *You're afraid he's making a sexual advance.* Apropos the main argument of this book, the latter comment derives from the same understanding as Poland's, but its potential effects could be quite different. Poland's comment permits the patient to take it at whatever level she is ready for. If she wishes, she will hear what he is implying; if not, she can ignore it (at least temporarily)—yet also let it have an impact unconsciously. This is a tactic that is probably used often by skilled therapists but is rarely explicitly addressed in the literature. When done appropriately, and with sufficient respect for what the patient is capable of dealing with, and—apropos Poland's aforementioned caveat about tone—when not employed in a superior or judgmental way, it can diminish considerably the likelihood of "tissue rejection."

Not surprisingly, Harry Stack Sullivan also provided a rich store of guidelines for the effective framing of therapeutic comments. From Sullivan's perspective of "participant observation" it was very clear that what transpired in the therapeutic hour was not the simple unfolding of something from within the patient while the therapist merely watched (cf. Wachtel, 1987, Chap. 3). The experience of the patient was a joint product of the patient's past history and present characteristics *and* of the therapist's participation in that history. That "the therapist speaks for effect" did not have to be told to Sullivan.

Numerous accounts, both by Sullivan and by others describing his work, illustrate his keen appreciation of the impact on the patient of precisely what he said and how he said it. As A. H. Chapman put it in his volume *The Treatment Techniques of Harry Stack Sullivan*, it was Sullivan's view that since words "are the implements with which therapists work, attention to their most effective use should be included in teaching psychotherapy" (Chapman, 1978, p. 17). In this context, Chapman goes on to comment that "It is an odd fact that most distinguished psychiatric innovators have paid little or no attention to *the precise verbal and nonverbal techniques* that therapists use to obtain and convey information with patients" (Chapman, 1978, p. 17; italics in original).

Chapman stresses Sullivan's concern not to pursue the task of therapeutic inquiry in ways that will lower the patient's self esteem, and provides numerous examples illustrating Sullivan's careful attention to the impact of the particular way of approaching any topic. He suggests, for example, that

> In discussing with a patient a problem she has with her husband, it may be an error to ask, "Have you talked this over with him?" If the patient has not discussed the subject with him, she may feel that the therapist's inquiry implies that she has blundered by not doing so. Indirect questions which do not undermine the patient's self-esteem may be much better. "What

does your husband think about this problem? Has he brought the subject up with you? Has he in other ways made his feelings clear on this point?" (Chapman, 1978, pp. 16–17)

In this example, casting the inquiry initially as one in which the *husband's* behavior is first examined, in which *his* responsibility to discuss the issues between them and to share feelings is the focus, enables the topic to be addressed without directly confronting the patient's vulnerabilities. As the inquiry proceeds, it gradually shifts toward enabling the patient herself to take responsiblity for communicating. Thus, the series of questions ends with "Do you think it would be advisable to get this problem out into the open between the two of you?" (Chapman, 1978, p. 17), but this point is reached only after preliminary work designed to protect her self-esteem and, we may add, to enable her really to hear what her therapist is saying.

Alexander and French (1946) also showed an uncommon appreciation for how the specific features of the therapist's communications can influence their therapeutic impact. Although endorsing the commonly held goal of avoiding both criticism or praise in what they say to the patient, they note that we "deceive ourselves . . . if we hope thereby to keep the patient from reading praise or blame into our interpretations." And they argue that although transference influences certainly account for a good part of this tendency on the patient's part, "It is not only as a result of such transference mechanisms that the patient may get an impression as to how the therapist evaluates the motives he interprets" (p. 93). By way of illustration, they offer the following example:

> If . . . a young man has just formed an attachment for a young woman, who in many ways resembles his mother, and if his therapist decides to call attention to this resemblance, it is by no means a matter of indifference just how he shall go about it. If he tells the patient that he is attracted to the young woman because she represents his mother, the implication will be that the patient should inhibit any sexual impulse toward the young woman as he would toward his mother. On the other hand, if the therapist waits until the patient has already begun to react with guilt to his sexual impulses toward the young woman and then points out to the patient that he feels *guilty* because he identifies the girl with the mother, the implication of this interpretation will tend to diminish the patient's guilt feelings because the patient will feel that the therapist is reminding him that the girl is really *not* his mother. It is evident, therefore, that it is a matter of great importance to the advancement of the therapeutic process in which way the therapist chooses to make the interpretation. (Alexander & French, 1946, pp. 93–94; italics added)

COUNTERTRANSFERENCE INFLUENCES AND COUNTERVAILING LINGUISTIC STRUCTURES[3]

The nature of the meta-messages conveyed to the patient is rarely a matter of technique alone. It is crucial that the therapist be alert to her emotional response to the patient's communications and to what has transpired between them. One's attitude is conveyed not only in one's words, but in one's tone, rhythm, posture, and so forth, and it is virtually impossible to disguise over the long run how one feels about the patient or about what he is saying. Especially if a therapist consistently makes comments to a patient that, however accurate, convey critical meta-messages, an examination of the therapist's personal reactions to the patient, of how the patient evokes feelings in her that stem from her own past or from her own unresolved conflicts, is clearly in order. Nothing in this book's agenda is intended to slight this critically important task of self-examination by the therapist.

It is important to be clear, however, that countertransference considerations and the considerations of proper phrasing and therapeutic communication that are the primary topic of this book do not constitute two clearly separable realms. On the one hand, the feelings evoked in us by the patient are a function not only of our personal history but of our set as we approach the patient and the therapeutic task. This set, in turn, depends on how we conceptualize the nature of psychological difficulties and the therapeutic process. Whether we experience the patient as manipulative, for example, depends as much on our theory as it does on more personal and idiosyncratic influences. For some therapists, the behavior that might be described as manipulative is understood instead as the patient's trying, imperfectly and largely self-defeatingly, to gain some measure of self-esteem in a life clogged with faulty assumptions about human interaction and consequent unpleasant experiences. Moreover, how manipulative, or resistant, or hostile or inaccessible the patient feels to the therapist will depend as well on how competent and prepared the *therapist* feels. When one feels competent in the presence of a patient, when one feels one knows what to say and how to be therapeutically effective, the patient is likely to seem more

---

[3]The term "countertransference" is of course a technical term from a particular orientation, the psychoanalytic or psychodynamic. I use it in this heading as a quick shorthand to orient the reader to what I will be discussing in this section. But since this book aims to reach clinicians of a wide range of theoretical persuasions, I wish to point out here that although the *term* is specifically psychoanalytic, the issues it points to are far from the exclusive province or exclusive concern of that orientation. Here, as elsewhere in this book, the actual unfolding of my argument will proceed with a minimum of jargon and with an eye to communicating with therapists of varying points of view.

likeable, and it is easier to empathize with whatever emotions he is manifesting.

On the other hand, in a field such as ours, one's theory itself is far from independent of who one is. That is, the same background personality factors and life experiences that are the soil for specific countertransference reactions to the patient provide as well much of the basis for our choice of a theory. With so many competing theories, there are many justifiable ways of conceiving both the therapeutic task and the psychological foundations of our patients' problems. Which one we choose to ally ourselves with will at least in part depend on which fits our personality and our own life experience.

Thus it is never an either/or question of whether one's reactions result from countertransference or not. Certainly the therapist must continuously monitor her participation in the therapeutic process with the patient and attempt to understand the contribution of her own history and vulnerabilities to what is happening and to how she understands it. But it is important to appreciate as well that the degree to which countertransference influences will markedly skew the therapeutic process can depend quite substantially on the kinds of considerations at the heart of this book. By closely studying effective modes and structures of communication, by making them "second nature," the therapist can at least temper the distorting role of countertransferential reactions.

In general, the influence of unconscious conflicts and of residues from one's early history is most evident where ambiguity is greatest. Structure, in turn, helps to keep such influences in check and to create a relatively conflict-free zone. This is true as well for one's functioning as a psychotherapist. Attention to the phrasings and communicational strategies described in this book is no substitute for the therapist's continuing examination of her emotional reactions to the patient's characteristic ways of experiencing and interacting. But it can provide a structure that can help keep untoward reactions within reasonable limits as well as provide a further dimension of skillfulness in the conduct of the therapeutic work. As Poland (1986) has suggested in a somewhat different context, when one reaches for something to say to the patient, one is likely to "pull from the top of the pile." If, as a result of the kind of careful study advocated here, therapeutically facilitative phrasings are naturally at the top of the pile, what one says to the patient is much more likely to be what one might later wish one had said.

The skills of the therapist in effectively framing therapeutic communications tend to be particularly vulnerable to countertransference influences because few therapists have studied the topic closely and explicitly. To be sure, many therapists achieve a fairly good sense of these principles intuitively and, without giving the matter too much thought, come up with therapeutically helpful phrasings a good deal of the time. But because it is not based on the same kind of reflection and careful study that other aspects of their therapeutic skills are, this capacity is particularly vulnerable to the stresses and pressures that are an inevitable part of therapeutic work and to the winds of countertransference. Moreover, for the same reason, this aspect of therapeutic functioning is more likely to be influenced without the therapist's even being clear that such influence has occurred.

One aim of this book is to help the reader be more focally aware of the words she chooses in communicating her observations to the patient. I hope to bring to the reader's attention considerations that, even if frequently successfully negotiated in an intuitive fashion, have not been submitted to close study and reflection. I aim as well to provide a host of concrete examples that can provide the reader with a kind of warehouse of well-honed tools for clinical work.

Some of the examples will feel quite familiar to the experienced therapist. They are representative of the kinds of observations and reflections one learns to make on the intuitive basis noted above. But though familiar, they nonetheless merit close attention. In this way, the reader can increase the likelihood of their availability in her consciousness when they are needed.

The need for continuing work in this regard is underlined by a second sense of familiarity that the reader is likely to experience: The "bad" examples that are the starting point for a number of the discussions in the book are likely also to feel familiar. It is virtually impossible to do therapy day in and day out without finding oneself periodically making problematic comments to patients of just the sort I will focus on here. And this not because one is incompetent or sloppy but simply because the work we do is difficult, and it never can be perfect. Indeed, even after engaging in the kind of intensive scrutiny provided by the analyses presented here, the reader will not completely eliminate such unfortunate phrasings. I do hope, however, that their frequency can be considerably reduced and that, furthermore, the overall approach described here will make it easier to recoup rather than compound the difficulty.[4]

---

[4]In this regard, we may note that another benefit of studying closely the subtleties of the therapist's metamessages is that, in addition to any assist this may give to *avoiding* countertherapeutic communications, attending more closely to the form and tone of one's comments in the way stressed here can also be helpful in *alerting* the therapist to emerging countertransferential reactions. That is, if one learns to be more attentive to the way one phrases one comments, they can be a sensitive indicator or early warning system pointing toward countertransferential feelings and attitudes of which the therapist has not yet become clearly mindful.

In contrast to the ring of familiarity that many of the examples will have for most readers, some may feel like comments one has perhaps groped for but not quite been able to articulate, and still others may seem rather novel. They are the result of many years of active reflection on this dimension of therapeutic work and of being stimulated and encouraged to do so by students and supervisees who found this focus both intriguing and a useful supplement to the perspectives that more typically occupied their supervisory experiences.

The examples and discussions offered throughout the book overlap considerably. Principles mentioned in one chapter inevitably turn out to be significant in the formulation of comments in another. The division of the discussion into different types of comments or different principles of formulating comments is somewhat arbitrary, reflecting the necessities of the linear nature of books. This caveat notwithstanding, I will discuss in each chapter a somewhat different aspect of the process of communicating one's understanding to the patient in a therapeutically useful way. If the reader is aware that many of the examples, though discussed under one particular rubric, in fact reflect *several* of the principles addressed here, he or she will gain a richer understanding.

The understanding of principles, of the *thought process* behind the comments made, is central to what I wish to convey in this work. Although the volume is unusually rich with concrete clinical detail, equally central is its concern with clinical strategies and principles. In the next three chapters, I turn to a consideration of the theoretical foundations of therapeutic work and to the underlying principles that give coherence to the various concrete illustrations that consititute most of the body of book. Having done so, I then turn to a number of specific challenges encountered in therapeutic practice and to the examination of particular ways of intervening and communicating that I believe can be helpful for therapists operating from a wide variety of therapeutic persuasions.

CHAPTER 2

Cyclical Psychodynamics I
Vicious Circles

The principles offered in this volume are largely independent of any particular theoretical orientation. To a significant degree they are a distillation of what skilled clinicians, regardless of their identified orientation or school, have come to recognize are the most effective ways to communicate in the therapeutic session. Indeed, to a considerable degree what this book does is to spell out the implicit clinical wisdom that, if not often fully articulated, is nonetheless evident in the work of experienced therapists of quite varied persuasions. Research has shown that practitioners of different schools tend to be more alike after practicing for some years than they were as beginners and, indeed, that experienced clinicians of differing schools are more like each other than they are like neophytes of their own school (Fiedler, 1950a, 1950b). There seem to be some important skills and general principles that characterize the work of most effective clinicians and that are at least partly independent of the theoretical orientation with which the therapist identifies (cf. Frank, 1973).

Inevitably, of course, the particular way in which these general principles are given expression, the "flavor" of the actual comments the therapist makes, will be shaped both by her personality and by the theory from which she operates. In the next few chapters I try to convey briefly the theory that guides my own work and its bearing on the approach to therapeutic communication discussed throughout this book. The clinical discussions that constitute the heart of the volume however, do not require adherence to all the particulars of the theory outlined below. I think it likely that even therapists who disagree strongly with me about one or another of the theoretical points in this and the following chapters may nonetheless find quite congenial many of the book's clinical examples and recommendations. In any event, the reader will find that examination of the rationale behind the therapist's choices will not be limited to this chapter. Throughout, it is my aim not merely to consider what the therapist might say in any particular clinical situation but, rather, to explicate as well the thought processes on her part that prompt the choice of one particular comment over another.

The theory that guides my work is one that I have come to call cyclical psychodynamics (see Wachtel, 1977, 1985, 1987, for a fuller description of the theory and its implications). As will be apparent, the name derives from two central features of the theory—its origin in the psychodynamic tradition, and the central role it gives to repetitive cycles of interaction between people and to cycles of reciprocal causation between intrapsychic processes and the events of daily living.

Cyclical psychodynamics is strongly rooted in the interpersonal stream of psychodynamic thought and in aspects of what Greenberg and Mitchell (1983) and Mitchell (1988) have identified as a broader relational perspective in contemporary psychoanalytic theorizing. It has been shaped as well by my participation in the movement toward integrating the disparate theoretical approaches in our field and my efforts to incorporate, within a psychodynamic framework, many of the key methods, ideas, and discoveries deriving from the behavioral and family systems traditions (e.g., Wachtel, 1977, 1987; Wachtel & Wachtel, 1986). As that movement has grown, and given rise to an international association—the Society for the Exploration of Psychotherapy Integration (SEPI)—it has brought me into closer contact with still other schools of thought and has resulted in still further (and currently ongoing) modifications in the theory.

Finally, the theory has been increasingly influenced by my efforts to address, via psychologically oriented social criticism, a number of features of our society that have seemed to me especially problematic—in particular its isolating individualism; its encouragement of consumerism as a substitute for the relational bonds of family and community that it systematically weakens; the impact on the environment of the insatiable demand for growth that develops as a compensation; and the increasing difficulties it has had in maintaining its commitment to the principles of equality and social justice on which it was founded. In exploring the psychological impact and psychological sources of these developments (e.g., Wachtel, 1989), I have found my thinking about clinical matters influenced in turn. In subtle but significant ways, what I have learned from these inquiries into our social system about the myth of autonomy and the denial of interdependency in our society is reflected in the clinical recommendations offered in these pages.

FIXATION OR DEVELOPMENT?

At the heart of the cyclical psychodynamic point of view is an alternative to the widely influential concepts of fixation and developmental arrest.[1] Psychoanalytically oriented therapists have repeatedly been struck by the apparently primitive or archaic quality of some of the fantasies their patients reveal in the course of treatment. The various wishes, images, and affects that emerge in the sessions often seem out of touch with the patient's contemporary adult reality, and this has led analysts to posit that key aspects of the developing personality are somehow split off from the main line of development and rendered impervious to the modulating and modifying influences of encounters with reality. In contrast to social learning theories, for example, which see adaptive and maladaptive outcomes alike as deriving from the actual events and contingencies we confront, psychoanalytic accounts have usually posited that psychopathology is a result most basically of psychological processes whose impact is largely independent of the actual events and relationships that characterize our daily life. Central to most versions of psychoanalytic thought has usually been a picture of development as in some way short circuited.[2]

In classical Freudian theory, what was short circuited were certain sexual and aggressive urges and their associated fantasies. These urges and fantasies, driven by peremptory biological promptings, were seen as exerting a continuing influence on the personality that was largely unmodified by later experience. Maintained in a state of repression, they function apart from the evolving organization of the ego, the sector of the personality that is in touch with perceptual reality and capable of

---

[1]Mitchell (1988) has also recently challenged the concepts of fixation and arrest in a valuable contribution that complements, and is largely consistent with, the point of view presented here. Zeanah, Anders, Seifer, and Stern (1989), reviewing the developmental implications of recent advances in research on infancy, have similarly highlighted the limitations and contradictions of a fixation-arrest model. Proposing a "continuous construction model" as a "major paradigmatic shift away from the fixation–regression model of psychopathology and development," they suggest that in such a model "patterns of internal subjective experience and patterns of relating to others are derived from past relationship experiences but are continuously operating in the present" (Zeanah et al., 1989, p. 657).

[2]This is not to suggest that social learning accounts posit a simple one-to-one relationship between behavior and environmental events. Expectations, schemas, and other such cognitive mediators can lead to persistence in old patterns even as contingencies change (see, for example, Bandura, 1969, 1977; Mischel, 1973; Seligman, 1975). But these theories clearly do not conceptualize portions of the psyche that are split off and rendered impervious to further influence.

adapting to it. Whereas our more conscious ideas and desires are capable of being modified as we encounter new experiences and learn more about the opportunities, frustrations, and dangers that the world presents, these repressed urges are viewed as inaccessible to such modification. Persisting in their original archaic form, they exert their influence as a kind of supremely independent variable, a wild card in the psyche incapable of being tamed by reality.

More recent variants of psychoanalytic thought, such as object relations theory and self psychology, stress as primary the sense of relatedness or the evolution of a stable and coherent sense of self, rather than the playing out of biological urges for pleasure or aggression. But in certain aspects of their theorizing, both schools retain the central emphasis on unmodified fragments of early experience that exert a direct influence on the personality largely unrelated to later experiences. In these more recent theories, the influences that persist in their "archaic" form are either the voices, images, scoldings, and seductions of early "objects" or images of the self that are characterized by an unstable combination of untempered grandiosity, extreme fragility, and feelings of worthlessness and fragmentation. It is these representations of self or other that are seen as primarily responsible for the distortions in our relations to others and in our orientation to the world.

Cyclical psychodynamic theory is attentive to the same set of observations that have led other psychodynamic theorists to root their thinking in ideas of fixation and arrest, but it understands those observations quite differently. Like other psychodynamic theories, it emphasizes the roles of conflict, defense, and unconscious processes more generally. As will become apparent shortly, however, the cyclical psychodynamic perspective directs the therapist to pay far greater attention to the precise details of how the person is presently living his life and to how unconscious psychological structures and the patterns of daily life reciprocally interact with and maintain each other. It points to an understanding of how those deeper structures not only *influence* daily interactions and experiences but are *influenced by* them and/or symbolically represent them. And, as will be apparent, it leads the therapist to be much more receptive to the patient's question "now that I understand, what do I do?" and to root her explorations of transference and countertransference in an appreciation of the subtleties of the patient's daily life.

The key to the cyclical psychodynamic reconceptualization of the phenomena observed by earlier generations of analysts lies in examining the connection between the *seemingly* out of touch fantasies, wishes, or images of self and other and the actuality of the person's present way of life. Through the lens of a cyclical psychodynamic analysis, the apparently archaic processes and structures are revealed as not nearly as anachronistic as they are depicted in most psychoanalytic accounts. Rather, they can be recognized as both symbolizations and consequences of the very way of life of which they are also a determinant.

The contrasting focus of exploration of the cyclical psychodynamic approach and more traditional psychodynamic perspectives can be illustrated by considering how one might attempt to understand the sort of patient whose meekness and inability to assert himself might be seen, from a traditional psychodynamic perspective, as a consequence of his defending against rather primitive, and potentially disorganizing, rage. Rather than viewing the patient's anger as primary—as an archaic impulse from the past—and the defense as a reaction to it, a cyclical psychodynamic analysis illuminates how both the anger and the defense are continually regenerated in response to each other. A common consequence of defensive efforts that too rigidly and singlemindedly repel all hints of possible anger is that the individual is handicapped in asserting his rights and needs. In the effort to bury the forbidden feeling, to banish aggressiveness from the visible psychological landscape, such an individual is led into a position of helplessness and an inability to protect or even to represent his interests effectively. The result of such a state of affairs is some mixture of being taken advantage of, being overlooked and dismissed, or simply not having one's needs noticed by those toward whom one has gone out of one's way to be accomodating, helpful, and considerate.

Such experiences are likely to stir anger in the patient, as they would in almost anyone; but being particularly unable to tolerate anger, he redoubles his efforts to push the anger back by again being self-abnegating, unassuming, excessively cooperative and inoffensive to a fault. As a consequence, he sets the stage for still another experience of not getting his due or not being treated with respect, generating still more anger in response, necessitating still further efforts to hide that anger from himself and to push it back with behavior that is its opposite, and creating yet another repetition of the pattern that has dominated his life.

Thus the anger that he struggles against now is not "old" anger that has been "in" him since childhood, although it is very likely that the struggle *began* back then and that the pattern has been in force for many years. Rather, the anger he struggles to keep at bay today is anger that was generated quite *recently* and, ironically, that was generated by the very efforts he has made to purge himself of anger. A self-perpetuating process has been established that maintains itself by the consequences it repeatedly generates.

A similar kind of dynamic can be seen in many patients who manifest the alternations between grandiosity and feeling pathetically insignificant that are characteristic of individuals diagnosed as narcissistic personalities. The origins of this pattern might well include the sorts of experiences depicted by Kohut and other authors who emphasize the crucial role of the earliest years in generating such difficulties; but *whatever* happened in the first few years of life, there is usually an *ongoing* dynamic, involving a transaction between the patient's inner state and the overt events of his life, that is much more germane to understanding how *change* can be brought about. Such patients, for example, as a way of dealing with their fragile and fluctuating self-esteem, feel a need to present themselves as much more than they really are. Either gross and obvious braggadocio or more subtle forms of exaggeration and image management (or sometimes one and sometimes the other) are likely to be common, and the consequences of this effort to feel better about themselves are likely to be mixed. On the one hand, at least some people are likely to be impressed by the story of himself that the patient presents and to provide at least short-term bolstering of his more grandiose image of himself. On the other, precisely because he *has* been exaggerating, because he has not really gained admiration or acceptance for who he truly is, this pattern of self-misrepresentation is likely to generate feelings of hollowness and fraudulence.

The balance between these two poles keeps shifting, accounting for the shifts in self-esteem that can be observed clinically. Sometimes the grandiosity is predominant, the "strokes" are effective, and he feels expansive (and possibly aggressive and contemptuous as well). At other times, the sense of hollowness and fraudulence is at the fore. In either case, though, the instability of the pattern, the sense of precariousness, leads to redoubled efforts to be what he desperately feels he *must* be— that is, something more than he *really* is. As a consequence, no matter how many genuine strengths the patient may have—and patients of this sort are frequently reported to have considerable talents and proficiencies—those strengths can never form the basis for a solid, dependable, and realistic sense of self because the patient is always selling himself (to others and also to himself) as something more than that, is always trying to be and to seem what he is not.[3]

---

[3]Daniel Wile points out (personal communication) that another pattern is implicit in this description as well, paralleling what has been spelled out thus far. For many people with whom such an individual interacts, his bragging and overbearing manner lead them to experience him as tedious, unpleasant to spend time with, and unworthy of respect. He is thus deprived in his interactions with them of what he desperately craves, the interest, admiration, and engagement of others. Here too, as compensation for this defeat, more of the same is the likely result. -

VICIOUS CIRCLES

It should be evident in both the illustrations just presented that the patient's difficulties are seen as deriving from a vicious circle. In the first instance, the more afraid the patient is of anger, the more he tries to bury it and to act unaggressive in the extreme. In turn, the more he buries his own healthy aggressiveness and assertiveness, the more likely he is to be frustrated, ignored, overshadowed, and treated as insignificant. This in turn makes him angry (though likely unable to let himself be *aware* of the anger), and the anger requires still more efforts to disguise and control it. Over and over, anger generates defenses against it whose consequences generate still more anger, still more need for the same defense, and still further perpetuation of the already problematic pattern of living.

A similar circularity is evident in the case of the "narcissistic" patient.[4] Fragile self-esteem and a sense of hollowness and fraudulence lead to compensatory efforts to boost self-esteem through bragging, dominance, exaggeration, and an aggressive self-presentation. The consequence of these efforts, however, is to heighten the patient's sense of fraudulence, as he gilds the lily until it droops under the weight, and attempts to meet a standard that has no place for his human limitations. In defending in turn against the pain of his now further exacerbated feeling of fraudulence and inadequacy, he repeats the pattern once more, and sets the stage for still another repetition of the cycle.

Whatever the patient may learn about how the pattern got started, it will perpetuate itself so long as he keeps *living* the way he does. And (as will be elaborated shortly) he keeps living that way because he is *afraid* not to. He cannot give it up, even if it no longer makes sense to him, because the intensity of the anxiety is such that it overrides whatever understanding he may temporarily achieve. Only if the anxiety itself is addressed and overcome—if, to anticipate the fuller discussion of anxiety below, the aim of helping the patient become less afraid takes precedence over the aim of helping him gain insight into how the pattern began—is he likely to take the *actions* necessary finally to make the problem a thing of the past.

---

[4] I am placing quotation marks around the word "narcissistic" because although the term has come into such common usage that it is the clearest way of conveying the sort of patient I am referring to, it also has unfortunate pejorative connotations of precisely the sort this book aims to counter. These individuals have enough troubles already without our diagnostic epithets adding to them. Moreover, the term originates in a libido theory context that has been stretched to fit new theoretical schemes until it practically groans. The adoption by our profession of a new terminology to refer to these patients (perhaps "self-esteem disorder?") would be a boon to them and to us.

As illustrated in these two examples, the common denominator underlying cyclical psychodynamic accounts of people's difficulties is that they depict the patient's psychological state not as a direct expression of a childhood mental state or process, but rather as an element in a vicious circle in which both the defense and the defended against, both the unconscious psychological forces and the way of life with which they are associated, determine each other in a continuing cycle of confirmation and reconfirmation. From a cyclical psychodynamic perspective, the vicious circle is the basic psychological unit and the basic source of dynamic continuity. The relevant causal processes lie not in the distant past but in the interactive present.

To be sure, the origins of the pattern can be *traced* to earlier events. But from a cyclical psychodynamic perspective, those events are no longer what is maintaining the process; and knowing how the pattern started can no more change what is presently amiss than knowing that years of smoking caused one's lung cancer or years of eating fatty foods caused one's cardiovascular difficulties can in itself undo the damage. One must change one's habits *now* and, very likely, must also receive some additional treatment that has little directly to do with smoking or eating but rather with *their accumulated consequences*. Much the same is the case in the psychological realm.

UNCONSCIOUS PROCESSES AND THE CENTRALITY OF IRONY

It should be clear that not all aspects of the circular patterns described here are conscious. Clinicians from a wide range of viewpoints have recognized that key elements in people's psychological difficulties may not be represented in conscious awareness. Such influences are crucial in cyclical psychodynamic accounts as well. The ways in which those unconscious processes are understood, however—the routes by which they are thought to be maintained and to influence other aspects of our psychological life—differ significantly between cyclical psychodynamic accounts and those of other versions of psychodynamic thought.

A chief characteristic of the circular patterns described by cyclical psychodynamic theory is *irony*. With surprising regularity, the situation that the patient ends up in is precisely the one he is trying to avoid. He does not *aim* for the consequences he encounters; he produces them despite—yet because of—his vigorous efforts to prevent them. Thus, although a cyclical pschodynamic analysis points to how we actively bring about the patterns we have come to therapy to change, and do so repeatedly, such an analysis differs quite substantially from that embodied in the concept of "repetition compulsion" (Freud, 1920/1959). The latter concept imples that—either for reasons that are biological or even metaphysical or, more strictly psychologically, for the purpose of attempting to master a trauma by repeating it actively—we intentionally (if unconsciously) cause the trauma to recur again and again. In contrast, the cyclical psychodynamic account of how we repeat problematic patterns does not typically posit an intention to reproduce the offending situation. The intention, rather, is quite the opposite—to *prevent* the repetition. The irony in what ensues lies in how, by the very act of carrying out that intention, the patient contributes to the outcome he is trying to avoid.

This differing notion of the dynamics of repetition is the foundation for a number of the ways of approaching the patient that are advocated in the later chapters of this book. Enabling the patient to recognize the active role he plays in his difficulties is often hampered by the burden of guilt and self-blame that such recognition can generate. If the patient can be helped to appreciate the element of irony in his repetitive difficulties, a powerful impediment to his acceptance of responsibility for his life can be diminished. Through understanding how he consistently brings about certain consequences that he does *not* intend, he can be empowered to initiate changes without being simultaneously immobilized by guilt and self-accusation.[5]

THE CONCEPT OF "ACCOMPLICES"

In what I have said thus far, the role of other people in maintaining the problematic patterns in which the patient is caught has surely been evident. I wish now, however, further to highlight this role, for it is crucial both in understanding patients' difficulties and in understanding what is needed to help them change. People live in contexts, and our behavior, both adaptive and maladaptive, is always *in relation to* someone or something.

To be sure, our perceptions of what others are doing, of what they think or demand of us, of what the consequences might be of relating

[5]Obviously, many of the consequences people bring about *are* intended, either consciously or unconsciously. Cyclical psychodynamic analyses do not preclude such linkages between consequence and intention. In the realm of repetitive maladaptive patterns, however, the cyclical psychodynamic perspective points us to notice the surprisingly pervasive influence of ironic, *un*intended consequences. Although appreciation of conflict and ambivalence implies that many outcomes must be understood as both wanted *and* not wanted, I believe that the case material presented in this book will enable the reader to understand why I emphasize irony more than other psychodynamic writers do.

to others in one way or another, can be quite far from veridical. However one prefers to conceptualize the psychological processes that make our behavior and experience considerably less than a one-to-one mapping of the actual events and figures in our lives—whether they be thought of as fantasies, schemas, representations, personifications, inner objects, or internalized working models—such processes are a crucial component of the dynamics of people's difficulties. But it is crucial as well that the therapist not retreat to a hermetic "inner world" in conceptualizing the issues. Understanding how people change requires understanding that in an odd way a neurosis is a joint activity, a cooperative venture of a most peculiar sort.

If one looks closely at the neurotic patterns in which the patient is entangled, one invariably finds that the maintenance of those patterns proceeds with the assistance of other people. As I put it a bit whimsically in another context,

> The sheer staying power of neurotic patterns is little short of miraculous, but we are prone to give the neurosis—and the neurotic—too much credit for this prodigious, if unfortunate, tenacity. . . . Maintaining a neurosis is hard, dirty work, that cannot be successfully achieved alone. To keep a neurosis going, one needs help. Every neurosis requires accomplices. (Wachtel, 1991a, p. 21)

Indeed, it is only when one understands how others are drawn into the pattern as accomplices, how they are induced to interact in ways that confirm neurotic expectations and perceptions, that one appreciates fully both the depth of the patient's dilemma and what is required to bring about change.

The people who play the role of accomplice in our lives are not necessarily malicious; most often they are not even aware that they are playing such a role. But their participation is crucial, and the therapist's understanding of it can make the difference between success and failure. Focus in the therapeutic work on how patients induce others to play a complementary role in their neuroses is in many instances the key element in understanding how the patient's difficulties are perpetuated. It has occurred to me, in fact, that it would not be far from accurate to say that the process whereby others are continually recruited into a persisting maladaptive pattern *is* the neurosis.

By way of illustration, let us return to the two prototypes cited above. In the first example (the individual who is conflicted about expressions of anger), the patient's behavior is likely, in dozens of ways, to induce behavior in others that does not meet his needs or is dismissive or frustrating. In many of these instances, the participation of the "accomplice" in the neurotic pattern is likely to be not only involuntary and unintended but unwitting as well. The patient may, for example, indicate to a friend who asks if he'd like to see a horror movie that he'd be happy to, even though in fact such movies give him nightmares; he doesn't, after all, want to offend or to put a damper on others' enthusiasms. The friend may thus be quite unaware that he has caused discomfort and may be quite puzzled at whatever fallout there might be as a result. Or the patient might go out of his way to extend himself to others the night before a big exam, leaving himself little time for his own studying. The others might be grateful for his willingness to help this way, and impressed with how on top of things he is that he can afford to do this, but have little awareness that they are participants in a drama that for the patient, rarely has a happy ending.

Perhaps if the potential accomplice is especially considerate or sensitive, he might ask, "Are you sure you have time to help me tonight?" or (in other situations) "Are you sure it's OK for me to go out with Jennifer? I had the impression you were interested in her?" or, "I appreciate your offer to pick me up at the airport, but don't you have a deadline to meet?" In these, as in countless other instances in which the patient, one might say, aggressively places himself second, it would take not only unusual sensitivity but also unusual persistence to resist the juggernaut of magnanimity that the patient mobilizes. It is as if all the warded off aggression is marshalled in the service of deference and self-abnegation. For the individual drawn into this pattern to avoid becoming an oppressor requires overriding the patient's disclaimers ("No, no, I'm happy to do it. No problem at all."), but after a while, doing *that* feels like being aggressive. And so, silently in most instances, with a feeling of discomfort or "stickiness" in others, each day a part of the standing army of accomplices is called to active duty.[6]

A somewhat different, but equally interesting, state of affairs holds when one examines the participation of accomplices in relation to the so-called narcissistic patient. Such patients tend to draw in as accomplices a more limited or specific spectrum of personality types than does the patient of the unassertive type just described. The latter, the person who is allergic to aggressiveness, is likely to encounter a fairly random mix of other people. Any of us may be prone to be drawn in as an accomplice to such a person. That is both because the patterns between the patient and the accomplice are relatively simple in comparison to those to be described next and because few people feel a strong need to

---

[6]The reader may find interesting parallels between the pattern just described and what Horney has discussed as the "moving-toward" neurotic trend or the "self-effacing solution" (Horney, 1945, 1950).

avoid such individuals at all costs. With the narcissistic patient, the situation is noticeably different. Many people will go out of their way to have little to do with such a person.

As a rule, two main types of individuals tend to get drawn in as accomplices in the narcissistic pattern. First there are those individuals whose own self-esteem depends very centrally on being associated with or attached to another person who can be looked up to. Whether for a sense of protection or safety, or for the bolstering of their own sense of self-worth that comes with a kind of narcissism—by identification, such individuals long (albeit ambivalently) to be connected to someone who is a bit larger than life. When the narcissistic patient comes on the scene, with his swagger and air of expansiveness and certainty, such individuals are drawn into his orbit.

At first the narcissistic individual finds this gratifying. Their admiration is just what he is seeking, and their using him to bolster their self-esteem serves to bolster *his* self-esteem. But their attentions usually turn out to be a mixed blessing. For although their manifest role in the relationship is as the underdog, there is also a way in which they become harsh taskmasters. As they insinuate themselves into the narcissist's life, they become increasingly essential for the regulation of his own sense of being adequate and worthwhile. He has become addicted, as it were, to their admiration, and as dependent covertly as they are more manifestly. But the needs of these accomplices are such that it is essential for their own self-regard that the person they admire be very special. If the patient, as a part of his groping toward greater psychological health, is tempted to present himself more realistically, to show himself more three-dimensionally, these accomplices recoil. Letting some of the hot air out of the narcissistic balloon may be better for our patient, who is struggling to get his feet back on the ground, but it does not feel to these accomplices like what *they* need. Thus, however fervent their admiration for the patient, it is also potentially fickle. And the experience that lies at the heart of their potential disaffection—that the patient turned out in the end to be quite ordinary, not nearly special enough—is the very judgment, the very pain that our patient has dedicated his life to keeping at bay.

A second sort who turns up regularly as an accomplice in the narcissistic pattern is other narcissists. Since their own needs drive them to try to be at the center of the action, they are drawn to others like themselves, who also give off an aura of being movers and shakers. The attraction, however, is highly ambivalent and likely to be painful to both sides. What often ensues is a kind of escalation of fraudulence, as each exaggerates just a bit in order to beat, or even just to equal, the other. Since each feels deep down like a faker who must cover his perceived inadequacy, each feels that to match the talents, attributes, or exploits of the other he must embellish. But the embellishments offered by each are perceived by the other as further proof that "really I am not enough," and so must be responded to with still further flourish and adornment. Thus does each up the ante for the other, setting an increasingly false standard as they mutually build the house of cards into an ever more precarious structure, whose periodic crumbling is better known to their therapists than to each other.

Appreciation of the role of accomplices in the patient's difficulties enables the therapist to be sensitive to the *reality* dimension in neurotic suffering. We are used to thinking of neurosis as entailing *needless* suffering, *unrealistic* suffering, suffering based on distorted perceptions, on misapprehensions of the reality the individual faces. And certainly this is largely true. But one does not sufficiently appreciate the challenge facing the psychotherapist if one does not also recognize that the very nature of neurotic ways of living creates what one might call a "neurotic reality"; that is, a reality in which the expectations and reactions the person encounters from others are, at least in certain respects, more in line with the assumptions that constitute the neurosis than they are with what one might describe (with apologies to Heinz Hartmann) as the average expectable environment.

Put differently, the patient's dilemma begins to take on a life of its own. Given the predicament he has gotten himself into, given the particular cast of characters who inhabit his life and the particular relationships and expectations he has established with them, there *is* a likelihood that relinquishing the neurotic pattern will result in some of the consequences he fears, or at least that the *process* of relinquishing, unless helped and guided by the therapist in certain ways, can be as much a source of pain as of liberation. Though the pain is likely to be temporary and the liberation more enduring, the former tends to speak in a louder voice. Unless its role is appreciated by the therapist, gains are likely to be short-lived or the struggle for change to be longer and more grueling than it needs to be.

When the narcissistic patient, for example, begins to confront and accept his own limitations (and, of course, thereby to lay the foundations of truly appreciating for the first time his real strengths), he does face the prospect of being diminished in the eyes of some people who have become important mainstays of his self-esteem. He has set up expectations in others that in some sense can't be met simply by "ordinary" competent performance. Even his job could possibly be threatened if he has sold himself as a Superman and must now defend a more reasonable standard. For not only must he make this transition with people who have admired him just a bit too much but perhaps also with people who have tolerated him because of his seemingly extraordinary talents but who have little love for an individual who has seemed relentlessly self-promoting and insensitive to the needs of others. Performance they would accept readily from someone else may seem insufficient to compensate for the hurt he has inflicted.

In the case of the meek and overly solicitous individual, a different set of expectations may present an obstacle to change. He is likely to be experienced as someone who is acceptable because he is so little trouble. He may not be very interesting or especially competent (see below), but he can be relied on to make life easy for others and not to make waves. That is his role in a variety of relationships and organizations, and that is the unstated social compact that is the basis for his acceptance. When he begins to assert himself, the unarticulated reaction of others may be, in effect, "We can accept that in other people, but from you we didn't expect this!"

Life, in other words, is not fair. The narcissistic individual may be most likely to encounter rejection just when he is beginning to be more genuine. The insensitivity and braggadocio that have characterized his interactions with others are *not* his essence, but their legacy interferes with the acceptance he needs to relinquish them; the perception by others that these *are* his defining qualities helps keep him locked into them.

Similarly, incompetence and lack of imagination or initiative are not the defining essence of the individual who has squelched his vitality in the relentless suppression of anger and aggressiveness. But here too his effort to transcend the strictures that have bound his life encounters the toxic residue of their previous operation. He can only become more alive and interesting and creative by being more assertive and at least somewhat less easy to get along with. But when being "easy to get along with" is perceived by others as his primary social asset, he may find himself encountering subtle sanctions that force him back into his prior mold. And in the process, the assumptions (both his own *and* others') that have been the foundation of that prior way of being—especially the assumption that he is not strong or talented enough to justify ever being "difficult"—may seem to be confirmed.

Appreciation of this reality basis for the patient's anxieties—of the ways in which the patient's neurotic patterns of living become self-perpetuating and draw out from others the very attitudes and reactions that will keep his neurotic assumptions intact—can enable the therapist to confront the patient's worst fears about himself without becoming one more accomplice in the patient's private rogues' gallery. The strategies and nuances of phrasing described in this book build on this foundation and extend it into the concrete details of clinical practice. If one recognizes the centrality of vicious circles, of irony, and of the role of accomplices in maintaining the patient's difficulties, it is possible to be much more effective in helping the patient to extricate himself from the web of influences that have maintained his neurotic misery and/or restricted his emotional freedom. It is possible, moreover, as the clinical examples in this book illustrate, to address the "deeper" levels of the patient's difficulties without inducing the guilt and shame that are a frequent accompaniment of conventionally phrased clinical interventions.

Cyclical Psychodynamics II
The Centrality of Anxiety

It has been clear to most psychotherapists for some time now that anxiety and related distressing affects usually lie at the heart of their patients' difficulties. In large measure, people seek psychotherapy because they have become afraid of aspects of the world or aspects of their own experience that seem relatively harmless to most people. The task of the therapist consists to a significant degree in helping them to overcome these fears and live more fully, freely, and enjoyably.

This is not to say that overt anxiety is always strongly present or that the patient necessarily understands his difficulties in these terms. Although the concept of defense is usually thought of as particular to the psychodynamic point of view, in fact the operation of defenses is but an instance of the more general tendency to avoid what causes anxiety; almost all theoretical perspectives recognize that because of the tendency to avoid what is anxiety provoking, anxiety often has its effects silently. If the person can help it, he does *not* walk around anxious all day. Rather, what happens is that his life is bounded by invisible markers that he responds to with exquisite sensitivity and with scarcely any awareness of being anxious or even of avoiding.

In the Freudian tradition this tendency is conceptualized via the notion of signal anxiety: at the slightest indication of the stirring of forbidden desires, the ego gives an almost imperceptible signal of anxiety, and that is enough to call the defenses into play; it is only when the defenses *fail* to head off the perceived danger that the full-blown experience of conscious anxiety comes to pass. In other traditions, from the Sullivanian to the behavioral, a similar idea is expressed via the concept of the anxiety *gradient*. Just the slightest increase in discomfort is sufficient to generate subtle avoidances, and in most instances the full experience of anxiety that would otherwise have ensued is prevented. (There may, of course, be further anxiety generated as a result of the avoidances themselves; as will be elaborated below, comfort of this sort is not usually achieved without a cost.)

Anxiety, then, has its impact not just in creating a state of distress but in the distortions of development and distortions of current functioning that are introduced by the efforts the person makes to *avoid* anxiety. Although sometimes, as in the phobias or in panic disorders, it is the anxiety itself that is the chief problem that the patient brings, most often the picture is more complex. Efforts to avoid anxiety begin to generate their own consequences: crucial skills in living, that in the normal course of development require countless experiences of practice and shaping, are impaired because the person is driven by anxiety to avoid the relevant experiences. Clear thinking is disrupted because anxiety-provoking *thoughts* are avoided, much as are overt behaviors. As a consequence, the patient's dilemmas are compounded by an inability to think them through or by a compelled reaching of false conclusions that temporarily reduce or avoid anxiety but in the long run generate still further problems. Finally, clear appreciation of one's own desires, aspirations, concerns, and subjective experience is disrupted, leaving the individual without a rudder and thus vulnerable to engaging in activities, or even to defining his values and aspirations, in ways that are antithetical to his deepest nature.

Interestingly, the structure of the interacting set of causes and effects just described can again be understood in terms of a vicious circle. All of the above-noted repercussions of the effort to avoid anxiety tend to generate still further anxiety as a consequence of the vulnerabilities and distortions in living they introduce; and the avoidance of these secondary anxieties in turn generates still more of the reactions and sequelae that exacerbate that vulnerability still further. Most experienced therapists, regardless of theoretical orientation, are acquainted with this set of interweaving influences and the central role anxiety plays in them, even if they do not necessarily focus on the vicious circular structure to the overall pattern.

In the cyclical psychodynamic approach to therapeutic change, this understanding of anxiety is especially crucial. The patient's problems are understood as deriving most fundamentally from his having learned early in life to be afraid of his feelings, thoughts, and inclinations, and the effort to help him overcome his problems is focused very largely on helping him reappropriate those feelings and incorporate them into a fuller and richer sense of self and of life's possibilities.

Not all of the early anxiety on which later neurotic structures build, of course, is thoroughly unrealistic. Parents often can be intolerant of developments and inclinations in their children that are part of the healthy, expansive expression of the child's vitality. The reasons for this intolerance can range from severe psychopathology in the parents, to more specific vulnerabilities or areas of conflict traceable to the parents' own childhoods, to the simple fact that raising a child is a demanding and stressful experience. Children's needs are intense and constant, and modulation is not one of their virtues; any parent who is honest with him- or herself will recognize feelings that the child-rearing manuals do not tout. Since the child is dependent on the parent—first for physical survival and later for a sense of connection and well-being and for the structure and support required to promote further growth and development—it is understandable that every child, at least to some degree, will trim his sails to suit the prevailing winds.

Often, however, the trimming is both more substantial and less discriminating than might be optimal. Several factors, rooted in the existential realities of human childhood, make it likely that in the course of development every one of us will impose certain blinders and limits on ourselves that have less to do with what the world requires of us than with the particular skew with which we have learned to view that world. This is why therapists tend to reject the simple dichotomy between normality and psychological disorder, and postulate instead that neurosis is a matter of degree. We all show the stigmata of the helplessness with which members of our species enter the world and the many years it takes before we achieve even a rough approximation to parity with those on whom we depend.

Add to this that the young child is not only extremely dependent on the giants that surround him but also only dimly able to comprehend their moods, motives, and guiding cognitive framework. This limited capacity to appreciate the reasons for adults' actions makes them seem more capricious—and hence more dangerous—than they actually are. It also makes it difficult to discriminate when it is appropriate to express an urge or a feeling and when it is best kept under wraps—that is, when an inclination the child experiences is safe and when it is dangerous. Moreover, the child is also less able to *control* his behavior than an adult can (or than the adults around him, when they are feeling stressed, wish he could). The line between impulse and action and between affect and outcry is thin in childhood, and, as a consequence, impulses represent far more of a threat than they will when the child grows up.

In the course of development, these difficulties in comprehension, control, and discrimination, combining toxically with extreme dependency, yield the phenomena that are the seeds of later neuroses. The anxiety-driven protective efforts of early life—and indeed of adult life as well—are characterized not by conscious and specific choices to inhibit particular behaviors or avoid particular situations, but by wholesale flight from anything having to do with the feelings and experiences that are being defended against.

Loving support, dependability, and encouragement of gradually increasing growth and independence from the parents can help to mitigate these unfortunate regularities of human childhood, permitting the attainment of workable compromises in which the sense of safety and the capacity to expand and express oneself are in a reasonably satisfactory balance. In combination with satisfying and age-appropriate interactions with peers, these mitigating factors can enable maturation to proceed and provide a foundation for making corrections later in life. But the adaptiveness and attunement to reality that we achieve will always be partial and relative. For all of us there remain significant areas of conflict and significant ways in which experience is restricted and distorted (and indeed, restricted and distorted in ways that prevent us from noticing that they *are* restricted and distorted).

As a consequence, one of the chief aims of the psychotherapist is to help the patient overcome the fears and inhibitions that have led him to react to his normal and healthy feelings as if they were a threat; to help him reappropriate parts of himself that have been dissociated from full awareness, that have motivated avoidances, and that are likely to generate still further areas of vulnerability, deficits in crucial skills in living, and impediments to the very relationships that could in principle be correctives to the debilitating anxiety. As the reader proceeds in this book, it will be apparent that many of the formulations and phrasings described are designed to accomplish precisely this task—to help the patient become more comfortable with his own thoughts and feelings, to see that he has been unnecessarily afraid or repelled, to create an atmosphere in which this reappropriation is possible.

THE RENUNCIATORY VISION OF THERAPEUTIC CHANGE

By now most therapists understand the role of anxiety in much the fashion just described, and understand their own role in terms that are consonant. It is possible, however, in many aspects of stance and tone that are still common in the practice of psychotherapy, to see the influence of other conceptions that contrast quite sharply with what has just been described. As Wile (1985) has put it, many features of the practice of psychotherapy are based on a view—sometimes held quite consciously and explicitly, sometimes operating silently and without the therapist being fully aware of all its ramifications—that the primary task of therapy is to bring to awareness impulses and fantasies that the patient has persistently kept hidden, and that the means of doing so is to intensify the wishes to the point where they break through into the patient's awareness. This requires the therapist "to frustrate the wish and to maintain an adequate . . . level of anxiety. Gratifying the wish is thought to be incompatible with analyzing it" (Wile, 1985, p. 794).

In a similar vein, Aron depicts an "atmosphere of renunciation and mourning" that is frequently evident in psychoanalytically grounded therapies and suggests that this atmosphere is

> exacerbated by the rule of abstinence. The patient must give up infantile wishes, renounce unconscious longings, abandon strivings after childhood sexual objects, and all of this must be done in an atmosphere of deprivation. The analyst must always be careful *not* to gratify transference wishes, because if gratified these wishes would no longer push for satisfaction (discharge) and therefore there would be no motivation (energy) with which to uncover repressed memory. (Aron, 1991, p. 91)

Addressing a related aspect of psychoanalytic practice, Leo Stone, a highly respected Freudian analyst who has contributed significantly to modifying the harsher overtones of classical technique, notes that the older point of view is still prevalent. As he puts it,

> To be "tough" with a patient is regarded as all right. To be a little gentle with a patient is always suspect. To raise a fee is natural, good analytic work. To lower a fee is, a priori, dubious indulgence. To withhold information is, a priori, good. To give a little information because you think it, as a matter of judgment, desirable at the time is, a priori, bad. (Langs & Stone, 1980, p. 9)

Summarizing some of these themes, Wile notes that

> Analysts have classically refrained from answering clients' questions, giving advice, and so on for fear that such actions would violate the rule of abstinence, interfere with the development of the transference, constitute an acting-out with the client of the transference, and, by indulging the client's infantile fantasy wishes, gratify or traumatize the client. (Wile, 1985, p. 797)

As will be apparent shortly, these views and attitudes are not in fact confined to therapists explicitly identified as psychoanalytic in their orientation. They have permeated therapeutic practice to a far greater degree than is usually recognized and, in an unnoticed and unexamined way, have shaped the practices of a broad spectrum of psychotherapists.

As part of his critique of these views, Wile advocates an approach he calls ego analysis, following the terminology of Fenichel (1941) and Apfelbaum (1966). The viewpoint of ego analysis (which as both Wile and Apfelbaum point out is not the same as ego psychology—indeed is sharply divergent from it in certain respects) has important similarities to that of the cyclical psychodynamic perspective on these matters described above. As Wile puts it,

> The ego analyst attributes clients' defenses against awareness of their impulses to their *distress* about these impulses, that is, their worry what it means that they have such impulses. The way to raise the impulse or feeling to consciousness, accordingly, is not to frustrate it, but to *decrease clients' alarm about it*, to enable clients to view themselves in a way that makes these threatening contents less threatening. The precondition for the emergence of warded-off contents is, as Weiss (1971) argues, safety rather than frustration. (Wile, 1985, p. 795; italics added)

This view of the therapist's role contrasts sharply with those approaches in which the emphasis is on the "austere and demanding discipline of psychoanalytic practice" (Stein, 1979) or on corresponding caution about "gratifying" the patient's infantile desires lest he sabotage the therapy by evading the difficult task with which it confronts him. It contrasts as well with conceptions in which an arms length approach to the patient is a necessary caution because the patient is viewed as "manipulative" or as trying to "control" the session. And it challenges the tendency to regard as the standard and appropriate stance of the therapist one of silence, anonymity, and hesitancy to ask or answer questions.

Perhaps most of all, the cyclical psychodynamic view of anxiety, like the viewpoint of ego analysis described by Wile, Apfelbaum, Gill, and others, challenges the notion, still prevalent in psychoanalytic circles, that the patient's basic impulses are essentially antisocial and regressive and that therapeutic change entails their renunciation. This latter view, evident in a wide range of psychoanalytic writings throughout the decades, is particularly highlighted by Aron:

> Freud often wrote that once the unconscious conflicts between impulses and defense were made conscious, then, in the light of secondary process thought, the patient would have to *renounce* or *condemn* the infantile wishes. Waelder (1960) wrote that once the drive was recognized as part of oneself, it would be condemned, "consciously denied gratification," so that after a while it would gradually be "given up." . . . This is consistent with references in Freud's writings to the analyst's having to "persuade" patients to "abandon" particular infantile strivings, as well as to his description of the need to induce the patient to "adopt our conviction . . . of

the impossibility of conducting life on the pleasure principle." (Aron, 1991)

Aron adds that in the classical psychoanalytic view there is an unrecognized paradox. The ego, he suggests,

> must gain the strength to tolerate increasingly clearer derivatives of the drives, only so that it will be able to consciously and willfully condemn and renounce them. The analytic atmosphere must be safe enough to convince patients that they have nothing to fear in allowing impulses access to consciousness; on the other hand, the time must come when the patient, now with conscious insight and knowledge of these infantile strivings, condemns and renounces them, and instead seeks out aims more appropriate to adult life. (Aron, 1991, p. 88)

The pervasiveness of this point of view is particularly highlighted by the following passage from Fenichel (1941), whom both Wile (1984) and Apfelbaum and Gill (1989) cite as one of the primary early proponents of the newer and *less* harsh version of psychoanalysis:

> I believe that in respect to [the rule of abstinence] no misunderstanding is possible. *A symptom is a substitute* for something repressed, and when in place of it another substitute a little more pleasant beckons to the patient, he gladly accepts it and is content with it. . . . If the daily hour is in itself some satisfaction for the patient, then he will only hold on to this bit of satisfaction and nothing drives him further. Therefore the analyst must not offer his patients any *transference satisfactions*. The fulfillment of what the patient longs for most in the analysis serves as a resistance to further analysis and therefore must be refused him. (Fenichel, 1941, p. 29; italics in original)

Such a view, largely anomolous in the context of the overall thrust of Fenichel's effort to depict an enlightened and progressive psychoanalytic technique, derives ultimately from the theoretical tendency critically examined in Chapter 2—the notion that the feelings and impulses involved in the patient's conflicts are not truly contemporary, but, rather, are "infantile" or "archaic" residues of early psychic life that have been rendered inaccessible to the maturational processes that enable us to become reasonable adults. Given such a view, it is not surprising that the assumption would evolve that these wishes and feelings must be renounced once they are identified and recognized. If they are as primitive and anachronistic as this conception implies, then of course they have no place in healthy adult life. The more accepting stance toward repressed feelings and wishes depicted in this book thus derives in good part from the alternative understanding of these wishes and feelings that is embodied in the cyclical psychodynamic point of view.

IMPLICATIONS OF THE REVISED THEORY OF ANXIETY

As Wile, Aron, Stone, Gill, Apfelbaum, and others have pointed out in one way or another, the result of these conceptions of abstinence and renunciation is an atmosphere that is considerably more adversarial and even accusatory than therapists are likely to realize. There is a danger that the patient will feel more "caught" than understood. Indeed, as Apfelbaum (1991) notes, citing Sterba, the analyst's role has even been described, presumably as a *positive* description, as that of a "libidinal detective!"

Much of the difficulty derives from a failure of therapeutic technique fully to capitalize on modifications in theory that contributed to a more satisfactory understanding of the processes leading to and maintaining patients' difficulties. As a consequence, the potential of newer understandings to generate a more accepting and humane approach to therapy was not realized. The most significant of these changes was Freud's recognition, only late in his career, that he had misunderstood the role of anxiety. Although Freud recognized from the first that the motive for his patients' defenses was some kind of intense discomfort, he did not see clearly for some time that that discomfort and the anxiety so often evident in his patients' complaints were one and the same. The influence of what is sometimes called the hydraulic model in Freud's thought—the images of substances under pressure, dammed up and pushing for release—led him for a long time to think of anxiety primarily as a *discharge* phenomenon: when the pressure of repressed libido became too great, some of that force was discharged in the form of anxiety.

Only after considerable other recasting of his theory had been achieved did it become clear to Freud that rather than being an epiphenomenon of repression, anxiety was the basic *cause* of repression (Freud, 1926/1959). People defended against certain aspects of their experience in order to avoid the terrible distress of anxiety. When anxiety appeared together with repression, that was not because repression had been so severe that there was no way to release the pressure except by turning libido into anxiety (a kind of psychoanalytic alchemy that was never really explained in any event). Rather, manifest anxiety was a sign of the *failure* of repression. It occurred when the forbidden impulse had been *insufficiently* repressed and thus when the danger it represented was close enough to make the individual quite uncomfortable.

The implications of this reformulation were—or should have been—momentous. Freud had said on a number of occasions that repression was the very "cornerstone" of psychoanalysis (e.g., Freud, 1914/1959). By now identifying anxiety as the motive underlying repression, Freud had in effect shifted the cornerstone. Anxiety, lying beneath and causing repression, should have been the new candidate for the central grounding concept.

The cyclical psychodynamic view of the role of anxiety in psychological disorder and distress—in which the patient's difficulties are seen as very largely a result of his having learned to fear some of his most fundamental and powerful inclinations—is rooted in this newer understanding of the central role of anxiety. So too is the less adversarial approach to therapy that is advocated in the pages of this book. The task of therapy, it appears in the light of these new formulations, is not so much to bring to light what the patient has wanted to keep hidden as to help the patient to overcome the anxiety that made the hiding feel necessary.

THE PERSISTENCE OF OLDER MODELS

To be sure, many therapists do not endorse the ideas about abstinence, frustration, silence, renunciation of impulses, and so forth that were depicted in the preceding pages. But as will be apparent as I proceed, in subtle and sometimes indirect ways these ideas have significantly influenced therapeutic technique. And this notwithstanding the fact that even among therapists explicitly identified with the psychoanalytic point of view there has been a considerable modification and evolution of the positions I have just discussed. In recent years, a number of leading figures in the analytic movement (e.g., Stone, 1961; Schafer, 1983) have struggled to introduce a more flexible and humane version of psychoanalytic treatment, and the recent turn toward object relations and self psychological approaches has further promoted this "softening" and "warming" of the analytic model of treatment. Moreover, Freud himself would probably not recognize some of the strictures that have been advocated in his name. Certainly his own technique included considerably more flexibility and genuine human interaction than what became for many years "standard" or "classical" technique.

Nonetheless, in significant ways the older models and images have continued to influence practice even among practitioners who no longer adhere to them, and indeed even among therapists who in no way think of themselves as psychoanalytic in orientation. The reason for this is that many aspects of daily clinical practice are not so much a product of explicit theoretical considerations as of incorporation, with relatively little awareness or reflection, of the attitudes and practices of one's own therapist.

Thus many of the features that give the therapeutic interaction its particular relational structure and emotional shadings are conveyed from generation to generation of psychotherapists by a mode of transmission that largely eludes reflective examination. The way one deals with patients' questions, whether and how one offers advice or opinions, how much or how little one reveals about oneself, and a host of other dimensions of the work that shape and influence the tone of the relationship are based very largely on an inner sense of what feels "right"—a feeling that derives significantly from the therapist's experience in her own therapy. But *her* therapist's practices themselves were likely to have been influenced, in an equally unexamined way, by *her* experiences in *her* own therapy. What results is what Wile (1985) has called "psychotherapy by precedent," a way of practicing rooted in ideas that once were widely and explicitly held in the therapeutic community and that has persisted even as those ideas have been superseded in the conscious thought of the therapists who implicitly perpetuate them.

The sway of these unrecognized and unexamined influences is, of course, not total. Practices are indeed shaped and changed by new ideas. The practice of psychotherapy today differs in significant ways from that of the early pioneers. But in certain crucial aspects of tone and emotional import—aspects of the therapeutic process and relationship that will be a primary focus of this book—change has been much slower and more limited. Through the medium of the silent transmission processes just described, the influence of early ideas has been maintained in practice even as some of these ideas have largely disappeared or been dismissed in explicit theoretical accounts.

Moreover, this influence is evident well beyond the confines of the theoretical orientation in which it originated. If we trace back the transmission of therapeutic practices from contemporary therapists, to their therapists' therapists, to their therapists' therapists' therapists, one need not go too far back to find a "grandparent" or "great grandparent" who was a Freudian. Earlier in the history of our field the influence of psychoanalytic ideas was far more pervasive than it is today, and indeed approached a virtual hegemony. Thus, even therapists who in no way think of themselves as Freudians, and who know that their own therapists were not Freudians either, may be unwittingly evidencing, in the tone and structure of their daily interactions with patients, the influence of early psychoanalytic ideas. (We may note here, by the way, that the tendency to underestimate the influence on daily practice of ideas from the early history of psychoanalysis is by no means limited to therapists who reject identification with psychoanalysis. It is also evident, for many of the same reasons, among therapists whose identification is with one of the modern variants of psychoanalytic thought, such as object relations theory or self psychology, that in their explicit formulations depart from classical Freudian theory in significant ways.[1])

THE OVERCOMING OF ANXIETY

If one attempts to construct a therapeutic approach more thoroughly rooted in modern understandings of anxiety, the crucial questions become not what is the patient hiding, but why is he so afraid and how can he be helped to become less afraid? Thus, one's attention naturally turns to how anxiety can be overcome. A great deal of evidence suggests that one of the most powerful correctives—if not *the* most powerful—is exposure to what has been fearfully avoided (e.g., Butler, Cullington, Munby, Amies, & Gelder, 1984; Emmelkamp, 1982; Marks, 1989). If the person can have the direct experience of safety in the presence of what he fears, his chances of recovery are greatly enhanced.

Precisely what it is that the patient must be exposed to, and how the exposure is to be brought about, differs from one therapeutic approach to another. For the behavior therapist, the most common application of this principle may be the rather straightforward exposure represented by systematic desensitization or flooding, with the focus being on an external stimulus toward which the patient has a phobic reaction. In the more insight-oriented therapies, both the medium of exposure and the choice of target are likely to be more complex and indirect. (Part of this complexity and indirection, of course, results from the fact that "exposure" is not likely to be the concept that these therapists think of when they approach their work.)

[1]Some readers may wonder if tracing these influences back from contemporary therapists, to *their* therapists, to their *therapists'* therapists, and so forth does not lead us into an infinite regress. The reason it does not is that the history of modern psychotherapy has a strong element of discontinuity. Modern psychotherapy essentially has its origins at the end of the last century. The profession as we know it today scarcely existed before then, and the tendency for professional psychotherapists to have undergone their own therapy as part of their training—the medium of unwitting transmission being discussed here— was almost certainly a product of that era. Although Freud, to be sure, drew on ideas that were already "in the air" at the time he began his work (see, for example, Ellenberger, 1970; Whyte, 1960), his influence was so powerful and pervasive that it is appropriate largely to take his ideas as the starting point in tracking the influences upon modern psychotherapists.

In the psychodynamically oriented therapies, a primary means by which the patient is exposed to previously avoided experiences is through interpretations. Interpretations are usually discussed in terms of clarifying meanings or conveying empathic understanding, and these functions of interpretations are certainly of considerable importance. But—and this may actually be the most important way in which they contribute to therapeutic change—interpretations serve as well to bring the patient into contact with experiences he has been fearfully warding off and enable him to reencounter them in a setting that is safe and controlled. These warded-off experiences are very largely "inner" experiences—that is, the patient's own thoughts, wishes, and feelings, which he has dedicated much of his energies to avoiding. There is much reason to believe that just as exposure facilitates the overcoming of fears of external stimuli, so too is it a crucial factor in mastering the anxieties associated with inner cues, anxieties that are at the heart of the psychodynamic understanding of people's psychological difficulties. It is when the person can feel the emotion he has been afraid to feel, or experience directly the wish or thought he has regarded as unacceptable and kept at bay, that he can begin to surmount the anxieties that have limited his life.

Interpretations facilitate exposure to these forbidden inner experiences in a number of ways. To begin with, by naming the implicit thought or inclination, the interpretation brings it into sharper focus and thus contributes to its entering the patient's experience more directly. Much of the warding off of conflictual experiences occurs through "not noticing" what we are doing or feeling, and the fact that the interpretation calls the patient's attention to what is going on, and implicitly directs the patient to notice, is one of its important features.[2]

Interpretations also facilitate exposure, and contribute to the overcoming of anxiety, by rendering the "unspeakable" spoken about. They bring out into the open what has had to be kept in a dark psychic closet. In the very process of doing so, they contribute to making the previously forbidden thought or feeling seem more acceptable. Moreover, the naming of the experience by the interpretation serves as a *stimulus* to the experience, calling it forth in somewhat the fashion that "fee fi fo" calls forth "fum." That is, when the therapist says "it sounds like you were angry at Bob," that comment not only clarifies what the patient was

---

[2]This is not to suggest that interpretations always directly name the forbidden wish or feeling. More typically, such direct interpretations of warded-off content are preceded by interpretations that call the patient's attention to his fear of approaching and exploring certain topics and to the various ways he characteristically avoids them. The clinical rationale and utility, as well as certain pitfalls, of such "defense interpretations" are further discussed in the chapters that follow.

feeling but also contributes to the patient's *experiencing* the anger a bit. It will not do this if the interpretation is off the mark (either because it misreads the patient's feeling about Bob or because it is premature). But if the patient is *ready* to confront his anger at Bob, the interpretation can evoke and intensify the incipient feeling so that it becomes a more complete experience. It is, after all, the patient's reexperiencing or feeling of the feeling, not the therapist's saying the words, that is the primary curative factor.

Furthermore, the therapist's speaking directly about what the patient had felt necessary to hide also conveys a readiness to address the feeling that can bolster the patient's courage to do the same. In effect, the therapist models lack of fear of the thought or feeling simply by speaking about it. Such modeling has been found in a variety of realms to contribute significantly to people's overcoming of troubling fears (Bandura, 1977), and it is almost certainly a contributing factor in the success of interpretive therapies as well.

Interpretations also contribute to promoting exposure to warded-off experiences by calling attention to and interrupting the defensive efforts that have enabled the patient to avoid those experiences in the past. The blocking of defensive efforts is perhaps most directly evident in approaches such as Gestalt therapy, especially as practiced by Fritz Perls, but it is clearly a key feature of all interpretive or insight-oriented therapies. Defense interpretations, after all, are never just "informational," nor are they really legitimately understood as neutral (see Wachtel, 1987, Chap. 11). Such interpretations, by calling the patient's attention to the defensive activity, serve to interrupt it, to prevent it from being run off smoothly and silently. As a consequence, they increase the likelihood that the patient will experience the thought or wish or feeling being defended against.

Effective Exposure versus "Mere Words"

In further considering the concept of exposure, and determining what kinds of comments and interventions by the therapist best bring it about, it is necessary to recognize that precisely what constitutes exposure, and especially what constitutes *effective* exposure, is a more complicated question than might at first appear. There are many ways in which exposure to a situation or stimulus can be attenuated, even if one is nominally in its presence. Determining how to bring the patient more fully into contact with the experiences he has avoided or warded off is much of the art of the practice of therapy.

Even in the relatively simple case of a patient with a bridge phobia driving across a bridge as part of a regimen of in vivo densensitization or flooding, there is ambiguity. Is the patient looking around and allowing himself to notice and experience as many as possible of the phobic cues—the color and pattern of the cables; the way the water looks as seen through the bridge railings; the vibrations of the car as it passes over the seams on the bridge roadway; the changing relation to the shoreline; and so forth? Or is he keeping his eyes fixed straight ahead and being so self-absorbed or consumed by his fear that he hardly sees or notices anything? The nature of the "exposure" in the two circumstances is quite different.

In those more complex exposures required by a therapeutic effort that is guided by a psychodynamic point of view, the ambiguities are, of course, still greater. If the therapy's focus is on the patient's own thoughts, feelings, and inclinations, then assuring that the patient's exposure to the relevant cues is complete and full-bodied is particularly difficult. It is certainly not enough for the patient simply to hear the therapist's words (*I wonder if you're feeling X*, or *You seem to be feeling Y.*). The real target of the therapeutic effort is the experience that those words elicit in the patient. A good interpretation is very largely defined by how much it resonates with the patient's experience and evokes and amplifies that experience.

Moreover, not only are the *therapist's* words in themselves insufficient for a significant therapeutic process to be brought about; the *patient's* response too can end up being limited to little more than "mere words." That is, the patient may substitute words for experience and thereby be deprived of much opportunity for a significant therapeutic effect. He may say things either to himself or out loud that bear directly on what the therapist has just said, yet he may not feel very much while doing so and may thus not replicate in any significant way the experience the therapist's comment is addressing. Even a very skillful therapist has only limited control over how much the patient is able to go beyond "mere words." Moreover, not only is it difficult to bring about an effective evocation of experience, it is also quite difficult to assess whether it has occurred.

There are a host of ways in which the patient can attenuate the experience of the forbidden desire or feeling. The various defense mechanisms that have been catalogued and described by psychoanalytically oriented therapists roughly correspond to those types of attenuation. Therapists of all persuasions recognize that it is not simply awareness that promotes change but awareness that is part of an affective experience. It is not enough to "know" that one is angry at a loved one, or that one has been yearning for something one has learned one shouldn't yearn for; it is necessary to *feel* that very yearning, not just to be intellectually cognizant of it.

The issue I am addressing here has, of course, often been discussed in terms of the distinction between intellectual and emotional insight. But intellectual and emotional insight are often very difficult to distinguish as the work proceeds. If therapists listen to tape recordings of patients seemingly affirming an interpretation, there will not always be general agreement as to when the patient is really experiencing the feeling he says he now recognizes and when he is offering "mere words." And often, the patient himself does not know. Rather few patients consciously dissimulate, but many can offer the therapist what they sense she wants without being aware of doing so. Especially since the therapy is directed toward feelings the patient has dedicated much of his life to not knowing about, the patient is not necessarily in a good position to be clear himself about whether he is really feeling the identified feeling or is merely surmising. The ambiguity that is inherent in the realm of affect makes uncertainty about the degree of effective exposure almost inevitable.

Many of the nuances of phrasing discussed in this book are designed precisely for the purpose of promoting effective exposure. Conceptualizing the therapeutic import of the therapist's comments in terms of facilitating exposure to the forbidden, rather than exclusively in terms of insight or some other more cognitive consideration, provides the therapist with a different perspective on her efforts and makes more likely the effective fostering of therapeutically effective exposure. In some instances, the aims are to make the comment as vivid and image-laden as possible and to promote the evocation of multiple sensory modalities. In others, the key to fostering effective exposure centers on the therapist's recognizing and understanding the patient's motivation to avoid and attenuate such exposure. Since that motivation results from the patient's anxiety and low self-esteem, comments that address the forbidden thought or feeling in a way that does not increase his shame or guilt will also make it more likely that he will be able to bear facing what he previously could not.

Mastery and the Experience of Safety

It is not enough, of course, simply to be exposed (or even to be *effectively* exposed, in the sense of truly experiencing what one has been avoiding). One could, after all, be exposed to the source of perceived danger and have a bad experience—that is, be even *more* persuaded of the danger. What is crucial is *mastery* and the *experience of safety*. Many of the therapeutic strategies discussed in this book are designed to contribute to such an experience. It is essential, for example, to pay attention to the interpersonal and cognitive skills required for mastery of the life situations the patient encounters and to understand the ways in which these skills have been impaired by anxiety and avoidance. (See especially Chapter 12 for a discussion of how the therapist's following through or not following through on this dimension can make the difference between therapeutic success and failure.)

Also of considerable value in this connection is an emphasis on *gradualism*. Enabling the patient to be exposed to disturbing material only gradually and at his own pace contributes significantly to the experience of mastery, as does helping the patient to confront interpersonal challenges in a graduated fashion.

Perhaps most important of all, facilitating the patient's sense of mastery of the previously forbidden requires attention to the dimension of self and self-esteem. What is most often threatened by the possibility of certain thoughts and wishes becoming conscious is the patient's image of self. As a consequence, the therapist's comments cannot be limited simply to the task of confronting the patient with "the truth." Crucial is doing so in a way that enables the patient to maintain his self-esteem. Once again the task is not simply for the patient to "know" about himself but, in this instance, to be more *self-accepting*. Therapeutic aims are not achieved unless the patient begins to integrate into his evolving sense of self the experiences and inclinations he has been warding off. And that will not happen if the patient continues to feel threatened or diminished by those experiences. Many of the comments described in this book are designed to enable the patient to confront previously avoided feelings and thoughts in a way that does not feel demeaning. The capacity to facilitate this, as much as a facility at identifying what those thoughts and feelings might be, is the hallmark of the psychotherapist with true talent for this kind of work.

We may further note that it is not only the "goodness" of the self that is vigorously defended but its coherence as well. In order to confront effectively the booming, buzzing confusion of the innumerable stimuli we encounter in a day, we must introduce some order into our experience. Multiple possibilities always exist for organizing the input we are constantly receiving (both from the outside world and from deep within the self), and so we must to some degree always *impose* an order on the potential chaos. Central to achieving such an order, which is the key to any feeling of security and to any adaptive efforts, is the organization of a coherent sense of self.

As Erikson (1963) has articulated so effectively, we must discover the continuity amidst diversity that makes us the same person from moment to moment and day to day, and we must *re*discover (and *reconstruct*) that continuity constantly in order not either to experience fragmentation or diffusion or to freeze in a prematurely rigidified structure of identity. For many people, experiences that seem to contradict the evolving sense of self and identity can be threatening even if they point to "good" things about the self that had not been previously noticed. As Sullivan (1947, 1953), Kohut (1971, 1977, 1985), and Rogers (1951, 1959, 1961) have suggested in different ways, so crucial is the image we hold of ourselves to our sense that the world is predictable and can be coped with that experiences that might modify that image can feel like portents of chaos. The sense of coherence and stability of the self is so key to our adaptive efforts that we will even struggle to maintain a *negative* image of the self if that negative image has been integrated into the core of our sense of reality. It is not uncommon, for example, for patients to fearfully ward off evidence that they are smarter, more moral, or more attractive than they think they are.

Sullivan (1953) has captured an important dimension of this tendency in his concept of the malevolent transformation. As he points out, if a person who has thought of himself as hateful or as hated begins to feel love or to feel loved by the other, considerable anxiety can be stirred. Such a situation raises the risk that safeguards carefully constructed over the years to protect from disappointment or danger (and thus to diminish at least somewhat the pain that would otherwise ensue) might be foolishly or prematurely relinquished, exposing the person to even greater pain. Thus, some patients will become especially uncomfortable at just those moments of hope, fearing opening themselves to the increased vulnerability that hope itself creates, and they will react with a hostility or suspiciousness designed (usually unconsciously) to drive the other person away. In this way, they can reestablish at least the protection against unpleasant surprises that a cynical view of oneself and of others provides.

It will be apparent as the reader proceeds in this volume that a number of the phrasings and strategies that are discussed are designed to help the patient integrate into an evolving sense of self various experiences and characteristics—whether "positive" or "negative"— that had previously seemed essential to ward off because they seemed at odds with whatever coherence the patient had been able to achieve.

CHAPTER 4

Cyclical Psychodynamics III
Insight, the Therapeutic Relationship, and the World Outside

The emphasis in the previous chapter on exposure and on direct experience is clearly in some contrast to the traditional emphasis on insight, although it does not directly contradict it. The differences between the account of therapeutic change offered here and those of earlier psychodynamic perspectives center not on the question of whether the therapist should aim to facilitate the patient's insight into previously unrecognized aspects of his experience, but rather on how pursuit of that insight fits into the overall set of processes that constitute effective psychotherapy. Put differently, what is at issue is whether deep and enduring change is in fact best achieved by the therapist's attempting to confine herself exclusively to promoting insight. In the account presented here, insight remains an important component of the change process, but its significance is seen as best understood in relation to the other change processes described in these chapters. Too exclusive a concern with insight can lead to foregoing other important sources of change that contribute significantly to the patient's achieving his therapeutic aims.

Moreover, too exclusive a focus by the therapist on the promotion of insight can actually impede even the achieving of insight itself. As will be discussed further below, insight is often greatly enhanced by direct efforts to overcome the anxiety that motivates the patient's clouding and distorting of his experience (see, for example, Wachtel, 1991b). It is enhanced as well by the patient's being helped to take new actions in the world that bring him into a different position vis-à-vis his conflicts and provide a new vantage point from which to view himself and his feelings and aims. The synergistic interaction between achieving insight and taking active steps to change troubling life patterns renders anachronistic some formulations of the therapeutic process that cast the therapist solely in the role of furthering understanding and that eschew any other kind of assistance as interfering with that superordinate aim. In the light of the analysis offered here, quite the opposite appears to be the case. It is the *refusal* to offer any other kind of assistance that impedes the fuller development of self-understanding.[1]

The sharp dichotomy between insight-oriented approaches and approaches in which advice, direction, and the corrective influence of the therapeutic interaction may be employed is a false one. Therapy conducted from the standpoint of cyclical psychodynamics, although placing considerably less emphasis than other insight-oriented approaches on the need for neutrality, anonymity, and disavowal of active efforts to assist the patient, remains strongly committed to the promotion of self-awareness and self-understanding. This commitment derives both from ethical and value concerns and from considerations of therapeutic efficacy.

For the patient to take appropriate steps to achieve his therapeutic goals, he must be clear just what those goals are. The anxieties that lie at the heart of so many of the difficulties patients bring to therapy make such clarity unlikely. Self-deception and self-alienation are for many patients the very essence of what troubles them, and these phenomena play a role in almost all psychological disorder. Active intervention techniques to assist the patient in achieving his aims must be predicated on an accurate understanding of what those aims are, and such understanding cannot be taken for granted. In the course of a well-conducted therapy, the patient's picture of what he hopes the therapy will accomplish is likely to change considerably. And the greater clarity he achieves about his true aims and feelings is in most instances one of the most significant benefits of the therapy, quite apart from any relief from troubling symptoms or interpersonal patterns.

Furthering self-understanding is crucial as well to the aim, central to the therapy described here, of helping the patient become more fully an active agent in his own life. A person cannot experience himself as the vital center giving direction to his daily actions and choices, nor can he be a truly active participant in his own therapy (a major thrust in the cyclical psychodynamic approach), if he is engaged in substantial self-

---

[1]Since comments that are "officially" labeled as interpretations almost always contain other unacknowledged elements as well, one might alternatively suggest that it is the refusal to *recognize* the other sources of influence (and the consequent inability to think explicitly and intelligently about them) that is the primary impediment.

deception that alienates him from his experiences and desires. It is important to be clear, however, that effective pursuit of deeply felt engagement with powerful but buried yearnings and feelings may require at times that the therapist depart from traditional notions of neutrality and nonintervention. The achievement by the patient of a true sense of agency in his life often requires the therapist to confront actively the obstacles impeding the patient's self-acceptance and self-direction. Such therapist activity is by no means incompatible with a commitment to promoting deeper self-understanding. The hyperindividualistic outlook of our culture (see Wachtel, 1989) often leads therapists and patients alike to assume that a true sense of selfhood and agency can (even *must*) be achieved without help from others and to regard the changes attained in the therapy as somehow sullied if recognizable assistance is offered. Such a view, I believe, is deleterious to the patient's prospects for therapeutic gain and, indeed, even to the prospect for insight.

INSIGHT AND CORRECTIVE EMOTIONAL EXPERIENCE

One of the earliest modern therapists to suggest that the traditional focus on insight must be complemented by an emphasis on new experience was Franz Alexander (e.g., Alexander & French, 1946; Alexander, 1961, 1963). Alexander's concept of the "corrective emotional experience," however, was formulated in a way that seemed to many to imply a kind of disingenuousness incompatible with full respect for the patient. I think this view was partly accurate and partly an instance of selective perception that excluded other ways of understanding or reworking Alexander's innovations. Most importantly, it reflected an unfortunate failure of imagination. For it would have taken little to recognize that whatever the specific tone of Alexander's own utilization of this concept, the broader idea that it is a corrective emotional *experience*, and not just an "insight," that is curative was a significant and valuable recasting of Freud's account of how therapeutic change is attained. Gradually, this appreciation has reentered our discourse on processes of therapeutic change—through the concept of "encounter" among existentially oriented therapists; through the formulations of Weiss and Sampson (1986) regarding the patient's "testing" of the therapist; through Kohut's accounts (e.g., Kohut, 1984) of the curative power of certain experiences with the therapist quite apart from the insights that may accompany them; through the various discussions by object relations theorists of the therapist's role as a good, reparative parent; and from other sources as well.

Alexander observed, correctly I believe, that often insight *followed* change. If one attempts to live differently, not only is change effected by that very fact, but one also gains a new vantage point from which to examine one's life. As a consequence, new insights are promoted, insights that are a *product* of change rather than its cause.

This does not, however, make insights simply an epiphenomenon. To begin with, insights help to consolidate and deepen the changes brought about in other ways. Moreover, though not the be-all and end-all of therapy, they are part of a back and forth loop between insight and behavior change in which both are genuinely causal. This loop can be interfered with if the emphasis on insight is too exclusive or too narrowly construed. If the therapist, in the name of promoting insight, refrains from pointing the patient toward the new behavior that will afford him the new vantage point, the synergy is disrupted. The result is likely to be an overestimation of the power of resistance, based on phenomena that are the product not of the patient's inherent oppositionalism or noncompliance but of avoidable therapeutic error.

THE THERAPEUTIC CONTRIBUTION OF THE PATIENT–THERAPIST RELATIONSHIP

The contribution of the therapeutic relationship has been emphasized increasingly by therapists of widely varying persuasions (e.g., Goldfried & Davison, 1976; Jacobson, 1989; Kohut, 1984; Rice, 1983; Safran & Segal, 1991; Weiss & Sampson, 1986). Systematic research too has highlighted the importance of the quality of the therapeutic relationship and, indeed, the literature on relationship influences and contributions in recent years is much too large to review in the present context (see, for example, Bergin & Garfield, 1986; Harvey & Parks, 1982; Lambert, 1983; Lambert, Shapiro, & Bergin, 1986).

The work of Alexander described above provided one impetus for this emphasis on the relationship, but there were many others. The findings of Jerome Frank (e.g., 1973, 1982), one of the earliest influential psychotherapy researchers, highlighted—as have many studies since—the roughly equivalent results obtained by therapies with considerably different procedures and rationales, and it suggested that certain common factors might be at work in all of them. Among these, the quality of the relationship between patient and therapist seemed an especially promising candidate.

In the development of the psychoanalytic approach in these years, although the primary thrust was on the relationship as a screen for the patient's fantasies rather than as something real and significant in its own right, there was increasing reference to what was called "the real relationship," "the therapeutic alliance," and "the working alliance" (Greenson, 1965; Zetzel, 1956), all of which in one way or another stressed that certain aspects of what was really transpiring between the persons in the room were crucial.[2] Stone's (1961) emphasis on physicianly concern and Schafer's (1983) on creating an atmosphere of safety similarly highlighted dimensions of the actual qualities of the relationship—apart from whatever distorting fantasies could be interpreted and explored—that contributed to therapeutic results. Kohut's (1984) notion of "transmuting internalization," though lacking in clarity, seemed to point in a similar direction.

Among psychoanalytic writers, the British analyst Peter Lomas has been particularly critical of the notion that meaningful psychological change can result from interpretation alone, and he has argued for emphasis on the impact of the therapeutic relationship per se. In Lomas's view, although psychoanalysts "have increasingly become aware that the consulting room contains two human beings who have strong feelings about each other, and that the practitioner needs to be more than an interpreting machine . . . little attempt has been made to acknowledge that it no longer makes sense to depend on a theory based on the paradigm of interpretation" (Lomas, 1987). Lomas argues that patients "will accept what is said only to the extent that it matches their experience of the therapist. If this is so, the therapist cannot sit back, believing that, as a professional, all she has to do is make 'correct' interpretations. She has to *act* in a healing way" (Lomas, 1987, pp. 5–6; italics in original).

Consonant with the main themes of this book, Lomas notes that "Interpretations are not isolated, discrete little bits of discourse, but manifestations of an overall message to the patient," a message that includes not only the content of the interpretation but the *manner* in which the interpretation is given and the quality of the relationship that is its context.

In considering the various relationship qualities that can be healing, Lomas acknowledges the therapeutic value of interpretation but places it in a larger context in which it is but one of many sources of therapeutic change:

[2]As I have discussed in more detail elsewhere (Wachtel, 1981), as useful as these notions are, they are problematic because they have been insufficiently integrated with the understanding reflected in the concept of transference. As I suggest below, a more comprehensive and coherent account of *all* these dimensions of the relationship between patient and therapist, and of the patient's perception and experience of the therapist, can be provided by utilizing Piaget's concepts of schema, assimilation, and accommodation.

> There are many possible ways besides interpretation in which one person may act therapeutically upon another. . . . They include understanding, listening, sharing, criticizing, comforting, stimulating, moving and allowing oneself to be moved, encouraging, provoking, tolerating; and perhaps above all, being as authentic as one can manage. (Lomas, 1987, p. 69)

Appreciation of the impact of the therapeutic relationship in its own right as a potentially corrective experience (as well an experience which, with the wrong kind of therapist input—or an improper *absence* of input—can unwittingly *maintain* the patient's difficulties) underlies many of the formulations presented in this book. Overemphasis on the patient's getting to "know" something about himself can lead to a failure to consider in sufficient detail the emotional impact of what the therapist says and of how she says it. If the therapist is too concerned about *what* point she is getting across, and insufficiently attuned to *how* she is conveying it, the crucial distinction between addressing difficult truths and actual harshness can become blurred.

NEUTRALITY, TRANSFERENCE, AND ANONYMITY

The foregoing discussion suggests that the contribution of the relationship to therapeutic change has frequently been underestimated or misunderstood and that this tendency to minimize its import is evident not only among proponents of therapies that rely heavily on active techniques, such as cognitive-behavioral and family therapies, but among psychoanalytic and psychodynamic therapists as well. At the same time, it will be obvious to most readers that the therapeutic relationship is by no means ignored in psychoanalytically oriented therapies. Indeed, it is not unreasonable to suggest that attention to the relationship is at the very heart of the psychoanalytic approach.

The apparent contradiction is readily resolved. Psychoanalytic therapists indeed see the relationship as central—but primarily as something to *examine*, not to be utilized as itself a lever for change.[3]

Central to this approach to the relationship, of course, is the concept of transference. The patient is understood as perceiving the therapist in terms of earlier experiences and relationships and as unconsciously attributing to the therapist characteristics that in fact derive from early figures in the patient's life or from his fantasies about them.

[3]As noted above, analysts representing interpersonal, self-psychological, and object relations perspectives have increasingly departed from stricter versions of this paradigm, but generally with at least some degree of ambivalence and some continuing adherence to the views described below.

By helping the patient to recognize the distortions in his perception of the analyst, the analyst promotes the patient's insight into the unconscious mental processes that guide his interactions with the world.

From a traditional psychoanalytic perspective, in order to facilitate this process of gaining insight, the analyst must keep to a minimum those actions that might reveal her true characteristics. Remaining as anonymous and ambiguous as possible is seen as having two salutary consequences. First, it increases the likelihood of the patient's *revealing* his unconscious biases and inclinations (since such characteristics are revealed most readily under conditions of ambiguity and lack of structure). Second, it helps the patient to *recognize* that he has in fact been under the sway of unconscious distorting processes: since the analyst has apparently done nothing to merit the patient's perception, the patient is more able to be persuaded that the perception comes from forces and memories within him rather than from what is "really" happening now.

In a classic statement of this position, Freud stated emphatically, "We overcome the transference by pointing out to the patient that his feelings *do not arise from the present situation and do not apply to the person of the doctor*, but that they are repeating something that has happened to him earlier" (Freud, 1916/1943, pp. 443–444; italics added). Elaborating on this theme, and explicating further its seeming implications for technique, Gill (1954) suggested in an influential and widely cited paper that

> The clearest transference manifestations are those which recur when the analyst's behavior is constant, since under these circumstances changing manifestations in the transference cannot be attributed to an external situation, to some changed factor in the interpersonal relationship, but the analysand must accept responsibility himself. (Gill, 1954, p. 781)

Gill himself has changed his views regarding transference quite significantly, as I shall discuss shortly. Many psychoanalytically oriented therapists, however, have remained fixated, as it were, on this earlier position, striving to intervene as little as possible and to reveal as little as possible about themselves in order to assure that the patient cannot attribute his experience of the therapist to something really about the therapist and that he must therefore accept that the reaction comes from within him.

In another influential presentation of the standard psychoanalytic view, for example, Greenson (1967) states that "transference reactions are always inappropriate" (p. 152) and that transference feelings and reactions "do not befit" the person in the present toward whom they are directed "but are a repetition of reactions originating in regard to significant persons of early childhood unconsciously displaced onto figures in the present" (p. 155). Langs (1973), taking this still further, claims that "to identify a fantasy about, or reaction to, the therapist as primarily transference . . . we must be able to refute with certainty *any* appropriate level of truth to the patient's unconscious or conscious claim that she correctly perceives the therapist in the manner spelled out through her associations" (p. 415; italics added).

It is interesting to note here Langs's use of the rather revealing word "refute." Such terminology betokens a rather adversarial conception of the relationship between therapist and patient. The patient is wrong and must be argued out of his error.[4] The word refute implies as well, apropos the discussion above of the difficulties with overly cognitive notions of how change is brought about, that therapeutic change is based on persuasion, on who has the more convincing argument.

The cyclical psychodynamic understanding of transference and of how to work with it in therapy is quite different from the views just cited. It rejects the either–or approach in which establishing the contribution of the patient's past and of his personality structure seems to require that the transference reaction be seen as having nothing to do with the reality of the ongoing transaction with the therapist. The cyclical psychodynamic conception of transference, in contrast, emphasizes the ongoing transactions, in *all* aspects of the person's functioning, between internal processes and previous history on the one hand, and the events and persons encountered at the moment on the other. The influence of the psychological processes (both conscious and unconscious) that leave the individual's unique imprint on every act of perception, every thought, and every action, is not somehow abrogated by the fact that there is some basis for the experience in what is actually transpiring; nor is the therapist's *access* to that personal equation interdicted by acknowledging that basis.

There is *always* some basis in reality for our experiences. *And* there is always a significant contribution that reflects the active, constructive nature of all perceptual processes. Our thoughts, our perceptions, our associations, our actions, are always a joint product of "internal" and "external" influences and processes. They reflect in every instance our particular way of organizing, construing, and reacting to the events of our lives; and our appreciation of that fact is enriched, not diminished, by extending that appreciation beyond the mythical notion that a spe-

---

[4]A central theme of the chapters that follow is the examination of how the therapist's communications may be unwittingly skewed, by a variety of assumptions and ingrained clinical habits, toward a needlessly adversarial tone.

cial subset of reactions comes only from "inside" and recognizing, instead, that "inside" influences are evident in *all* experiences, not as an alternative to "outside" influence but, on each and every occasion, alongside of them. Indeed, it is only our language that even separates them into "internal" and "external." In reality, they are part of one unitary flow of events and part and parcel of each other. "Internal" processes can only unfold and have meaning in relation to "external" events, and such events can only have psychological meaning as they are actively interpreted by "internal" processes and structures.

Gill (1984) has pointed to similar considerations in his own reworking of how to understand and work with transference. Explicitly modifying his earlier position cited above (Gill, 1954), he states unequivocally that "the notion of an 'uncontaminated' transference is a myth." Moreover, he adds,

> The belief that the analytic process has a kind of automaticity which takes over once it is set in motion fosters [a] reluctance to interact. But such reluctance implies a failure to be fully aware that because analysis takes place in an interpersonal context there is no such thing as non-interaction. Silence is of course a behaviour too. Nor can one maintain that silence is preferable for the purpose of analysis because it is neutral in reality. It may be intended to be neutral but silence too can be plausibly experienced as anything ranging from cruel inhumanity to tender concern. It is not possible to say that any of these attitudes is necessarily a distortion. (Gill, 1984, p. 168)

In a statement even more fully resonant with the cyclical psychodynamic perspective, Gill also comments,

> The individual sees the world not only as his intrapsychic patterns dictate, but also as he veridically assesses it. Furthermore, the two kinds of determinants mutually influence each other. The intrapsychic patterns not only determine selective attention to those aspects of the external world which conform to them, but the individual behaves in such a way as to enhance the likelihood that the responses he meets will indeed confirm the views with which he sets out. This external validation in turn is necessary for the maintenance of those patterns. It is this last insight that psychoanalytic theory often ignores, postulating instead an internal pressure to maintain the intrapsychic patterns without significant reference to the external world. (Gill, 1982, p. 92)

TRANSFERENCE AND SCHEMA

The issues discussed above can be further elucidated by addressing them from another direction. Considerable clarity can be brought to our understanding of transference reactions, and of the possibilities they present for the advancement of the therapeutic process, by examining them in the light of Piaget's concepts of schema, assimilation, and accommodation. As Piaget describes it, the psychological structures by which we apprehend and act upon the world are always characterized by two opposing, but complementary, tendencies. Assimilation is the process by which we make the unfamiliar familiar, enabling us to approach new situations in a way that allows us to bring to bear what we have learned from our previous encounters with the world. When we assimilate new experiences to our existing schemas, we discover the meeting ground between those experiences and what we can already do and comprehend. We enable ourselves to approach the world not as a *tabula rasa* but as an individual whose experiences have relevance in addressing the new challenges and possibilities we encounter.

Any new situation, however, is never *exactly* the same as those we have encountered previously. All require some adjustment to their difference, some *accommodation* to the variation. Often, as in a perfunctory "how are you?" while passing someone on the street, the degree of accommodation is rather small. We assimilate the experience to our previous "passing greeting" schemas and run off a sequence that seems largely preformed. But even here, some degree of accommodation is necessary. The loudness of our voice must be matched to the level of noise on the street (and to how eager we are to be heard and noticed by this particular individual at this time); our speech must be timed with regard to the speech of the other or to eye contact; our making of eye contact must be coordinated with the need to notice whether we are about to bump into someone or walk into a hole in the sidewalk. In other words, even the simplest act, even the most familiar "here we go again" situation requires us to do something which, in the total of all its details, is something we have never done before. *Never* is it *exactly* the same as another time. And, of course, in more complex acts, such as engaging in a conversation, teaching a class, or playing in a tennis match, the variation from occasion to occasion is considerable and significant.

No act or experience is ever completely new, uninfluenced by previous schemas. And none is ever completely the same. Assimilation *and* accommodation are, as Piaget put it, invariants. Though the balance between them can vary considerably, neither is ever completely absent in anything we do. As Piaget scholar John Flavell put it,

> However necessary it may be to describe assimilation and accommodation separately and sequentially, they should be thought of as simultaneous and indissociable as they operate in living cognition. Adaptation is a unitary event, and assimilation and accommodation are merely abstractions

from this unitary reality. As in the case of food ingestion, the cognitive incorporation of reality always implies both an assimilation *to* structure and an accommodation *of* structure. To assimilate an event it is necessary at the same to time to accommodate to it and vice versa. . . . [T]he balance between the two invariants can and does vary, both from stage to stage and within a given stage. Some cognitive acts show a relative preponderance of the assimilative component; others seem heavily weighted toward accommodation. However, "pure" assimilation and "pure" accommodation nowhere obtain in mental life. (Flavell, 1963, pp. 48–49)

Transference reactions, from this perspective, are best understood as the product of schemas in which assimilation predominates over accommodation. When we describe a patient's reaction as transferential, we are essentially saying that he accommodates only minimally to the specific qualities of the analyst that differ from those of his parents, and that the readiness to assimilate the experience with the analyst to schemas associated with previous experiences with early figures in his life can override many fine (and even not so fine) points of difference. But the perspective provided by considering transference in the light of Piaget reminds us that the transference reaction cannot be purely assimilative. There *must* be some degree of accommodation as well.

Most accounts of transference do not seem to recognize this. As the examples cited earlier show, they describe transference reactions as if they were exclusively and inexorably assimilative. In the process, they in effect lose the therapist. Transference appears, through their lens, to have nothing whatsoever to do with what is actually transpiring. No accommodation is occurring at all. The transference wells up exclusively from within, bubbling up like vintage champagne.

To some degree, of course, almost all analysts recognize that transference reactions, no matter how distorted or fanciful they might appear, are never made up out of whole cloth. It is usually acknowledged that there is some "peg" or "hook" on which the transference is hung, some actual characteristic or action that provides the initial basis for the patient's perception. Acknowledgment of this reality basis for the transferential experience, however, is often rather perfunctory. Lip service is paid to there being *some* basis for the patient's reactions, but essentially that reality foundation is treated as the husk, to be cast aside in the search for the kernels that constitute the focus of psychoanalytic exploration. It is seen, essentially, as an only *seemingly* relevant factor in the generation of the experience, as a kind of "excuse," in much the way a rationalization is an excuse that provides a plausible sounding but misleading explanation for the person's behavior or experience.

What the schema perspective points to, in contrast, is a recognition that however idiosyncratic the patient's response to the therapist, however much it is influenced by earlier experiences that cast their imprint on the new situation, it is nonetheless the patient's way of experiencing *this* situation. It is not necessary to deny the role of the context in order to help the patient understand his own contribution, to help him to see how selective, and even distorted, his experience of interpersonal events can be. Nor is this necessary in order to help him appreciate the shadow that his past casts upon his perception of the present. One needn't pretend there is no present to do that. Indeed, if one does, much of what needs to be understood is lost. When the transference is described, in a rhetoric designed to hide the therapist's contribution, as simply "emerging" or "unfolding" (see Wachtel, 1982), what happens is that the detailed and differentiated understanding that the patient *ought* to be able to gain from his therapy experience is blurred.

Far from obscuring the nature of the patient's internal processes, depictions that include the therapist's role in the process articulate them further and provide greater specificity. We learn *more* about our psychological proclivities when the role of ongoing events in eliciting the transference reaction is taken into account than when it is omitted or denied.

It is only a partial understanding for the patient to recognize that he has a tendency to see others as hostile, or seductive, or distant, and that this tendency comes from his past. If he also understands *when* such a tendency is most likely to be evoked, what behaviors or characteristics of others tend to elicit this particular proclivity, his understanding is much more precise and differentiated. And since precisely when the perception that someone is being seductive is due to transference, and when it is because that other person really *is* being seductive (or hostile, or worried, or only superficially attentive, or whatever) is not always easy to tell, such a more differentiated appreciation of his transference proclivities can aid the patient in negotiating the inherently ambiguous waters of interpersonal exchange.[5]

There is another crucial advantage as well to the more differentiated and context-related view of transference described here. By articulating when and where the patient is particularly prone to distort (through excessive assimilation and selectivity), one is then also in a position to appreciate where, in contrast, he distorts less. That is, one is directed to recognize the patient's *strengths* as well as his shortcomings

[5]More accurately, one needs to determine *to what extent* the perception is need-driven and transferential and *to what extent* it is caused by the other person's behavior and intent. As the foregoing discussion indicates, transference reactions almost never reflect a complete and total misreading of the other person. Rather, it is the extreme *selectivity* of perception, and the construction of a highly personalized and tendentious picture of what is transpiring, that renders the transference reaction a distortion.

or pathology. By relating the more distorted functioning to specific eliciting events and contexts, one becomes more aware of where they are *not* elicited, of where the patient's functioning is relatively intact and attuned to consensual reality.

This focus on strengths, it will be apparent, is a central theme of this book. So too is examination of the various ways in which therapists may unwittingly demean or devalue patients via pathologizing formulations and comments, and the provision of alternative ways of thinking and speaking that have quite different connotations and implications. As Gill has pointed out, these matters are by no means unrelated to the question of how the patient's transference reactions are conceptualized. As he puts it,

> The change in atmosphere [when one takes into account the analyst's contribtion to the transference] is one from the patient being wrong and misguided to one in which his point of view is given initial consideration. In other words his rational capacity is respected rather than belittled. It is in such an atmosphere, after his point of view has been acknowledged, that he is more likely to be willing to look for his own contribution to his experience. The position is of course contrary to the one which argues that to acknowledge the rationality of the patient's point of view is to confirm his belief that his experience is fully accounted for by the current behaviour of the analyst. (Gill, 1984, p. 173)

The aim of keeping the transference pure or clear, "unmuddied" or "uncontaminated" by the distortions that are supposedly introduced by the therapist being too active or too self revealing, has led many therapists to impose quite severe constraints upon their participation in the therapeutic process and on the possibilities for intervention they allow themselves. I have addressed this issue elsewhere (Wachtel, 1977) and will not be focally concerned in this book with the issue of active intervention. Since the focus of the present work is on the therapist's *language*, on what she *says* to the patient and how she couches what she says, I will concentrate here on the implications of the way the therapist understands the phenomena of transference for how she talks to the patient.

The aim of remaining as anonymous and unreactive as possible so as to be able to demonstrate to the patient that his experience of the therapist comes from his past and from within him, and the corresponding downplaying of what has actually transpired between them, can lead the therapist not to pay much attention to the particulars of what she is saying. By rendering the therapist's contribution to the transference reaction largely invisible—to the therapist as well as the patient—this viewpoint introduces a significant impediment to the therapist's careful consideration of the wording of her comments to the patient. As Gill has put it, such downplaying of the therapist's role "is a persistent remnant of the false precept that the analyst can indeed be only a reflecting mirror. An effort to deny the real impact of the analyst can only result in its remaining implicit so that it exerts its effects without being understood" (Gill, 1982, p. 86). Put differently, why bother to look carefully at what you are saying if you believe that the patient's response to it is essentially independent of what you have actually said?

Gill notes as well the unfortunate restrictions on their activity to which analysts are led by their denial of the role of their own behavior in their patients' reactions and fantasies. He argues that "no matter how far the analyst attempts to carry this limitation of his behavior, the very existence of the analytic situation provides the patient with innumerable cues which inevitably become the rationale for his transference responses." The analytic situation, he argues, *cannot* be made to disappear, adding that "It is easy to forget this truism in one's zeal to diminish the role of the realistic situation in determining the patient's responses" (Gill, 1982, p. 86).

One major consequence of this analysis is an appreciation of the impoverishment of the therapeutic relationship that can result from the therapist's having to pretend that the impact of her particularity is minimal. Gill notes that one aim of his reworking of the standard ideas about transference is to "loosen the atmosphere of an analysis from a rigid avoidance of doing the wrong thing to a more relaxed spontaneity with attention to the possible effects of whatever one does" (Reppen, 1982, p. 182). Elsewhere he adds:

> If the analyst remains under the illusion that the current cues he provides to the patient can be reduced to the vanishing point, he may be led into a silent withdrawal, which is not too distant from the caricature of an analyst as someone who does indeed refuse to have any personal relationship with the patient. What happens then is that silence has become a technique rather than merely an indication that the analyst is listening. *The patient's responses under such conditions can be mistaken for uncontaminated transference when they are in fact transference adaptations to the actuality of the silence.* (Gill, 1979, p. 277; italics in original)

Mitchell, addressing another dimension of these considerations, observes:

> Unless the analyst affectively enters the patient's relational matrix or, rather, discovers himself within it—unless the analyst is in some sense charmed by the patient's entreaties, shaped by the patient's projections, antagonized and frustrated by the patient's defenses—the patient is never

fully engaged and a certain depth within the analytic experience is lost. (Mitchell, 1988, p. 293)

The relevance of these observations by Gill and by Mitchell to the clinical suggestions and formulations offered in the remainder of this volume will be obvious to the reader. Understanding, for example, of the vicious circles in the patient's life is greatly enhanced by attending carefully to how they are manifested in the therapy room and—very importantly—by attending openly and nondefensively to the ways in which the therapist is herself drawn into the pattern. It will be apparent to the reader in the clinical discussions that follow this chapter that this inclusion of the therapist's participation is in many instances a key both to illuminating more fully the issues in the patient's life and to doing so in a way that is nonaccusatory and less damaging to the patient's self-esteem.

THE OVERESTIMATION OF THE RELATIONSHIP: THERAPY AS CATALYST

Notwithstanding all of the above considerations that highlight the importance of the therapeutic relationship and indicate the range of ways in which it can be influential in therapeutic change, I think a case can be made that modern psychoanalytic therapists *over*estimate the importance of the relationship. Put differently, the contemporary emphasis both on the analysis of transference and on the mutative properties of the relationship per se places too great a burden on what transpires in the consulting room. It is more accurate, I believe, and more likely to generate maximally effective therapeutic strategies, to view the relationship largely as a *catalyst*, mobilizing and guiding the patient toward taking the actions *in the world* that are necessary for change to be extensive and enduring.

To be sure, the corrective experiences that can occur in the relationship between patient and therapist are of enormous value. They permit a kind of relearning and of reorganizing of assumptions and experiences that is alive and vivid and that has the added advantage of taking place right before the therapist's eyes. This provides the therapist with a uniquely favorable vantage point from which to evaluate the changes that are occurring and the processes that both facilitate and impede those changes.

Thus, the experiences with the therapist are not only frequently powerful in their own right but also an invaluable source of data for further therapeutic work. There are few better ways of understanding the subtleties of how the patient operates in the world and of the emotional reactions he evokes in others. But that understanding is seriously incomplete if it is not integrated with understanding based on knowledge of the events of the patient's daily life. It is particularly in noticing the consonances between the way she feels with the patient and how other significant figures in the patient's life react to him that the therapist gains the most useful insight into the causes of the patient's difficulties. And it is in the search for those consonances, in the continuing shift of focus between in-session and outside-of-session occurrences, that the therapist most effectively gains deep understanding of what the reactions and experiences of those significant others are likely to be.

Although the therapeutic relationship is an important key to therapeutic change, its power to fuel the change process has limits, and recognition of those limits can help the therapist develop a more comprehensive and more effective approach. To begin with, we may remind ourselves just how small a portion of the patient's waking life the time with his therapist actually represents. Now, to be sure, the time spent literally in the therapist's presence is not likely to be the only time that the patient is thinking about what has transpired between them. (Indeed, the process is unlikely to be successful at all if the therapy is so encapsulated, and the therapist who does not attend to whether the patient thinks about the sessions outside the office is not likely to be very effective.) But the point remains that a great deal of living goes on outside of the context of the therapeutic relationship, and what transpires between the patient and other important people in his life can make the crucial difference between whether change is maintained or is continually undermined and short-circuited.[6]

Of special concern is the way in which good work in the therapeutic session can be undermined by what transpires with others after the patient leaves. Consider what happens, for example, when a patient who has been deeply conflicted and inhibited with respect to the expression of anger begins to express such feelings in the session. The therapist, who has been working hard to facilitate just such expression, is likely to be pleased at this occurrence and to experience it quite differently from the way she would experience other people getting

---

[6]Recognition of this fact points the therapist toward concern with the "cast of characters" in the patient's life and with the systems (family and other) in which the patient participates. Addressing the systems dimension is not the focus of the present book, but readers interested in how the cyclical psychodynamic perspective dovetails with perspectives deriving from family systems approaches can consult Wachtel and Wachtel (1986).

angry at her in other contexts. Here she is likely to be receptive and even in some respects welcoming of the patient's expressions of anger.[7]

From such experiences, the patient can begin to get more in touch with his feelings (not only of anger but of dependency, anxiety, affection, or what have you). He can learn that perhaps the expression of his feelings is not quite as dangerous, not quite as forbidden, as he has long feared. This is the sort of corrective emotional experience—not necessarily in Alexander's sense, but in a broad and general way (cf. Gill, 1982; Weiss & Sampson, 1986)—that is a central feature of the process of therapeutic change. But that new learning can be quickly undermined when the patient then goes out and applies what he has learned to the world outside. For unless sufficient attention is paid to *how* the patient expresses his feelings, and to the difficulties he may encounter and the discriminations he must make outside the therapy room, he is likely to encounter a far less receptive response to his behavior than he received from his therapist.

Others in the patient's life will have different standards and a different intent in their relation with the patient. In comparison with the therapist, their concern will not be nearly as centered on simply understanding him and fostering his development and self-awareness. Even those well disposed toward him will expect a considerably more balanced give and take than his therapist will. A way of expressing himself that felt like a liberating opening-up in the therapy room may prove either too intense and undiscriminating or too weak and ambiguous to yield salutary results when speaking to his boss or his wife.

The good therapist ignores to some degree the adequacy and appropriateness of the patient's initial expressions of a previously wardedoff feeling.[8] As noted earlier, it is the general *direction* of the patient's movement to which the therapist should primarily be attending. If new territory is being reappropriated for the expanding conscious self, that

---

[7]Obviously this is true only up to a point. Not *any* kind of anger in the session will be welcomed or accepted. But the threshold for counterannoyance is likely to be quite different in the session than elsewhere, as will the experienced personal meaning of the transaction to the therapist.

[8]Here again, it must be stated that the therapist's tolerance has—and should have—limits as well. If the patient's way of expressing himself is *too* inappropriate, this must be addressed in some way, even if it does represent a step toward greater openness on the patient's part. Nonetheless, the point remains that the threshold for experiencing a particular expression as inappropriate is quite different in the context of therapy from what it would be in other aspects of the patient's life. Indeed, within the parameters that I am discussing here, that is precisely what is therapeutic about the experience and relationship with the therapist.

is what is most important at first. Later there will be time for the fine tuning.

But that does not mean that the fine tuning is irrelevant or unimportant. Indeed, it is usually crucial. If a patient has spent most of his life suppressing and disguising from himself certain of his feelings, he has been deprived of the opportunities to shape their expression that are available to those who have more ready access to that feeling. The expression of anger, or love, or dependency has a normal developmental sequence. What is appropriate and interpersonally effective at age 5 is not at age 10, and what is appropriate at age 10 is not at age 20. Learning to give expression to one's feelings in an age-appropriate and context-appropriate way is a life-long process in which trial and error, feedback, and gradually increasing standards ordinarily play a role. When that process is impeded by the person's avoidance of *any* expression of certain feelings, it is likely that when the patient begins to overcome some of his repressions and inhibitions the initial expressions will show the effects of having been deprived of the thousands of shaping experiences that others have encountered. His expressions will be lacking in grace, subtlety, or some other dimension that is central to their being effective in daily living. As a result, there is a real danger that when he extends into his everyday life the lessons he has learned in the therapy, he will once again learn that expressing such feelings is dangerous after all.[9]

Sometimes what happens is that the patient instead learns a discrimination—it is safe to experience and express such feelings with the therapist, but not in the rest of his life. Such learning is not necessarily conscious, and if the therapist is too focused on the therapeutic relationship alone, she is likely not to know about it. What she sees is that the patient appears to be improving considerably. He is increasingly able to express feelings he once had repressed, and he is more and more open in the relationship. If she is not carefully attending to the patient's dealings with the world outside the consultation room, the therapist will not notice that this salutary process has not carried forth effectively into daily living. Perhaps this is one reason why therapists sometimes have a conviction about the efficacy of what they do that is not consonant with the much more modest effects that are revealed by systematic research: the therapist sees great improvement with her own eyes and does not

---

[9]Although not directly germane to the main focus of this book, the considerations just advanced point to the importance of the therapist attending to, and working to help the patient develop, the crucial *skills in living* that have been impaired by the patient's anxieties and attendant avoidances. For more on how to work with the skill dimension in the context of a therapy that attends as well to unconscious motivation, conflict, and fantasy, see Wachtel (1977, 1985; Wachtel & Wachtel, 1986).

have as clear a picture of what is happening in the 95% or more of the patient's waking hours that is spent with others.

This may also be why some of us may notice that our friends and acquaintances sometimes rave about how wonderful their therapists are, while we observe that their lives seem no less problematic than they were before. The patient's experience is not necessarily a distortion. His relationship *with the therapist* may really be quite good, perhaps better than any he has ever had. What is not sufficiently noticed is that this wonderful relationship has not contributed much to changing or enhancing his *other* relationships.

Also frequently placing limits on the impact of the relationship with the therapist is that significant others in the patient's life may be ambivalent at best about the changes that the patient is striving for. The therapist is not the only significant figure in the patient's world. Parents, spouse, friends, boss, colleagues, children, teachers all can have a powerful emotional impact on the patient's life and on the status of his internal conflicts. Unless careful attention is paid to their role and to how the patient interacts with them, once again the therapy may stagnate *even if* the relationship is a good one. Many facets of this dimension of the therapeutic process are discussed in detail in Wachtel and Wachtel (1986).

The point of the foregoing discussion is by no means to belittle the importance of the therapeutic relationship, either as a medium for learning about the patient's emotional life with unrivaled immediacy or as a powerful source of change in its own right. Rather, the point is that to expect the relationship alone to do the job is to place an unfair burden on an experience of great potential value. If the therapeutic potential of the relationship between therapist and patient is to be fully realized, it is crucial that the therapist develop skill in assuring that the patient's daily life is on the side of the therapy rather than in opposition. Life, ultimately, is more powerful than therapy. When the patient's life has been enlisted as an ally in the struggle against the neurosis, when the daily interactions that fill the patient's days begin to be a source of change rather than a contributor to the perpetuation of his difficulties, the change process is likely to be successful. It is when the relationship facilitates such a state of affairs that it is truly therapeutic.

THE PHRASING OF COMMUNICATIONS AND THE LARGER CONTEXT OF CHANGE

As the theoretical discussions in the past few chapters should make clear, the view that guides my work is a multiprocess view of change.

Numerous influences contribute to patients' progress in psychotherapy, and when one is treated as preponderant, it is likely that therapeutic effectiveness will be restricted. In that sense, the considerations advanced in these theoretical chapters point not only to the foundations for the clinical recommendations that follow in the rest of this book but also to their limits. The way the therapist phrases her communications to the patient is by no means the only dimension to her skillfulness or lack of skill. The range of processes and procedures mobilized in a successful psychotherapy is quite considerable.

I have chosen nonetheless to focus on this particular dimension of therapeutic technique for several reasons. First, although the matters of phrasing and connotation that are the object of inquiry here represent just one facet of psychotherapy, these matters are quite crucial. Frequently they are the decisive factor weighing in the direction of change or of therapeutic failure. Second, this facet of the work has tended to be rather *neglected,* both in the literature and—judging from the comments both of students in my graduate seminars and of experienced therapists in the workshops I have given on the topic—even in the face-to-face supervision that is supposed to convey to therapists in training the art and the craft of therapeutic practice.

To be sure, the meta-messages one conveys in one's remarks to the patient are not embodied in the words alone. Matters of timing, tone of voice, inflection, and body language all contribute substantially to the overall impact of what is said, and further study of these dimensions is greatly needed. But our words are what we have the most control over, and we are more able to notice and reflect upon our words than upon our tone. In what follows, it will be apparent that the comments examined in the text serve multiple purposes. Notwithstanding the many important contributions that reflect the development of an action approach to the therapeutic process (London, 1964), psychotherapy very largely remains what it always has been—the talking cure. It will be apparent to the reader who keeps in mind the theoretical principles offered in the past few chapters that those principles are reflected in varying ways in the different kinds of comments that the book addresses. Whether the focus is upon exposure to the previously avoided, the further development of skills in living, the experiencing of a sense of safety, the taking of action in daily life, or the experience of a facilitative relationship, this is most often conveyed in words. Our words, ultimately, are the primary medium for our participation in the therapeutic process. They must not be an afterthought.

CHAPTER 5

Accusatory and Facilitative Comments
Criticism and Permission in the Therapeutic Dialogue

We are accustomed to thinking of therapists' comments as neutral, as conveying neither approval nor disapproval but simply truth. As a group, therapists are perhaps the most devoted proponents of the ancient precept that "the truth shall set you free." But much more than simply "truth" is conveyed by most comments that therapists make. Truth is always multifaceted, and any particular comment necessarily captures only a certain portion or perspective. There are *many* true interpretations of what is going on that could potentially be conveyed. The epistemological foundations of psychotherapeutic work are better captured by Kurasawa's classic film *Rashomon*[1] than by Platonic notions of a single reality obscured by shadows or by overreaching attempts to reconstruct what "really" went on in a patient's childhood (cf. Spence, 1982).

For a variety of reasons, the truth that therapists seek tends often to be one kind of truth in particular—the *"deep, dark"* truth that the patient has been hiding from himself for many years. Leston Havens, one of the relatively few writers to concern himself explicitly with the uses of language in psychotherapy, has put it this way:

> In the current interpretive climate of much psychotherapeutic work, patients sit waiting for the next insight with their fists clenched. Small wonder, for it is rarely good news. (Havens, 1986, p. 78)

---

[1]*Rashomon* is most famous for its telling of a story from the perspective of several different characters. Each gives us a different picture of the "same" set of events, and the idea of a single, perspective-free reality is thereby challenged.

Havens's description may be a bit overdramatic, but it points to a problem that does indeed pervade the clinical enterprise. It is easy to assume that *unpleasant* truths about people are more "profound," and that what the therapeutic work must get to is bound to hurt. As we shall see as we proceed, this instinctive hunch on the part of therapists is not always sound. Indeed, quite often it is the very fact that people believe that the truth about them is unpleasant—even if this belief is kept out of consciousness—that is at the heart of their difficulties (cf. Wile, 1981, 1985).

Now of course therapists must often help their patients confront truths that are uncomfortable and that have been denied or warded off for that very reason. No good therapist promises a rose garden. But all "truths" are not equally therapeutic. It is often in the patient's *framing* of the truth, in the particular way he organizes, categorizes, and gives emotional meaning to what has transpired, that his difficulty lies. And it is the therapist's new and different—and generally less accusatory—framing of the truth that can open the possibility for cure.

PERMISSIONS AND REBUKES

The strategies of communication described here do not abandon the search for truth; but they seek to go beyond the naive view of a single truth that is simply "discovered" and instead to point to a version of the truth that will help the patient to see new possibilities for his life and to change the life patterns that have been the source of his troubles. Crucial to this effort is appreciation of the surplus meanings borne by the therapist's remarks. Far more than is usually recognized, therapists' comments, especially those addressing feelings or intentions that the patient has not fully admitted into consciousness, are likely to be experienced by the patient as either permissions or rebukes. On close analysis, they can be seen to convey either that what the patient has fearfully avoided is more acceptable than the patient has thought, or that the patient has been "caught" doing or thinking something he shouldn't (or, as discussed below, that he has been caught *avoiding* thinking something, which, by the ground rules of therapy, is just as "bad").

To be sure, the patient's experience of the therapist and her attitudes is hardly an objective matter. Perceived connotations of criticism or acceptance can be greatly influenced by the patient's transference to the therapist. But it is a great mistake to attribute *all* of these connotations to transference. A hefty portion of the variance in how the therapist's remarks are experienced lies in the remarks themselves. There are a variety of ways of conveying to the patient any particular focal message (to use the term introduced in Chapter 1), and the differences among them can be crucial.

Good interpretations tend to be permission-oriented. They address an aspect of the patient's experience that he has disavowed or obscured and convey the message that it is all right to be more accepting toward that experience. They expand the patient's sense of entitlement with regard to conflicted aspects of his psychic life. They point out to the patient in one way or another that he has been afraid to acknowledge something about himself and that perhaps this anxiety is no longer necessary, if indeed it ever was.

Not infrequently, however, if one looks closely at how interpretations are actually worded, one finds that they contain an implicit rebuke. Consider, for example, the following bit of therapeutic work that was reported in a supervisory group I conducted some years ago[2]:

The patient, a painfully shy young woman, had been sitting for a long time in an uncomfortable silence, occasionally adding that she just didn't have anything to say. Finally, at one point the therapist said to her, "I think you're silent because you're trying to hide a lot of anger." We had been discussing in the group for several weeks the issues addressed in the present chapter, and the therapist herself raised the question in the group discussion of whether this had been the best way to make the interpretation. She recalled being unhappy with her comment even at the time, but for a variety of reasons she felt that some comment was called for to break the impasse, and no other way to phrase it had occurred to her. In the class discussion, she added that she had felt, and still felt, that what she had to say was basically accurate even though she was displeased with how she had couched it. (The entire group, myself included, concurred on this latter point.)[3]

---

[2]The reader will find that throughout this volume many of the examples of problematic ways of putting things are drawn from experiences in supervising other therapists. The conclusion should not be drawn from this that I do not make such mistakes myself. Certain authors in our field have made a career out of writings that seem to distinguish their exemplary functioning from the far less satisfactory efforts of their supervisees. I regard such invidious comparisons as both destructive and, almost certainly, far from accurate. The explanation for my use of bad examples from others is simple and not particularly flattering: it is easier to see others' mistakes than one's own, especially when one is also afforded the safety and distance that supervision or teaching affords in contrast to the hotseat of the therapist.

[3]Apropos the discussion of countertransference in Chapter 1, I should note that there also seemed to me little indication that the therapist was reacting out of a strong personal reaction to the patient. Indeed, she seemed to like the patient a good deal and to have a strong empathic sense of the patient's dilemmas.

In the group, a number of alternative ways of conveying the interpretive message to the patient were suggested. Interestingly, the first few that were put forth were not very different in spirit. They all omitted the implicitly accusatory word "hide," but to at least some degree, they conveyed the same tone. One softened the comment somewhat by substituting for the word "hide" the phrase "keep from yourself." Other suggestions included:

I think you're feeling very angry at me and the boredom is a cover.
Behind your silence is a great deal of anger.
I think you're really very angry.
You're denying how angry you are.

The reader can readily see that these alternatives, the first ones that the group generated, share the problematic tone of the original. Contrast them, for example, with some of the versions that were generated as we kept at it:

I have the sense that you're angry but feel you're not supposed to be.
I wonder if you're staying silent because you feel you had better not say anything if what you're feeling is anger.

What makes these latter two statements a significant improvement is that they carry a much clearer implication that it's *all right* to be angry. They emphasize not the hiding or denying, but rather the patient's fear, and they carry the message that maybe the fear is unnecessary. Comments phrased this way, I believe, get across to the patient what is needed with far less damage to his self-esteem, and they permit him to pick up on them without reacting as defensively.

Put differently, the problem with the original comment and with the first few alternatives generated is not that they were wrong—recall that the entire group of therapists regarded these observations as accurate. The problem, rather, is that the particular version of accuracy that they embody contains—as all versions do—normative as well as descriptive elements. That is, the particular way the therapist chooses to express what she has observed will carry other messages as well, what I have called meta-messages. Most likely they will in particular either tell the patient about something that is wrong—for example, a wish or fantasy that is unrealistic or antisocial, or an effort to hide from himself or others what he is really thinking or feeling—or they will indicate to the patient that what he is feeling is in fact acceptable, and that the problem is that he has been excessively afraid of these feelings. They will, in other words, convey either criticism or permission.

Now clearly few therapists *intend* to criticize their patients with their remarks and, indeed, many therapists are scarcely less uncomfortable with the idea of giving permission, viewing it as "supportive," manipulative, superficial, or as intruding on the patient's autonomy. "Who am I to give permission?" some therapists ask. "It's not mine to give."

I am sympathetic to the intent behind such a view, and as the reader will see, there are significant aspects of it that, in my own way, I endorse. But I believe that close examination of the implications of what therapists actually say reveals the impossibility of real neutrality (cf. Wachtel, 1987, Chap. 11) and the necessity to take responsibility for—and attend to—the meta-messages that accompany our efforts to communicate our understanding of the patient's experience.

In the great majority of clinical situations, it is useful for the therapist to think quite explicitly about couching remarks in a context of permission and to avoid forms of expression that are more readily experienced as critical. Beginning students frequently phrase their comments in forms such as those just noted: "You are trying to hide . . . ," "You are avoiding . . . ," "You're denying how . . . you are," "You're really very . . . ," " . . . is a cover for . . . ," and so on. Indeed, in the seminar described above, as the students proceeded in generating alternatives, they found themselves smiling embarrassedly and literally wincing as they discovered how readily accusatory phrases came to mind, even as they were working on trying to avoid them.

Experienced therapists, we may expect, manifest these problematic phrasings less frequently. But even for them, the examples cited above are likely to have a familiar ring in two different senses. On the one hand, no effective therapist is unable to formulate comments of the sort I am recommending; without a considerable capacity to do so one would have long ago become a shoe salesman or a computer programmer. On the other hand, the examples are likely to evoke a sense of familiarity in another way as well: no therapist I know can truthfully say that the less salutary comments described are completely absent from her repertoire. The difficulty the group had at first in producing a better version was not just a matter of the students' inexperience. When I have given workshops on these issues to groups that included quite experienced therapists, they too could recognize the "bad" examples as far from absent in their work. And in my own work, despite years of writing and lecturing about these very issues, I find that such phrasings still sometimes creep in. These are, as it were, the unwanted "tics" of our profession.

The main cure for these "tics" is the firm possession of a set of alternative forms of expression, particularly of ways of framing comments whose meta-message conveys permission for the patient to reappropriate previously warded-off feelings. Among the sorts of phrasings that are of rather wide applicability in therapeutic work are the following:

> *You seem rather harsh with yourself when you sense any hint of sexual feeling.* [*instead of* "You avoid acknowledging sexual feelings."]
>
> *You seem to expect something terrible to happen to you if you have any wish to be taken care of.* [*instead of* "You're defending against feelings of dependency."]
>
> *I have the sense you're angry at your mother but think it's awful of you to feel that.* [*instead of* "You're a lot angrier at your mother than you realize."]
>
> *I think you're feeling critical of Susan because you're afraid if you get too close to her you'll get "mushy" and she won't think you're a man; maybe that kind of caution isn't really necessary.* [*instead of* "You ward off feelings of closeness with Susan and cut off any of the softer feelings."]

FURTHER EXAMINATION OF THE ACCUSATORY IMPLICATIONS OF THERAPISTS' COMMENTS: THE CONTRIBUTION OF DANIEL WILE

The ways in which therapists' comments can be critical and accusatory, and the antitherapeutic effects of such comments, have been a particular concern in the writings of Daniel Wile (e.g., 1984, 1985). At the extremes, Wile suggests, the rules and proscriptions that commonly define the role of the therapist can lead to a therapy characterized by "inhibition, silences, nonengagement, monologues, unanswered questions, unasked questions, and wariness" (Wile, 1985, p. 797).

In Wile's view, this state of affairs is not simply a matter of technique but also of the theory that guides and shapes both the therapist's stance and the form and nature of the interventions she chooses. According to Wile, when patients are primarily conceptualized as gratifying infantile impulses, as having developmental defects, as manipulating and trying to control or resist the therapy, it is difficult for the therapist not to communicate a view of them that is accusatory or pejorative.

In making his case, Wile illustrates and elaborates his position by examining published case reports by prominent psychoanalysts. He cites, for example, a case of Otto Kernberg's (Kernberg, 1977), in which the patient got increasingly angry at Kernberg and was viewed by Kernberg as unwilling to listen and as trying to control the therapy.

Rather than viewing the anger as a reflection of the patient's personal psychopathology as Kernberg did, Wile suggests it was an understandable response to the way Kernberg thought about her and talked to her. Looking closely at the interpretations Kernberg described making before the patient became angry and unreceptive to him, Wile suggests the following alternative understanding of what transpired:

> Kernberg had been telling her that she is masochistic, defensive, and infantile and that she wanted to have intercourse with her father. He *now* tells her that she wants to have intercourse with *him*. Although this may be everyday common sense talk to psychoanalysts, such statements may seem strange and accusatory to many others. It is understandable that she might develop "an incapacity to listen" and a growing sense that Kernberg's understanding of her was "terribly incomplete, imperfect and arbitrary." (Wile, 1982, p. 1)

Kernberg reported that the patient expressed "a strong wish to shift to another, presumably warmer and more understanding therapist" (Kernberg, 1977, p. 98), and that she later insisted that he say nothing to her other than comments that clearly reflected how she felt at the moment and/or that reassured her that he was with her. Kernberg did so reluctantly, seeing this behavior on the part of the patient as "an effort at omnipotent control" and wanting to interpret that to her. He refrained from doing so only because she had made it clear she would not listen to such comments. Consequently, at this point in the therapy Kernberg made different, uncharacteristic comments to her, such as indicating that he understood that she was terribly afraid his comments might be attempts to overpower, dominate, or brainwash her. To his surprise, these empathic comments about how she experienced him led to the patient's feeling a lot better.

In Kernberg's understanding of the case, Wile notes, what had transpired had primarily to do with the patient's defensive splitting in her perceptions of him and with a regression to a psychic state of affairs dating from the second or third year of life. Wile's understanding is quite different:

> Kernberg attributes the patient's behavior to her psychopathology. She has shifted to a "very early state of separation–individuation from mother . . . as a regressive escape from the oedipal aspects of the transference." My explanation is different. I see her as having finally found a way of establishing some sort of relationship with a man (Kernberg) who keeps criticizing her. She reports that she experiences Kernberg's interpretations as "harsh" and "invasive," a description of them with which I would

agree. Her solution is to get him to stop making these interpretations, to limit what he was to say. (Wile, 1982, p. 6)

The patient's problem, Wile argues, "is not her wish for omnipotent control, but her *inability* to control. She feels and is out of control of her life, her relationships, and the therapy" (p. 7). Consequently, the interpretations that would be therapeutic are not those that tell her how she is being manipulative, controlling, and infantile but those that address her sense of being invaded and overpowered and that address the feelings of unentitlement that lie behind that sense. In general, Wile suggests, it is primarily feelings of unentitlement and self-disparagement, rather than hiding from oneself infantile or antisocial inclinations, that are the source of psychological difficulties.

Wile views Kernberg's approach as lying toward the extreme accusatory end of the spectrum and thus as permitting us to view under greater magnification tendencies that are evident in milder forms in the work of many therapists. In contrast, Heinz Kohut's emphasis on empathic understanding of the pain behind the patient's demands, and his conception of the drives of classical psychoanalytic theory as "disintegration products" (Kohut, 1977) rather than as the primary sources of people's motivations, have some important affinities with Wile's own views (and with the views presented in this book). The problems Wile sees with Kohut's approach are more subtle, and in examining Kohut's work, Wile extends and clarifies his analysis of therapeutic and countertherapeutic communications.

He begins by noting and further examining Kohut's own critique of accusatory and pejorative formulations, especially as they are conveyed in Kohut's famous case of Mr. Z (Kohut, 1979). Mr. Z was a patient seen twice in analysis by Kohut, once at a time when Kohut was still practicing primarily from a classical psychoanalytic model and once after Kohut had substantially modified his approach. Kohut discusses the problems in his first treatment of Mr. Z as a way of illustrating his modifications of psychoanalytic treatment and theory.

In discussing his first treatment of Mr. Z, Kohut states,

> The theme that was most conspicuous during the first year of the analysis was that of a regressive mother transference, particularly as it was associated with the patient's narcissism . . . with his unrealistic, deluded grandiosity and his demands that the psychoanalytic situation should reinstate the position of exclusive control, of being admired and catered to by a doting mother who . . . devoted her total attention to the patient. (Kohut, 1979, p. 5)

Wile notes that Kohut goes on to describe how the patient "opposed these interpretations with intense resistances," how he blew up in intense rages at Kohut, rages which arose frequently in response to Kohut's interpretations "concerning his narcissistic demands and his arrogant feelings of 'entitlement'" (Kohut, 1979, p. 5). Elaborating the perspective that he developed in examining Kernberg's work, Wile suggests that the reasons for Mr. Z's "narcissistic rages" can be understood quite differently.

> Kohut is suggesting that Mr. Z has arrogant feelings of "entitlement," narcissistic demands, a regressive mother transference, unrealistic and deluded grandiose expectations, and that he was spoiled as a child and is trying to exert exclusive control in the psychoanalytic situation and get the therapist to act as an admiring and doting mother. Such a statement made in the course of common social discourse would immediately be recognized as an accusation. Mr. Z is being criticized and, as people sometimes do when they are criticized, he becomes angry and defensive. (Wile, 1982, p. 3)

Interestingly, Mr. Z himself attributed whatever gain he made in his first analysis to Kohut's introducing an interpretation on one occasion with the preliminary comment "Of course, it hurts when one is not given what one assumes to be one's due," and Kohut himself later gave some credence to this view of Mr. Z's.[4] Wile suggests that such a statement was relieving to Mr. Z because

> Mr. Z has been picturing himself, and believing that Kohut has been viewing him, as unlike other people—*as defective and pathological—and as having deviant and unacceptable feelings.* (Wile, 1982, p. 4; italics added)

Wile sees Kohut's later views, with their emphasis on empathy and their implicit acknowledgment of the accusatory aspects of standard psychoanalytic technique, as a definite advance. But he finds significant residually accusatory aspects even in Kohut's later work, a tendency important to recognize especially because Kohut has been viewed as advocating a kind of "kinder, gentler psychoanalysis." As Wile puts it, Kohut

> replaced the drive-and-defense psychology of classical psychoanalysis with the concept of developmental arrest. Narcissistic individuals are now seen

[4]Havens (1986) has called attention to a similar kind of comment as therapeutically useful. He notes that in a number of circumstances phrasings such as "No wonder you were frightened!" help to convey to the patient the naturalness (and hence the acceptability) of feelings the patient may have found threatening, unacceptable, and perhaps even proof of his lack of genuine humanity.

as fixated at an early stage of self development. The problem is that the resulting interpretations, based as they are on a picture of these indviduals as being *developmentally stunted or immature*, still have a pejorative tone. (Wile, 1982, p. 4; italics in original)

Indeed, such a tone is evident, says Wile, in the work of a great many therapists of widely varying orientations, who, he suggests, frequently view patients as

dependent, manipulative, narcissistic, hostile, symbiotic, controlling, masochistic, regressed, resistant, dishonest, irresponsible, pathologically jealous or competitive, engaged in game playing, or as refusing to give up their infantile gratifications and grow up. (Wile, 1982, p. 9)

Interpretations made from this frame of reference, Wile argues, are "inherently pejorative."

Wile's cautions, it seems to me, are well taken and alert us to a crucial dimension of therapeutic work. How we speak to patients is clearly not just a matter of technique but depends quite crucially on how we *think about* them. As we proceed, however, we shall see that it is possible to convey to the patient observations that might be thought of as at least cousins of the formulations Wile regards as "inherently pejorative" and to do so in a way that both furthers the process of exploration and maintains the patient's self-esteem. Sometimes it is quite essential to be able to accomplish this, because as a part of the vicious circles that people get caught in, they do begin to act controlling, dependent, masochistic, and so forth, even though they are not *inherently* that way. It is crucial to be able to explore these more problematic aspects of the patient's functioning and character, lest he feel the therapist is avoiding the real truth about him and thus find ironic confirmation of his fear that the real truth is too terrible to face. In doing this, however, it is essential as well to enable the patient to see that these observations address only a partial truth, and that the fuller picture provides a far less harsh view of his character. To accomplish this, both the explication of vicious circles and the articulation of conflict are of great value. Much of what follows will offer guidelines and illustrations elaborating on precisely how this can be done.

CONNOTATIONS AND "EXCULPATORY INTERPRETATIONS"

An interesting complement to Wile's discussion of accusatory interpretations is offered by Shawver (1983), who centers her analysis on the connotative dimension of the therapists' remarks and on the therapeutic value of what she calls "exculpatory" interpretations. Shawver argues that adequate appreciation of the connotative impact of therapists' comments has been impeded by a conception of the therapy process that views the therapist as uncovering, in neutral fashion, the secret contents of the patient's mind. This conception, Shawver suggests, leads to a view of the therapist's task as largely a diagnostic one, concerned with "the denotative accuracy of hypotheses," rather than with the creative utilization of the connotative dimension.

Although such a characterization may seem more clearly pertinent to older models of psychoanalytic practice than to more recent versions, in which relationship (and hence communication) is as much of concern as denotative accuracy, we shall see that the influence of the older model is more substantial than one might think even in the work of therapists who regard themselves as following a basically relational model.

To be sure, skillful therapists of any persuasion are likely to attend to the connotative element in their communications, and many therapists recognize that what they are conveying is not the simple and literal truth about what "actually" happened in the patient's past, but rather a *version* of the patient's life story that enables him to reconstitute his life in a different way (cf. Schafer, 1978, 1981; Schimek, 1975; Spence, 1982). But explicit discussion of the connotative dimension of therapeutic remarks remains a relatively scarce commodity in the therapeutic literature.

Shawver, in contrast, places connotation at the very center of the therapeutic process. Our interpretations, she argues, are never simply "dictated by the facts." Reality, especially subjective or interpersonal reality, is inherently ambiguous, and the task of the therapist is not only to gauge accurately the patient's circumstances and psychological make-up, but to convey to the patient a way of understanding himself that enables him to experience change. It is of particular importance that the therapist be aware when her interpretations are unnecessarily critical or confrontational and that she learn how to generate alternative ways of conveying the same denotative message that have less critical connotations. Shawver suggests that framing interpretations in an "exculpatory" way can enable patients more readily to accept responsibility and to do so in a way that does not do needless damage to their self-esteem.

To illustrate, she discusses how a therapist might respond in a case of an adolescent who has been getting into tangles with her mother over cleaning up her room. The patient tells the therapist that her mother's demands are unreasonable, that she has too much to do already, that her mother is herself a poor housekeeper, and so forth. Shawver contrasts two different ways of bringing to the patient's attention that she is not just a passive victim of her mother's demands but (for reasons it would be the next task of the therapy to explore) has herself actively participated in the tension between them by not cleaning her room.

In the confrontational version, the therapist says: You know, I think you're working awfully hard to avoid looking at the fact that your room is messy and that it's your fault. If you put half that much energy into cleaning your room it would be spotless (Shawver, 1983, p. 8).

Few readers, I expect, will have much difficulty in seeing that comment as critical and problematic. The patient is very likely to perceive it as but one more example of others picking on her and to withdraw or ward it off rather than really listen. Moreover, the consequence is likely to be that she is confirmed in her already low self-esteem or continues to be unable to see a way out of the dilemmas she faces.

Indeed, Shawver may have made an unfortunate choice of her "bad" example in this instance because the comment is so clearly countertherapeutic that the reader can too readily disavow it: "*I* would never say something like that to *my* patient."[5] Yet who of us cannot imagine, at the end of a long day and in a moment of frustration, saying something uncomfortably close to this. And indeed, with just a slight bit of "cleaning up" (say, leaving out *it's your fault*), the comment could be seen as an instance of the therapist's "telling it like it is."

In any event, the contrast is certainly very sharp with Shawver's alternative comment: You know, I think you really want to please your mother, to keep your room clean, to do good schoolwork, but you really feel unable to do everything it would take to please her, so you've just given up trying (Shawver, 1983, p. 8). Shawver notes that this version too is in some ways critical (it points out that the patient has "given up trying" to do the right thing and that she plays an active role in the situation she confronts). But it is also, Shawver notes, "exculpatory" and thus provides "a context in which a sense of responsibility and a sense of control over one's life can grow."[6]

Shawver notes that many therapists worry that exculpatory interpretations will have the opposite effect—contributing to complacency or denial on the patient's part, and hence to a *diminishing* of the sense of

---

[5]There are, to be sure, occasionally times when a confrontational comment is called for. But it should be clear that generally comments such as this are likely to do little to help someone feel better about himself and are likely to be regarded by most therapists as an error.

[6]Anticipating a later discussion, we may note that it is not only, in Shawver's terms, exculpatory; it is also empathic, stating things in a way that demonstrates understanding of and respect for the patient's experience and point of view. When put this way, the comment is easier for the patient to be open to and potentially to accept, notwithstanding the disagreement and questioning that it also contains.

responsibility—and she agrees that such can be the case if the exculpatory comment simply externalizes blame and encourages the patient to stop worrying about it. (This, she suggests, might be the case in the present example if the therapist were to say something like Your mother is too strict and too inconsistent. Don't try to live up to her demands; it'll drive you crazy [Shawver, 1983, p. 8].) Such a comment, however—which simply closes the conversation rather than promoting further exploration—is more likely to result from the therapist's inability to find a way of addressing the issues in a nonaccusatory way, rather than from an excess of concern in that direction. When one knows how to address difficult issues in nonaccusatory ways, one is less likely to have to avoid them or cover them over.

"ENTRY PHRASES": GETTING THE MESSAGE HEARD

In efforts to enable patients to hear messages that address areas of conflict, sometimes just a slight change in the framing of the comment, or the use of a particular phrase that provides a kind of entry point, can make the difference between increasing resistance or providing an opening wedge into greater insight and self-acceptance. The examples that follow illustrate what might be called "entry phrases," figures of speech that serve to lead the patient into experiences he usually keeps at bay. Although the examples cited here are specific, it should be readily apparent to the reader that the forms of each of these comments have wider applicability.

"At Least"

The first example of an entry phrase deals with a patient, Iris, who seemed repeatedly to take on the role of victim in her interactions with other people and in some sense to cultivate that role and embrace it as part of her identity. Such a state of affairs poses a dilemma for the therapist alert to the issues being addressed here. To view the patient as seeking out, and even getting gratification from, being a victim is one of the conceptualizations noted by Wile as having a considerable potential for being derogatory and demeaning; yet it is also at times a genuine and significant facet of the patient's difficulties, which must be addressed if the patient is to be helped.

Iris found herself with great regularity in situations and relationships in which she was exploited, mistreated, or victimized. When she talked about these experiences in therapy, it was not so much with a sense of outrage or complaint but, rather, as if this was simply her lot in life. Indeed, her presentations of her victimization had a subtle but distinct air of pleasure about them. It was hard to escape the conclusion that there was something gratifying to her about relating these events and that being the victim of others' shallowness, insensitivity, and lack of consideration was in some respects a part of her identity that she valued and nurtured.

The challenge here was to point this out to the patient without it being experienced as an accusation (and as one more instance of victimization). The tack taken emphasized an empathic appreciation of the patient's experience, expressed in such a way that it also had the effect of starkly holding that experience up for examination: *I guess concentrating on how people mistreat you feels like the best deal you can get. If you can't have what you want, at least you can feel you are due the sympathy of someone who has been wronged.*

Such a message is most useful when linked to other comments that highlight the consequences for her of this way of protecting herself from pain. Thus on another occasion one might say to such a patient something like, *I am hopeful that you can in fact be treated a lot better than you are. But it's understandable, given your life experiences, that you'd be skeptical; and I can readily see why you'd at least want to be able to feel whatever little comfort comes from the sense of knowing that it's not your fault, that it's they who are being unfair. But the problem is that this then becomes a self-fulfilling prophecy. People pick up that you don't expect very much of them or that you're resentful, and then if they respond to that, it seems to prove you were right not to expect much of them.*

"Even More"

Just as "at least" is a phrase that can provide an opening wedge into material otherwise unable to pass through the patient's psychic Iron Curtain, so too can variations of the phrase "even more."

In one instance a patient I will call Richard had been having considerable difficulty coming to grips with his wish for greater intimacy with his wife, Diana. He would minimize both his desire for the intimacy and his dissatisfaction with the rather distant equilibrium they had established. Athough the sessions were filled with hints that this was an important issue for him that contributed significantly to his feelings of depression, the topic seemed to be too threatening for him to acknowledge.

On one occasion, Richard began the session by talking about something Diana had recently revealed to him about her past. It seemed that this revelation (of a relatively minor event) was tantalizing to him, but its limited nature also registered for him as a sign of what was missing (as if he felt "*This* is what has to be regarded as a revelation in our relationship"). Initial probes into his feelings about this event led to considerable vagueness and evasion, and it was clear that he was once again giving out hints that he was hesitant to follow up on. What I finally said that did open things up was: *You've been noticing how much the intimacy you and Diana have means to you, and it's stirred the wish in you for even more.*

This way of phrasing it emphasized the positive rather than the negative pole of the tension Richard was experiencing. At the same time, though clearly a version of the experience tailored for therapeutic purposes, it was also accurate and true. Even the rather minor revelation she had shared with him *did* represent an increase in intimacy between them, and it did as well make him notice that intimacy between them meant more to him than he usually acknowledged. But this recognition threatened to go undergound, like most other intimations of this feeling, because Richard felt unable to cope with the feelings of disappointment and humiliation he experienced if he let himself realize how much the level of intimacy they had achieved thus far fell short of what he wanted and of what he felt a "healthy and normal" person should have. His difficulties and disappointments were thus being maintained by his shame that he had such difficulties, and thus his possibilities of doing anything to change this state of affairs were severely curtailed.

One could, to be sure, describe this latter state of affairs differently as well. Indeed, it would not be inaccurate to say that it stirred in him a feeling of "how pathetic is it for this to be what constitutes intimacy in our relationship!" But a comment directed to this dimension of Richard's experience, although not inaccurate, would be countertherapeutic. Most likely it would lead him into further labyrinths of evasiveness and denial. Addressing the same issue from the positive side, that he wished for "even more" intimacy, was not only more delicate but less confronting and shaming as well. It also accurately addressed the experience of having tasted a bit of intimacy, of having come into contact both with what it felt like and with the wish for more. It cast the wish for more intimacy not in terms of the failures of the past but rather of the possibilities for the future.[7]

INTERPRETING THROUGH QUESTIONS

In Chapter 6 we will be concerned with the process of inquiry, and naturally the questions asked of patients will be of considerable interest. But before we proceed to that discussion, we may note here that at times

---

[7]See Chapter 7 for a more extensive discussion of the therapeutic value and importance of building on positives.

questions are asked in therapy primarily as a means of getting a point across rather than for the purpose of inquiring (though that purpose is not entirely absent). The following two examples illustrate the use of questions to convey an idea to the patient that might be experienced as too confrontational or threatening if stated directly. The first involved another case in which the problematic dimension involved the patient's apparent need to fail. The therapist, a supervisee of mine, was quite struck by this tendency on the patient's part but, alerted to the issue of accusatory interpretations by our work together, she felt uncomfortable with the comment it occurred to her to make ("You are working very hard to fail.") She came to the supervisory session to discuss how to get this idea across to the patient in a less accusatory way.

There are, of course, a great many ways one could accomplish this. Two, however, that seemed to fit particularly well with this patient's psychology turned out to be in the form of questions. The first was a bit more declarative, with the question only a portion of it: *There seems to be something potentially uncomfortable about actually succeeding, and even though you come very close to succeeding on many occasions, and clearly are capable of it, somehow something happens to interrupt it. Do you have any idea why you might want to avoid succeeding, what it might be that would be scary about that?* Adding the question to the declarative statement in this instance softens and extends it. The patient's curiosity is enlisted in the therapeutic process, and the patient is invited, as a collaborator, to explore the question together with the therapist. As a consequence, the element of accusation that the patient might feel about being told she is intentionally failing is diminished quite considerably. Framing the comment in terms of something being potentially uncomfortable, instead of simply stating that she is avoiding, has a similarly antiaccusatory implication.

We may also note that to some degree the structure of the question *assumes* the patient's acceptance of the statement that precedes. She is, of course, free to say that she *doesn't* think she's avoiding succeeding, but the way the entire comment is constructed encourages the patient's exploration of the matter. To ask "Why do you think this might be?" implies that it *is*. In effect, the question credits the patient with already appreciating something that she may actually only really attain any clarity about once she engages the question.[8]

An alternative approach to addressing the patient's apparent need

---

[8]Some therapists may have concerns about attributing to the patient a clarity of feeling or understanding that the patient has not yet reached. These concerns, as well as the unique therapeutic opportunities introduced by such "attributional" comments are taken up in detail in Chapter 9.

to fail was designed to capitalize on her somewhat whimsical sense of humor. It too approaches the issue in question form, in this instance via two linked questions: *What is it that you do that, if you weren't careful, might have the danger of letting you succeed? And what do you do to pull the fat out of the fire, to make sure that doesn't happen?*

In contrast to a direct statement that she seems to be working hard to fail, this (logically equivalent, but connotationally different) set of questions conveys that "if you are not careful, you will succeed." In its details it serves several functions. First, it is a supportive rather than a critical comment; it includes very centrally a message of confidence in the patient's abilities, a message, one might say, that success is her natural state. Moreover, it does this in a way that does not simply offer bland reassurance, but rather points her to look at what she *does* that, if followed through, would lead to success, and it points her as well to look at what she does that disrupts the path toward success.

Second, it addresses implicitly that success is in some way a threat to her. "If you're not careful" implies a perception of danger on the patient's part, and "pull the fat out of the fire" implies a sense of relief. One would, of course, want as well to follow up this line of inquiry with a more direct examination of what the danger is, of why she might be afraid of succeeding; but the set of questions, with its appeal to her absurdist sense of humor, is designed to intrigue her, to draw her into an issue which, if addressed as a direct declarative statement about her avoidance of success, might be viewed as an attack and warded off.

Another way of using a question to make a point is illustrated in the case of a patient, May, who fit in many ways the picture of the classic hysteric patients reported in the early psychoanalytic literature. May suffered from a vaguely defined "leg problem" that had developed shortly after she was in an automobile accident. No medical basis for this problem was apparent, but it prevented her from walking more than a few feet. Her therapist felt that the symptom was likely related to a number of challenges she was on the verge of having to face that were able to be avoided by the symptom. Shortly before the accident, she was being confronted with some difficult career-change questions and with other "what will I do with my life" issues.

Her therapist wanted to address with her the idea that the symptom was a way of avoiding these challenges and conflicts, but he had been unsuccessful in finding a way to do so that did not feel accusatory to her. The comments he had thought to make (interpretations of how the symptom was a way of avoiding something) felt to him that they would evoke considerable anger and hurt on her part. I suggested he address the matter via the route of inquiry, saying to her something such as *When you get better, you're going to have to deal with a number of difficult questions, so we might as well begin working on them now. What are the challenges you're going to be confronted with once you can walk again?* This way of stating the problem does not challenge the "reality" of the symptom. Its thrust is not *you've developed the symptom to avoid something,* but *you'll have to deal with these things eventually.* Moreover, it conveys an assumption that the symptom *will* get better. It thus has a strong element of suggestion, but a suggestion that is not at all incompatible with the furtherance of exploration.[9]

At another point in the work with May, a different use of a question also helped to get a point across in a way that minimized resistance. May had done a variety of things to avoid letting the therapy have an impact on her, from missing sessions when the work was beginning to get somewhere, to coming late, to denying that the therapy or therapist meant anything to her. Efforts by her therapist to interpret in any way the avoidant nature of these actions met with incredulity of one sort or another. I suggested he draw her into an examination of her avoidance with a comment such as the following: *You know, therapy inevitably has to look at things that people are uncomfortable about. And so everyone has to have some way of keeping those uncomfortable things away. What do you think your ways are?*

This way of putting it had several aspects that probably contributed to May's response to it. (To the surprise not only of her therapist but of me as well, May responded by saying "I guess that's why I miss so many sessions and come late a lot. That's my way of keeping things safe." Moreover, with the therapist's guidance, she followed this up with further fruitful work on what she might be avoiding.) One key feature of the comment is that it "normalized" May's responses. They were not "resistances" that demonstrated her recalcitrance, her being a bad girl. Rather they were the almost inevitable response to this situation, and they were part of something that *everyone* did in one way or another. Moreover, they made her avoidant reactions meaningful and sensible. They weren't just indications of uncooperativeness or immaturity. They were an understandable reaction to a threatening experience. Finally, the question format served to draw her in. It invited a response and was couched in such a way that a response was *expected*; it would have seemed odd in this context *not* to respond. Moreover, the way the question was put indicated an interest in May's uniqueness—what is *your* way of doing this?—and invited her own curiosity to come into play.

---

[9]See Chapter 9 for a detailed examination of the role of suggestion in therapeutic work and its relation to exploratory psychotherapy.

The properties of the questions just cited are properties relevant to questions and inquiries in therapy more generally. Let us turn next to an explicit examination of the process of inquiry in general and its relation to the more declarative comments that we usually label as interpretations or interventions.

CHAPTER 6

Exploration, Not Interrogation

As therapists, we are often in the position of trying to help the patient become aware of or to explore something he has been trying hard not to see. Though our intended posture is one of cooperative exploration, of siding with the patient in the struggle against his neurosis, the interaction can at times become unintentionally and unwittingly adversarial.

In part this adversarial dimension is what Freud noticed when he developed the concept of resistance. Though he wants desperately to cooperate and overcome his neurosis, the patient nonetheless is also motivated to ward off the therapist's efforts in ways that are deleterious to the therapy. This is not because the patient is simply negative or misguided. It is because it is the very things that make him anxious that the therapist must uncover; and although it is in the long-range interest of the patient to undergo the experience of clarification and correction that therapy can offer, the short-term gain of avoiding anxiety has a powerful, if mostly unacknowledged, effect on his choices.

In large measure the therapist's expertise lies in dealing skillfully with the resistance, in finding a way to enable the patient to face those aspects of himself and of his life that are causing his difficulties. But the therapist is best able to accomplish this task if she recognizes that the patient's resistance is not the only factor that can contribute to an adversarial set in the therapy. The therapist's mode of inquiring can at times be equally responsible.

Even more than in making interpretations, therapists are accustomed to regarding their inquiries into the patient's experience and way of life as neutral. But as I will show in this chapter, in inquiring or "exploring" too there are meta-messages. Rarely is a comment "purely" an inquiry; the inquiry usually has a point to make.

Indeed, in insight-oriented approaches to therapy, one cannot really distinguish between separate stages of inquiry and of intervention. In large measure the inquiry *is* the intervention: therapy is viewed as a process of inquiring more and more deeply into the individual's experience in order to further his self-understanding. In such approaches in particular, it is essential to be clear about the ways in which what is conceptualized and discussed as a process of inquiry in fact includes a good deal of getting the therapist's point across.[1]

On close inspection, one can understand the process of inquiry in an exploratory psychotherapy as a kind of argument; and appropriately so, for the therapist's *task* is to change the patient's mind. Cognitive therapists do this very explicitly (indeed, sometimes too explicitly for my tastes). But dynamic therapists do it as well, if often subtly and without full awareness of doing so.

As with interpretation, so too with exploration or inquiry there are facilitative and nonfacilitative ways to say things. Comments couched in the form of inquiries, like any other comments therapists make, are capable of having accusatory (or exculpatory) connotations. The art of inquiry in therapy is one of leading the patient gently and gradually into territory he has heretofore been afraid to face. In doing this, the particular way the therapist couches his inquiry can make a crucial difference.

THE ART OF GENTLE INQUIRY

By the art of gentle inquiry, I mean the ability to inquire into aspects of the patient's experience and motivations that are troubling to him, into features of his sense of self or of his overall life structure about which he feels ashamed and which he tries to hide from himself and from others, and to do so in a way that is minimally accusatory or damaging to the patient's self-esteem. Effective inquiry increases the likelihood that the patient will experience the therapist's comments as an invitation to explore rather than take them as a challenge to be warded off or as a signal to hide.

Havens (1986) provides a useful example of the contrast between ways of inquiring likely to increase resistance and ways more likely to be therapeutically evocative. He compares the therapist's saying *Why didn't you call?*—which he sees as judgmental and inquisitive—with the em-

---

[1]After completing this chapter, I became aware of an excellent paper by Schneider (1991) that explores this latter point in some detail.

pathic comment *You must have had some good reason for not calling.* With the latter phrase the therapist "[puts himself] with the patient and extend[s] that empathy investigatively" (p. 78). A similar effect is achieved, Havens suggests, with a comment such as *It is easy to see why you might not call.*

In this chapter we look at a variety of ways of attempting to open doors that the patient has felt he needed to keep closed. The examples in this chapter differ substantially among themselves, but they all have in common that in some way the therapist is trying to introduce a topic that the patient could readily perceive as being forced on him and could respond to with a strong need to ward off the therapist's intrusion. How to open the topic without closing the door is the challenge to be addressed.

EXPLORATIONS OF CONFLICT

A key to conducting the inquiry in a way that does not create needless resistance or end up lowering the patient's self-esteem is to keep clearly in mind that the patient is most often in conflict. Often, the primary challenge facing the therapist is to find a route into the experience of conflict, to access the complexity beneath the apparently monolithic attitudes that (at a terribly high cost) protect the patient from the less acknowledged side of his conflict. Finding potential tiny chinks in the defensive armor without becoming adversarial is the key to inquiry that is effective and therapeutic.

The Sole Exception as an Opening Wedge

Consider, for example, the case of Joseph, a patient with an obsessional preoccupation with his mustache. Thoughts about his mustache filled Joseph's consciousness for an inordinate number of hours. Should he shave it? Should he let it grow longer? Did he look good with the mustache? Would women see him as more dashing with it? Would they see him as cold and aggressive? Did it make him look older? Was this (looking older) a good thing or a bad thing? The repetitive, preoccupying, and seemingly unresolvable quality that obsessions can have was apparent in abundance.

From numerous indications, it seemed clear to Joseph's therapist that a central dynamic in this obsession was Joseph's strongly conflictual feelings toward his father. Joseph's manifest attitude was unambiguous: he loved and admired his father and stated often that he wanted some day to impart his father's values to his own children. But there were many signs that in fact his immigrant father's highly authoritarian and paternalistic values were viewed by Joseph as constraining and old-fashioned and were regarded as much with contempt as with the exaggerated respect that was Joseph's manifest stance. The reader will surely not be surprised to learn that Joseph's father himself had a mustache and that indeed it was hard for anyone in Joseph's family to picture his father without it.

In attempting to explore Joseph's mixed feelings toward his father, Joseph's therapist ran up against a brick wall. It seemed the harder he tried to open up this question, and indeed the more Joseph seemed to be giving him broad, even exaggerated, clues as to the validity of this formulation, the more strenuous were Joseph's denials. Finally, I suggested to the therapist that he ask the following question in response to Joseph's ritualistic statements about wanting to impart his father's values and qualities to his own son: *If there were just one thing of your father's you were not going to impart, what would it be?*

Such a question seemed a good candidate for breaking the log jam for a number of reasons. To begin with, it operates from *within* the patient's conscious premises. That is, the idea of "just one" thing accords, in its surface meaning, with the assumption that almost everything else about his father would be valuable and worth imparting. At the same time, it is a question that, if at first only in a very limited way, opens up the issue of conflict. It implies that some things about father are admirable and some—at least one—might not be. Inquiring in this fashion does not (at least initially) challenge the basic structure of the patient's beliefs. It operates largely from *within* the patient's belief system, seeking out weak points, as it were, in the defensive structure. The patient is being enlisted in the effort to find the appropriate point of entry; he is being given an opportunity to explore his reservations about his father without having first to acknowledge explicitly anything questionable in what up until now has been an essential element in his identity and his sense of stability.

I can understand that some therapists might regard such a question as a kind of "trick." I would suggest, however, that in fact what such an inquiry establishes is a medium for cooperative exploration of issues that the patient finds it difficult to find a self-respecting way into. If the patient really experiences the question as manipulative, or really doesn't want to engage it, it is all too easy to find a way not to do so. But for many patients, such an inquiry provides a much needed lifeline to grab onto in the effort to pull themselves out of the quicksand of neurotic contradictions.

Who Wants It More?

In a case with quite different manifest issues, but where the resolution of an impasse lay in a closely related mode of inquiry, the patient, Margaret, was discussing her own and her husband's participation in an effort at in vitro fertilization. There were hints that the husband felt resentful that his wife was not "naturally fertile" and that he had to go through a process that involved a great deal of "hassle." There were also indications that *she* felt resentful and wished that her husband was less concerned with having a biological child and would settle for an adoption. She could acknowledge that she found the procedure unpleasant and that it scared her, but she had a great stake in denying that there was any conflict between her and her husband over the issue. The official picture, as it were, was that the two of them formed a solid front, that both of them wanted to have a child and were willing to go through whatever they had to in order to accomplish this.

Exploration of a number of issues important to Margaret's therapy was being blocked by the taboo that existed around examining Margaret's and her husband's attitudes more closely. It seemed likely that such an exploration would be useful in helping Margaret resolve a number of difficulties that seemed oddly resistive to her otherwise quite considerable analytic abilities. Finally, in an effort to lift at least a corner of the veil that covered this topic, I said to her: *In most couples, even if both want it, one wants it <u>more</u>. Which of you is that?*

This question was much more productive in beginning to open up discussion of the conflicts and tensions between them that had been sparked by the in vitro effort. What I think was crucial was that the question didn't imply that either of them didn't want the baby or didn't want the procedure, only that one wanted it more (and of course, logically but for the moment silently, that one wanted it less). Once the patient can identify who wants it more, then one can ask *What are the considerations that lead you [or him] to want it more?* This can then lead to asking what disposes the other partner to want it less, what are the other's reservations, etc. In this way, a topic that initially seems like it simply cannot be talked about becomes one that the patient finds herself talking about almost inadvertently.

When Is It Less? When Is It More?

Related considerations lie behind an odd, yet common and effective strategy in inquiring about the sources of anxiety with patients who claim to feel anxious "all the time." With certain patients of this sort, it is extremely difficult to get them to look at what is making them anxious, at how their anxiety is at least in part related to ongoing life events or to their thoughts or feelings. If one asks such patients if there are ever any times that they feel less anxious, one is met with a resolute no. "I'm *always* anxious." Yet if one asks instead, *Are there ever any times you are even more anxious?* not infrequently one finds that this logically equivalent question elicits a useful and illuminating response. It is as if the patient fears that any concession to the idea that he feels less anxious on some occasions will lead to his fears being ignored or minimized.[2] But if one acknowledges the side of his feelings that he is most consciously identified with, if he is reassured that you are not trying to wipe out his experience, then he can begin to explore his experience in a more differentiated way. Here too, then, beginning one's inquiry from an appreciation of the patient's frame of reference, and taking a step in the needed direction while keeping one foot planted where the patient still needs to be, can open up inquiry into questions that would be un-addressable if one were to attempt what would be in effect a frontal assault on the patient's defenses.

PROTECTED DENIAL AS A MEDIUM FOR EXPLORATION: TEMPORARILY SIDING WITH THE DEFENSE

Generally, psychotherapy aims to help the patient gradually relinquish the defenses that have obscured and distorted his perceptions of himself and other people. At times, however, a temporary siding with the defense on the therapist's part can promote the patient's efforts at self-exploration more effectively than can an interpretation designed to expose the defense more directly and immediately. Such an approach must be distinguished from what is typically described as "supportive therapy." In the latter, the aim is to enable the patient to feel less distressed by bolstering his defenses, and exploration of more conflicted material is discouraged. In the approach described here, in contrast, the aim is to *promote* exploration via a route that takes into account the patient's anxiety and vulnerability. Recognizing that the patient is in

---

[2]This may indeed be a useful clue as to one possible source of the patient's general sense of apprehension. After the patient has been helped to notice at least some variation in her level of anxiety, it may then be useful to make a comment such as: *I wonder if you've been afraid that if you acknowledge at all that you can feel less anxious at times, then I'll be less attentive to your feelings or won't take your anxiety as seriously.* Such a comment can be followed up both with questions such as "I wonder where this sense on your part came from" (seeking both historical origins and continuing experiences that seem to fit this perception) and with discussion of how having to maintain the view that the anxiety never varies gets in the way of understanding it and doing something about what is generating the anxiety.

conflict, the therapist sides with the defense only partially and temporarily, as part of an overall effort to help the patient reappropriate experiences and inclinations he has felt unable consciously to accept as his.

Consider, for example, the following illustration from a case presented to me by a supervisee. The patient, Arlene, suffered from anorexia, but an anorexia that differed some from the typical case. She did not experience herself as looking better being so thin, and seemed genuinely distressed at her emaciated appearance. Moreover, she felt uncomfortably hungry much of the time and even enjoyed food to some degree on those occasions when she did eat. The therapist had occasional tantalizing hints of the fears, fantasies, and wishes that lay behind Arlene's eating disorder, but mostly experienced little cooperation in his efforts to explore with her what her difficulties were about.

Arlene did refer periodically to concerns about "control," but when her therapist tried to get at what it was she was trying to control, or what going *out* of control would be like, he was not successful. She kept saying, "I don't know," or "I can't come up with anything." I suggested to the therapist that he ask instead, *What would you most want not to happen?*

This way of phrasing the inquiry has a subtly different implication from the questions the therapist had been asking. It permits inquiry to be pursued via a message that overtly supports *denial*. Rather than pointing the patient immediately toward exploring a conflicted *wish* (fear of which is very likely implicated in her fear of losing control), it instead acknowledges the part of her that does *not* want the event to happen. In this way it opens a somewhat protected path toward inquiry into a topic that would otherwise leave her feeling too exposed to pursue.

Such "protected probing" enables material to be brought forth in such a way that it is rendered safe by the structure of the question. One can conceive of this approach as one in which the therapist *uses a defense to breach a defense*. By circumscribing what the patient is revealing about herself at that point in the process of exploration, the process itself is permitted to proceed and in fact to deepen. The therapist's aim is to approach, not avoid, the more conflicted aspects of the patient's experience—but in a way that is sensitive to the patient's anxieties and need for at least temporary protection.

In a different context, Feather and Rhoads (1972) similarly found that they could reach material that the patient was otherwise unready to confront by asking such questions as "What is the worst possible thing you can imagine happening?" without pursuing the *wish* that they felt was strongly associated with the fear. They report that their patients (a group that, for various reasons, tended to be less psychologically minded than average) typically responded at first with thoughts of "going to pieces," "losing control," or "becoming totally paralyzed." The therapist then would follow up this response with questions about precisely *how* they would go to pieces, lose control, and so forth, still treating these fantasies solely as fears of undesired events, without implying that any wishes might also be involved. The fantasies reported in response to this next level of probing usually took the form of carrying out some violent or socially taboo behavior. The authors report, for example, that

> in 30 cases of speech phobia, nearly one half the patients fantasized such violent acts as kicking the lectern over, shouting obscenities at the audience, or physically attacking the audience; the rest fantasized exhibiting themselves by undressing, urinating, masturbating, etc. Five young men had the fantasy of their pants falling down. (Feather & Rhoads, 1972, p. 503)

Other patients, they report, were unable, even under these instructions, to fantasize how they might lose control, but (apropos some of the strategies described in this chapter) they were able to do so if asked how "*someone else* who has the same problem" might act.

Because of the particular focus and goal of the work Feather and Rhoads describe in that report, they did not attempt to undo their patients' defensive disavowal even at the end of their work with them. The patients they were treating had been suffering from a variety of unusually persistent and distressing symptoms that had proved intractable both to standard psychoanalytic therapy and to standard behavioral therapy. Their creative and fascinating work with these patients (see their original report in Feather & Rhoads, 1972) produced quite remarkable improvement in their symptoms, which, in light of the patients' previous treatment history, it was understandable they would not be inclined to risk by pushing the patients to acknowledge the previously unacknowledged wishes. They note that a frequent response to their eliciting these fantasies was that the patient would "quickly reassure the therapist (or himself?) that he would not really do such a thing" (Feather & Rhoads, 1972, p. 503; material in parentheses appeared in the original). Feather and Rhoads never challenged these statements by the patients and, indeed, attempted throughout to heighten the patients' sense of the difference between fantasies and actions.

That these psychoanalytically trained clinicians could put aside their usual definition of cure for the sake of the patients' well-being was most impressive, and the success of their work makes it clear that it is not always necessary for full insight to be achieved in order for treatment gains to be significant and lasting. The method of inquiry they employed, however, lends itself as well to being used as a *transitional* strategy, enabling the patient to begin confronting a set of issues indirectly at first and then, as described in much of this chapter, gradually to be helped to own more fully wishes and experiences that previously were inaccessible and unacceptable.

EXTERNALIZATION IN THE SERVICE OF THERAPY

Another means of doing a temporary end run around the patient's defenses entails helping the patient to attend to matters he would otherwise find too difficult to face by utilizing for the purposes of the therapy the patient's tendency to externalize responsibility for his experiences. Externalization is a common defensive maneuver which, in the ordinary course of events can keep people less clear about their own experiences and less able to deal effectively with the challenges their lives present. In a limited way, however, it can be used temporarily by the therapist as a means of gently moving *into* an area that the patient needs to explore but would be likely to be rather defensive about.

An approach of this sort was employed with a patient I shall call Janine. Janine had had the experience on a number of occasions of men leaving her without even talking to her about their discontent. Instead, she would wake up one morning and find a note on a table or a pillow. It seemed clear to the therapist, a supervisee of mine, that the reason these men left, *and* that they left in the fashion they did, was that Janine had a tendency to overreact enormously to upsetting events. The therapist surmised that these men just didn't want to face the very extreme emotional storm that would greet them if they actually tried to talk about the difficulties in the relationship.

What was very interesting from the point of view of technique, was that a version of the same dilemma encountered by Janine's boyfriends was experienced by her therapist. He feared that to raise with her his understanding of what went on with her boyfriends would lead to her becoming upset—in her characteristically exaggerated way—in the therapy too; and he sensed that like the men who left her, he too was hesitant to face that.

Moreover, although he recognized this hesitancy as something he

would have to deal with, and appreciated in principle that if her exaggerated reaction occurred right in the session it might provide an opportunity to explore this tendency in vivo,[3] he also felt, on the basis of his
previous experience with Janine, that her upset would be so disorganizing that she would in fact not learn anything from it; she would neither
hear what he was saying nor put it together with any other aspects of her
experience in a coherent and therapeutically useful way.

How, then, he asked, could he probe into this important pattern in
a way that might have a chance of being heard and being therapeutic?
Although I felt that eventually he would have to deal directly with the
transference and countertransference implications of his feeling that he
needed to tiptoe around with her, and that this would be a key element
of the therapeutic process, I suggested he begin the inquiry into this
pattern as follows: *Let me ask you about your boyfriends. Do you think they did
what they did because for some reason they felt you couldn't take the confrontation?*

Note that the comment did *not* say that she could not take the
confrontation. On its surface it was not about her at all. It was about the
men, how *they* would perceive the situation. In that sense it could be seen
as fostering externalization, turning the patient's and therapist's attention away from Janine's own experience and toward that of others. It
also, however, provided an opportunity to begin addressing a topic that
had been a source of great pain for Janine and that she had had great
difficulty in approaching.

In planning how to conduct the inquiry into this pattern, I further
suggested to the therapist that if Janine did acknowledge, even tentatively, that that might be how her boyfriends perceived things and why
they acted as they did, he might then ask her *What might have made them
think that?* and, if that did not prove fruitful, to follow it with the slightly
more pointed *What do you think they were afraid would happen if they said
something to you directly?* The latter version still focuses explicitly on what
they were afraid of, but pushes just a bit more for the patient to reflect
on what she does that conveys that impression.

The hope would be, of course, that she would begin to see that they
might have feared how terribly upset she got and that then a path would
be opened up for exploring this behavior—what it represented, where

---

[3]Here is one of those instances where the perspectives of behavioral and dynamic therapists can be seen to overlap. The behavioral concept of in vivo experience converges here
with the dynamic concept of transference. One of the key considerations that leads
dynamic therapists to emphasize exploration of the transference is precisely that it provides an opportunity for therapeutic learning to occur in the context of a vivid in vivo
experience.

and how it was learned, what were the thoughts and emotional assumptions that led to her reactions snowballing, and what were the consequences of her expressing her upset in the way she did. In such a way she might gain a better understanding of how her way of expressing herself appeared exaggerated to others and led them to retreat instead of taking her complaints seriously and of how her overwrought reaction increased her own sense of upset and vulnerability.

This latter focus would also require careful and delicate phrasing. It could easily be experienced by her as an accusation that she was just faking and wasn't really as upset as she appeared. In addressing this, one might speculate out loud something like *I wonder if part of the problem is that there have been many times in the past when others haven't appreciated how upset you were or haven't responded in a helpful way, and so you've come not to believe that others will even notice your upset unless you turn the volume way up.*

Then, depending on her response to that, one could further suggest, *I think what often happens is that even though what you're doing is trying to get them to notice, the result is just the opposite of what you want. What happens is that they experience your upset as exaggerated or as too much, and they back off. And then you're left feeling very frustrated and very abandoned, and so you try even harder to get across to them how bad you feel, and once more a very real and genuine upset gets expressed in such a way that people experience it as not as real as it is or as too much for them to deal with.*[4]

As exploration of this pattern proceeds, the therapist can begin to address how it is played out in the therapy relationship, how his and Janine's interaction replicates a key configuration in her life. The strategy offered here is not an alternative to this approach, but a complement. It opens up space for Janine to begin looking at what goes on rather than just reacting, and thus it fosters the necessary observing ego for the analysis of the transference to be therapeutically productive. If the focus on the transference is premature, if the patient has not been helped to reach a point where she can reflect as well as experience, then transference analysis is likely to be unproductive, a carrying through of a theoretical imperative rather than a sensitive response to the patient's needs.[5]

---

[4]This is, of course, an interpretation of one of the vicious circles in which she is caught and of the irony that characterizes it (see Chapter 2).

[5]In the view of some analytically oriented therapists, modes of interacting with the patient such as described here seem incompatible with effective exploration of the transference. For a detailed discussion of the conceptual foundation underlying the present approach to transference phenomena, and further consideration of how strategies such as those described here can be compatible with a meaningful and thorough analysis of the transference, see Chapter 4 of this book and Wachtel (1987).

Both the tenacity with which the patient clings to externalization and how thoroughly it obscures the patient's vision of his own actions and experiences vary considerably from patient to patient. With some patients, just a simple question such as *Is there any way in which you play a role in what happens?* or *What keeps things going this way?* can be useful. With others, more complex or indirect approaches are necessary. One way of combining the two to some degree—i.e., beginning to probe into the patient's responsibility while (for a very defensive patient) still offering some degree of temporarily reassuring externalization, would be to say *Is there something in what he/she does that draws you into it too, that gets you to act in ways that keep the whole cycle going?* Here we are moving into an inquiry about the patient's active role, but in a way that is almost imperceptible. The question seems at first to be maintaining the externalization (the patient's participation is itself the other's fault), yet the direction of inquiry is definitely opening up the topic of the patient's own role.

Something of this sort proved useful with Dan, a rather defensive man who tended to occupy his sessions with seemingly endless talk about how he was being treated by his father, with virtually no mention of how that felt to *Dan* or of what was stirred in him by his father's actions. Questions about Dan's own experience, or comments about how his tendency to focus on his father got him away from that experience, had little impact on the pattern. They were either essentially ignored or experienced as a criticism (and discussions of *that* pattern, between *us*, were similarly unproductive). The only path into his own experience seemed to lie *through* his preoccupation with his father. Questions such as *How have you adapted to [X, Y, or Z behavior by your father] over the years?* did point Dan toward somewhat greater self-exploration. After a while, especially if he at least temporarily became engaged by such self-examination, the process could be extended by questions such as *Does that show itself in any way* outside *of your relationship to your father?* This permitted the gradual accumulation of concrete details about his life and his experience, and it served as a kind of base camp for further efforts at interesting Dan in exploring his own experience.[6]

[6]We may also note that the phrase "over the years" served as a kind of bridge between Dan's defensive clinging to a focus on what his father did and entry into his current lived experience. It permitted an initial approach in terms that could be experienced as rather general and as distant in time, which later could be brought into closer focus by questions such as *And how do you experience that now?* or *What are the ways in which you do that now?* As in the discussion above, the aim is first to help him see how he got caught in something of external origin, then to let him see how *he* got caught in it, what *his* contribution to it was, and then to help him to appreciate its role in his life in the present.

Thus, with patients like Janine and Dan, one attempts step by step to address a matter that the patient feels quite defensive about, but in a way that is nonaccusatory and accepts the patient's way of constructing his or her experience even as one is working to question that construction. One understands how even maladaptive behavior can make sense from the patient's frame of reference, how given a particular set of experiences, and a particular way of interpreting those experiences, it may seem like just about the only avenue open to the patient. Starting with an acceptance of the patient's initially externalizing orientation, gradually one helps the patient to find his way deeper into his own experience.

EXPLORING THROUGH THE TRANSFERENCE AND THE IDENTIFICATORY TRANSFERENCE

Another way of exploring traits the patient may be defensive about without arousing excessive resistance or damaging the patient's self-esteem derives from a perspective on transference that has been only relatively occasionally addressed in the psychoanalytic literature. Most often, transference is adduced when the patient reacts to the therapist in ways that resemble his (the patient's) reaction to or perception of one of his parents: "You see me as depriving and nasty (or weak and needing protection, or self-absorbed, or intimidatingly perfect, and so forth) just as you experienced your parents that way."

But there is another aspect of transference, which I call the "identificatory transference," that is very useful in furthering what I have been calling gentle inquiry. That is the examination of ways in which the patient reacts *to you* as important others in his past have reacted *to him*. Thus, in these instances there is a kind of role reversal. It is not a matter of transferring childhood perceptions or reactions to new objects but, rather, of *reversing* the roles of childhood, of the patient's being the parent and, implicitly, placing the therapist in the role of the child—in *his* role (cf. Racker, 1968; Searles, 1965; Tansey & Burke, 1989; Weiss & Sampson, 1986).

What is learned here occurs largely via two kinds of identifications. First, the patient (at least implicitly) identifies with the parent, usually as a form of what Anna Freud (1936) called identification with the aggressor. Second, the therapist, in turn, identifies with the patient (as victim); she experiences in the counterrole of the transference (as distinct from the countertransference) what it must have felt like for the patient to be in the position he was vis-à-vis his parent.

A very valuable implication of this perspective is that the therapist, by regarding those behaviors as the patient's way (usually unconscious-ly) of demonstrating to the therapist how he was treated by his parents, is enabled to call the patient's attention to various behaviors that might otherwise be difficult to address without seeming accusatory.

In the case of Tina, presented to me in supervision, the patient was being unusually provocative with her therapist, challenging, disparag-ing, and invalidating everything the therapist said. She would cancel sessions, saying it didn't really matter much anyway, tell her therapist she was nice to talk to but didn't help very much, and indicate in various ways that the therapist's efforts were simply not important to her. Based on my understanding of the case, I suggested to the therapist that she employ the perspective of the identificatory transference and say to the patient, *I think maybe you're trying to convey to me as vividly as you can how your parents treated you; in telling me over and over again how unimportant I am, how little impact I have on you, you're letting me know that they conveyed something similar to you and letting me sense what that feels like.* In this way, the patient's behavior is being addressed directly, but without the pa-tient *being blamed* for it. Indeed, it is being addressed as a positive contribution to the task of the therapy, as a way the patient is getting something important across to the therapist.

It is essential to be clear that the *tone* of a comment like the one just described is crucial. If the therapist does not mean what she is saying, and is really being sarcastic (as such a comment *could* be), it is scarcely an instance of gentle inquiry. This type of identificatory transference interpretation should not be employed unless the therapist, based on substantial clinical evidence, genuinely believes that the parents did treat the patient this way.

It is important to add, however, that the perspective implied in the comment can be a valuable aid in *discovering* what the parents were like in relation to the patient. That is, by attending to one's experience with the patient from this vantage point (as well as from the more traditional standpoint in which the therapist is perceived as *like* the parent), one can gain valuable insights into the patient's psychological life and the in-teractions that shaped it. Quite apart from its value in helping the therapist address certain difficult events between them in a less accus-atory way, this perspective can also help the therapist generate clinical hypotheses regarding complex aspects of the patient's experience that had previously gone unnoticed.

In an interesting wrinkle, that points us to still another approach to the process of inquiry in apparently resistant patients, Tina's therapist told me she thought Tina's most likely response to such a comment would be to say something like "No, my parents were never like that. They were always very nice to me. If there was any fault at all, it was that they never could say no to me."

Now one of the central characteristics of this patient was that she was excessively bouncy and unable to be serious or reflective in any way. The therapist suspected that in fact this characteristic partly accounted for the great difficulty this attractive young woman had in maintaining a relationship with a man for more than one or two dates. Not only was the criticalness and dismissiveness implicit in her manner with her therapist likely manifested with men too, but her therapist wondered as well if her very bounciness, perhaps initially attractive, served very quickly to communicate an unwillingness or inability to take anyone seriously or to let anyone matter to her that men quickly recoiled from. Moreover, the seemingly lighthearted, frivolous, eager-to-please image initially conveyed by her bounciness also probably had the effect of particularly attracting men who would have very little tolerance for the faultfinding that was shortly to come.

Tina's unreflectiveness made it very difficult to raise or examine these questions. Efforts to inquire into the atmosphere of Tina's home in growing up, to see if there had perhaps been a ban or taboo on serious feelings, met with a flip, dismissive (though polite and nominally pleasant) brush-off.

When Tina's therapist told me what she thought Tina's response would be to the comment described above (suggesting that Tina's behavior toward her therapist conveyed something about how her parents treated her) I suggested she pursue the following line of inquiry with Tina. To begin with she would ask, *Do you think it could have been that your mother was always "nice" because she had difficulty ever acknowledging anything was wrong, that she felt compelled to be unwaveringly cheerful and upbeat all the time?*

In much the fashion of the earlier discussions of externalization, this line of inquiry can be seen as a first step facilitating the patient's eventually examining *her own* compulsively bouncy style, opening a door to doing so by describing the style as a family ethic she grew up with. Thus it would not have to be experienced as a personal failing but rather as a kind of loyalty and/or an almost inevitable consequence of growing up in the family she grew up in. (See Wachtel, 1991b, for another example of opening the exploration of a characteristic the patient was reluctant to acknowledge via first addressing related characteristics of the patient's family.)

From the vantage point of technique, there are a number of ways in which the above-noted question can be followed up. If Tina acknowledges some truth in this description of her mother, then of course one has made a step in the direction of exploring that tendency in the family. If, as seems more likely, she denies that mother had difficulty acknowledging the more serious or difficult side of life, one can then ask (following up on Tina's claim that mother had no difficulty addressing troubling matters), *Can you give me an example of some of the things that troubled her?* If the patient does, we again are on the way to going behind some of the compulsive bounciness and beginning some real therapeutic work. If she cannot give an example, it *also* points to something of therapeutic import, because she is brought somewhat closer to the reality of the pervasive denial and compulsive avoidance of unpleasant topics that reigned in the household.

That the foregoing addresses a version of the identificatory transference paradigm may be obscured because of the presence of other elements that enter into the formulation. What identifies the focus as the identificatory transference is that in Tina's manner of being light and pleasant but ultimately uninvolved, unengaged, and unwilling to share deep emotional feelings, she is relating to the therapist not as she related to her mother but as *her mother* related to *her*.

Taking this route into the patient's experience makes it easier for the therapist to be more empathic and less angry toward the patient. A therapist's anger toward a patient most often stems from frustration, from the feeling that she is impotent to help. As soon as one sees a handle, the anger is likely to subside, even if the patient's behavior continues to be outrageous. The premium in our work as therapists is so strongly on understanding (and the frustration and self-derogation that accompany our *not* understanding so substantial) that as therapists we are often able to tolerate acceptingly many behaviors by our patients we would never tolerate in others—*if* we can have the consolation, indeed, the pleasure, of understanding those behaviors (and thus of feeling effective).

Following the line of inquiry just described, the therapist can address, in an empathic and genuine way, behavior that would otherwise be experienced as frustrating and as a barrier to the therapeutic work. The identificatory transference perspective both illuminates and takes the accusatory sting out of the pattern of flip nonchalance that the therapist had found so maddening. Pulling it all together, the therapist could now say something on the order of:

It must be hard to have to follow that kind of implicit rule all the time, not to be able to say when something is bothering you; to have to be flippant and bouncy and not care all the time, even when you feel down or worried; and then to have to bear the consequences of other people's experience of that, such as guys shying away. I'm sure it wasn't easy for your mother to follow it either, but *nonetheless the example she set for you, especially when you were a little girl and very impressionable, made it necessary for <u>you</u> to follow it too. And now, you've become so used to it you hardly notice that you <u>are</u> following a rule, and especially that you're following a rule that actually goes against your grain in some ways, that keeps a real and important part of you locked up. I'm amazed you've been able to do it all these years, and I'm not surprised that you're now finding it a bit exhausting.*

This comment (a composite for expository purposes of several different things the therapist might have said at different times) is a complex one that incorporates a number of different therapeutic elements and perspectives. It reviews for the patient the price she pays for her bounciness (not being able to say when something is troubling her; men shying away) while presenting it sympathetically as something that "must be hard." It also casts the patient's engaging in such a pattern as something that is not her fault, suggesting this was almost inevitable given the home she grew up in; yet it manages not to blame mother either, noting that it must have been hard for her, too. Almost as an aside, it slips in an important message about this pattern going against the patient's grain and keeping an important part of her locked up, and it does so in a way that is difficult to challenge because it attributes that understanding to the patient as something she is already recognizing. The patient's "exhaustion" with the pattern, her being fed up with maintaining it and with its high toll on her life is similarly being attributed to her somewhat ahead of her having come to it fully on her own. Chapter 9 will discuss in more detail such "attributional" comments in which the patient is given credit for an insight, or for being ready and eager to change a problematic pattern, somewhat in advance of having consciously and fully reached the point of experiencing it. That credit, one might say, functions a bit like credit in the financial realm. Being lent to her before she is yet able to repay it, but as an indication of confidence that she eventually will be able to, it in fact provides her temporarily with resources that ultimately enable her to demonstrate that the credit given was a good investment.

INQUIRING INTO THE PATIENT'S BEHAVIOR IN THE SESSION

We are (correctly) used to thinking of the patient's behavior in relation to the therapist as providing a particularly valuable opportunity for therapeutic learning. But the very sense of immediacy that can make such a focus of great therapeutic value also leaves the patient potentially feeling more vulnerable and exposed. Consequently, attention to such behavior requires particular concern with tact and a nonaccusatory mode of communication. This is especially the case when the patient's behavior is annoying or provocative. The therapist, in trying not to be accusatory or critical, can feel boxed into a corner.

An especially ticklish instance of this presented itself to me in the form of a patient whom I'll call Martin. Martin quite frequently would "snoop" around my office at the beginning or end of sessions. He would look over anything that was lying on my desk, ask about various papers lying about, and generally behave in a way that felt intrusive and inappropriate. It was clear to me that this behavior was important and needed to be inquired into, but I delayed doing so both because I sensed Martin's vulnerability and because I felt irritated at Martin's behavior and felt that to inquire under such circumstances would be countertherapeutic. I kept it in the back of my mind to inquire about when I found an appropriate route into it.

The opportunity presented itself in the context of another discussion, and served to deepen that discussion as well as to permit the "snooping" just mentioned to be addressed more fruitfully. Martin was a very avoidant individual, who was always extremely vague and abstract (We had discussed in an earlier session his use of phrases such as "I'm almost ambivalent," in which even the ambiguity of experience implied by ambivalence had to be further hedged with an "almost," and he had been able to laugh appreciatively at the extent of his evasiveness.) In the session before the one under discussion here, it had come out that he knew extraordinarily little about his wife, Caterina, and her family. They had emigrated from South America, and it was not clear why they had emigrated, what social class they had belonged to there, how they felt about being here, and whether they regarded themselves as having come down in the world. It became evident in that session (to Martin as well as to me) that the gaps in his knowledge were highly relevant to some key issues in his present relationship with his wife, and he had a sharpened sense of the price he paid for his avoidant style.

In the session discussed here, however, he stepped back a bit from his newly gained appreciation of having avoided finding out about his wife's feelings. He said he had thought about it and realized that Caterina was simply a very private individual. *She*, after all, had said to him "I don't want to get psychoanalytical. My background is my background, I don't really want to go into it very much." The retreat was not total, however. Martin had begun to come to grips with his avoidant tendencies and couldn't ward off his complex feelings about her and their relationship as easily as he once had. He kept working on it, saying "Maybe I'm protecting her, or maybe, I don't know . . . "

At that point I interjected "or maybe that's why you married her. She was someone with whom you could have a relationship in which vagueness was part of the contract."

As I made the comment I became aware that, regardless of how accurate it might be, it could easily be experienced by the patient as confronting or attacking. A red light went off for me, and I thought about how to further develop the comment in a way that would be therapeutic. I decided that the most useful course would be to highlight the element of conflict. I felt he might be more able to grab hold of what I was trying to convey about his vagueness and avoidance if I also addressed the other side of the conflict—his wish to be clearer. As will be apparent shortly, in doing so I also found an opening to bring up the behavior in the sessions that I had been wanting to address for a while.

The full initial comment (including the possibly accurate, but none-theless faulty, beginning) was as follows:

"Maybe that's why you married her. Caterina was someone with whom you could have a relationship in which vagueness was a part of the contract. I'm raising this because I think you're feeling some conflict about this now. You're beginning to question whether this is really what you want your marriage to be like. I think you're wanting to be clearer about yourself, to see others more clearly, to get some clarity you haven't had."[7]

When Martin responded positively to this comment, and seemed to be more in touch with the side of himself that did want to see more clearly and directly, I went on to bring up his behavior at the beginning and end of sessions. In doing so, I had two aims. Not only did I feel that he would have a valuable learning experience in confronting and examining his behavior, but I viewed this as an opportunity as well to take up, in a nonaccusatory way, behavior that had been annoying me. For the therapist to be annoyed at or frustrated with the patient is clearly not a desirable state of affairs. Here was a chance to "clear the air" in a way that reframed his behavior (for both of us). As will be clear from the following comment, the same element served the furthering of both aims: the opportunity to cast Martin's behavior as a reflection of his curiosity, of his desire to know, rather than as a breach of some sort or as an intrusion that was "inappropriate." What I said to Martin was the following:

"One thing that comes to mind, now that I understand better your

---

[7]This last sentence not only addresses the other side of the conflict; as with the example cited earlier, it also has an attributional dimension, highlighting a side of the patient's feelings one *hopes* will grow stronger—his desire for greater clarity. See Chapter 9 for further discussions of the use of such comments.

wish to see more clearly, is something I've been aware of for a while but didn't comment on because I didn't have a sense of whether it meant anything or what it was about. Practically from the first day you came in here you did something fairly unusual. Almost every session, either at the beginning of the session or the end of the session, you look all over my desk and ask me questions: 'Who's that picture of?' 'What's that paper about?' You read pieces of paper lying on the desk, you're very curious, and you're looking at everything in a way that at first I felt a bit uncomfortable with. Now I think I understand it better, and I see it as part of something important and positive. I see it as your trying to break out of the fog you've lived in most of your life, and that you're looking around to see 'who *is* this guy I'm talking to, and what is this all about?' It's a kind of longing to know more about me, to get past the vagueness and the mystery, and I think that's because there's been so much vagueness and mystery in your life, so much that has not been clear, not been confronted, not been articulated in anything near the way your intelligence ought to enable you to articulate things."

The reader may note that here I am not just calling him vague or inarticulate. By *contrasting* his inability to articulate his experience here with his much greater ability in other contexts (e.g., business) I am, as it were, approaching the "negative" from the positive side.

One may also note that this comment is a rather lengthy one. In general, I agree with the common wisdom that it is best to keep one's comments relatively short. I suspect, however, that in fact therapists make longer comments in their daily practice than one would surmise from what is written about the therapeutic process. In this connection, it is interesting and amusing to note Racker's comment, regarding Freud's technique, that

> Freud interprets constantly, makes detailed and sometimes very extensive interpretations (speaking more or less as much as the patient), and the session is a straightforward *dialogue*. Those who link the concept of "classical technique" with a predominance of a monologue on the part of the patient and with few and generally short interpretations on the part of the analyst, will have to conclude . . . that in this aspect Freud was not a "classical analyst." (Racker, 1968, p. 35; italics in the original)

In any event, I am keenly aware that attention to the range of considerations presented in this book may at times be likely to make one's comments a bit longer than they otherwise might be. In my view, the overall trade-off is a positive one, but there will certainly be times when one is too long-winded,[8] and concern for brevity should not be ignored.

RHETORICAL QUESTIONS

One of the ambiguities in coming to grips with the meta-messages that are embedded in therapeutic inquiry is that therapists often make their points in a quasi-Socratic way. Interpretations or suggestions are not infrequently couched in the form of a question, and it is not always easy—for patient *or* therapist—to sort out precisely what function such a comment/question has in the therapeutic dialogue. If the patient notices the rhetorical nature of a question, I believe it is important to acknowledge his perception.[9] But often it can honestly be said as well that *Yes, you're right, I certainly was trying to get a point across and was not just asking a question; but I was also asking a question. I have a general idea of what I think is going on, but in fact exploring this together really will help me to understand it better.*

A good example of such a quasiquestion, and of how it can nonetheless be a "real" question as well, comes from work with a patient who suffered from an extremely harsh superego. Jennifer was enormously self-critical, holding herself to standards that were almost saintly. Efforts to point out how harsh she was with herself, to discuss her inordinately high standards, seemed to have little impact. I therefore took to asking, as a kind of point of information when she would talk critically about something she had done, *Is it just you who shouldn't do this, or would it be a terrible thing if anyone did it?* Or alternatively, I might ask, *If Bill or Marilyn or Ruth did this, would you feel the same way about it?* To be sure, part of my aim was to find another route into helping her to see how severe were the standards to which she held herself; but I was also genuinely

---

[8]The example just cited may indeed be an illustration of this. Although I believe that the comment contains the proper elements and the proper thrust, it may well be longer than it needs to be. Perhaps the message should have been conveyed in a series of statements rather than all at once. (The reader should note, however, that comments "feel" longer in print than they do as they unfold as part of a spontaneous process of communication with another person.)

[9]The therapist's mantle of ambiguity and neutrality, his refusal to acknowledge his participation in what transpires, can exacerbate the patient's lack of trust in his own perceptions and heighten the patient's tendency to invalidate his own feelings and predilections (see Wachtel, 1987, Chap. 11, "You Can't Go Far in Neutral").

interested in knowing the parameters of her criticalness, to understand better the standards to which she held *others*. The rhetorical question was no doubt rhetorical. But it was also a question.

ACCUSATORY INQUIRIES

On other occasions the therapist's questions are not rhetorical but are nonetheless a device for getting a point across. This is often not a very salutary situation, because it tends to occur when the therapist has a fairly clear view about potential actions that are in the patient's interest, but has a notion of the therapist's role that requires her to restrict her activities to "exploration" or "inquiry." Usually, the intent of the question is at least somewhat obscure to the therapist, which is of course one of the reasons that what results can be far from optimal. An interesting example of this came to my attention in a case seminar I was conducting.

A while back, the patient, William, had found his wife's diary lying around and had read it, confirming his suspicion that his wife was having an affair. On a number of occasions since, the diary was left similarly accessible, and William again read it, feeling ashamed of himself for doing so and upset about what the diary revealed. There were numerous indications that in fact William's wife had intended for him to read the diary and that the two of them were engaged in a quite counterproductive form of covert and unacknowledged communication. Moreover, there were indications as well that his wife was hoping that William would bring things out into the open so they could begin to address what was going on between them.[10]

William's therapist felt it was important for William to find a way to discuss with his wife his having read the diary, its contents, and his feeling that she had in fact intended for him to read it. He felt constrained in offering direct counsel in this regard, however, by an understanding of the therapeutic process that required him not to give advice but only to "inquire." He therefore put to William a question: "What makes it difficult to talk to her about the diary?"

At first glance the question may appear innocuous. It is, after all, an "inquiry," a question that encourages William to look more closely at his experience and at his motives and concerns. The question conveys, however, a subtle and problematic meta-message: as it is put, it seems

---

[10]They had earlier been in couples therapy together, but for various reasons such therapy was not an option at this point, despite indications that it might be the best prospect for both of them.

to imply that it should be *easy* to talk to his wife about what has transpired, that it is only William's subjective difficulties that stand in the way.

Much more helpful, I believe, would have been a comment such as *I guess at this point it feels kind of difficult to bring it up.* The connotation conveyed by this comment is quite different from that of the question the therapist asked. There is in this message too an implication that bringing it up might be a good idea, but it acknowledges that the patient's anxiety about doing so—especially in light of his having to admit that he himself had done something he was ashamed of in reading the diary—is understandable and expectable and that what he faces is by no means easy, even if it may be necessary. The "what makes it difficult" question that the therapist asked may be seen as a cousin of the "why didn't you call" example of Havens discussed earlier in this chapter, and it highlights for us once again that connotations and meta-messages must concern us in all aspects of the therapeutic process. Inquiry is not a protected province in which such concerns may be put aside.

CHAPTER 7

Building on the Patient's Strengths

Our efforts to help people change are rooted in an understanding of what is wrong. The theories that guide therapeutic work tend to be theories of pathology or disorder. In the history of our field, theories in which the individual's strengths take center stage have been relatively rare. One interesting, though problematic, exception was Maslow (e.g., 1962). Maslow called explicit attention to the prevalent tendency to root the study of personality in the study of pathology and chose instead to focus his work on the study of unusually healthy individuals. The study of health and of "human potential," Maslow thought, would reveal possibilities that are obscured by the pathocentric blinders worn by most workers in the field.

The general program of treating optimal functioning as a worthy focus of attention, and of building a theory of personality from the positive rather than the negative pole, remains a compelling and attractive alternative. Maslow's own work, however, was flawed by an individualistic bias that was uncongenial to a deep understanding of the interdependence that characterizes healthy human functioning. (See Wachtel, 1989, especially Chap. 6, for a critique of Maslow's approach to human potential.)

Maslow and other contributors to the human potential movement had considerable influence on practices that were, so to speak, first cousins of psychotherapy—for example, the various "growth," "encounter," and other groups that emanated from centers such as Essalen in California. They had relatively little influence, however, on the practice of psychotherapy per se. One notable exception in this regard was Carl Rogers, who was a leading figure both in the field of psychotherapy and in the human potential movement. Rogers's influential work in the field of psychotherapy proper, however (e.g., Rogers, 1942, 1951, 1961) largely preceded his participation in—indeed even the existence of—the human potential movement.

Rogers came closer than most other leading figures in the field of psychotherapy to building on the positives in the patient or client. In large measure his therapy was built on "prizing" the client, on respecting the client's humanity and viewing affirmatively his or her experience, without questioning it or diagnosing it. Indeed, one can see some affinities between Rogers's affirmative approach and the perspective of Wile that I discussed earlier as being so largely consonant with the point of view of this book. The particular approach to affirmation of the client advocated by Rogers, however, seems to me to place restraints on the therapist's intensive probing of issues in which anxiety and conflict have led to defensiveness and consequent distortion or self-deception[1]; and it certainly limits the kinds of active interventions that in my view are a frequently useful complement to the effort to understand.

In this chapter I want to consider how the therapeutic effort can be pointed toward affirming and building upon the patient's strengths. Such an agenda, it should be clear, in no way implies ignoring the difficulties, the weaknesses, the inhibitions, or the self-defeating and self-limiting character traits that are likely to play a central role in the problems that have brought the patient into therapy; only a clear-eyed confrontation with the realities of the patient's life can yield deep and lasting change. But it does imply that the overall vision of most psychotherapy is too one-sidedly focused on the negative. Effective psychotherapeutic effort must have an equally clear vision of the patient's strengths. It is on those strengths that change is built, and failure to see them clearly can make change extremely unlikely.

BUILDING ON VARIATIONS

Therapy is a process of change. When it is working as it should, any description of the patient is a description of a person in transition.

---

[1]To be sure, the Rogerian method is itself a way of delving more deeply into the person's experience, and in many instances the patient, empathic stance of the client-centered therapist, attending to and resonating with the client's account, can lead to a gradual increase in the ability to articulate experience and to clarifying and bringing into focus aspects of experience that were previously inaccessible. Indeed, in the hands of some of its practitioners, the Rogerian approach to exploration of experience and the interpretive stance of the psychodynamically oriented clinician are difficult to distinguish. Where differences can be found, however, it is my view that the latter is more likely to enable the patient to confront aims and experiences that were previously fearfully avoided.

Often, one of the major problems that must be overcome is the patient's tendency to think of himself in static terms, and it is one of the important functions of the therapist to help the patient see himself as changing and, indeed, as able to change (cf. Frank, 1973).

The therapist's comments can facilitate or impede the patient's sense that change is possible. Variant ways of communicating what is largely the same message can either contribute to the patient's feeling of being "stuck" or encourage him to project himself into a variety of alternative futures.

As an illustration, consider the following example: a supervisee said to a patient who was frequently silent, *You seem to have difficulty talking.* Descriptively, his comment was essentially accurate, but I raised a question about it in the supervisory session. It seemed to me that this way of phrasing it contributed to a self-attribution by the patient of "I am a person who has difficulty talking" and that the static ring of such a way of thinking could be discouraging.

I suggested that in the future it might be more useful to say something like *Sometimes you talk more easily than at other times.* Such a way of putting it addresses the same behavior on the patient's part—it considers the patient's silence at that moment, notes that the silence is not an isolated instance but part of a pattern, and implicitly invites the patient to reflect on that pattern—but it has the advantage of including a recognition that there are times when the patient *does* talk readily. It conveys that there is something to build on, that not-talking is not some kind of fixed attribute of the patient, which he must simply accept as "what I am like." There are times when he is quite capable of talking, and this too is part of who he is. Further, it encourages the patient (and the therapist) to try to understand *why* he has difficulty talking at some times and not others, to examine when (or to whom) he talks readily and when he has difficulty.

In principle, most if not all therapists are interested in such questions. But when we think of patients as silent patients, or as patients with poor reality testing (rather than as patients whose reality testing is impaired in certain circumstances), or when we think of them as seductive, or hostile, or unassertive, or masochistic, it is easy to lose track of the variability in the patient's manifestations of those qualities and to short-circuit the search for what accounts for the variations. When, in addition, such static characterizations not only enter the therapist's thinking, but are conveyed as well to the patient by the way the therapist's comments are phrased, the possibility of exploring how the experience in question is related to ongoing life events, and even the process of change itself, is further impeded.

Taking care to communicate that the problematic pattern or behavior the therapist is focusing on is not simply what the patient "is like," and to help the patient examine it as an understandable response to some situation he finds himself in,[2] can enable the therapist to get his message across to the patient with a minimum of resistance and distortion.

In the case of Rick, for example, a central part of the work involved helping him to recognize and come to terms with his feeling that his father did not love him. There were many indications that Rick felt this and that it had had a significant impact on how he felt about himself and on other aspects of his life. But he had largely kept himself from appreciating this by blurring over the issue, talking about other topics, and focusing, when he did discuss his father, on abstruse details of the trust fund and anticipated inheritance that tied him to his father. He was, however, rather resistant to grasping this until a simple variation was introduced in how this tendency was addressed. Instead of simply saying that he became vague and unfocused when he spoke about his father, the comment was made that when he spoke about his father's feelings toward him *he didn't see things with the clarity he usually did.* This explicit acknowledgment that he was perfectly capable of being clear in other situations enabled him to acknowledge that he did blur when it came to this topic, and indeed it seemed to spark as well a curiosity about why he should function so differently when thinking about his father's feelings toward him than he did in other contexts.

BUILDING ON STRENGTHS

A different perspective on how building on variations in the patient's functioning can be helpful is provided by the following case. A behavior therapist described to me a case of his in which the patient had great difficulty being open, direct, or expressive. He wanted to make some kind of interpretive comment about it, but felt, on the basis of his knowledge of the patient, that she would take any comment along these lines as critical, and would get angry and upset and perhaps leave therapy. He felt quite pessimistic about the case.

I suggested that he address this issue by making use of the varia-

[2]It is important to be clear that by "situation" here I do not necessarily mean an "objective" situation. It may well be that the patient is responding to the situation in a highly idiosyncratic way, and that someone else would respond to it quite differently. My focus is on what the situation *means* to the person. But nonetheless, it is essential to be clear that the response does not occur in a vacuum, that the patient's experience is a function not only of his history and his character, but of the present context; and that failure to include that context in one's formulation can create an unnecessary therapeutic impasse.

tions that existed in this pattern. I recommended that he wait until a point when she was being at least a bit more open and expressive than she usually was and then comment on this openness and wonder what enabled her to feel more comfortable in expressing herself on this occasion. Such a comment addresses the same issue, but it does so in a less threatening and challenging way. It enables the patient to reflect on the question of being more open or closed without pinning the label of "closed" on her or pointing to where she is falling short.

The comment also is designed to catch her at a point where she is likely to be more receptive. When the therapist shows he is attentive to positive change in her, she may be able to hear what he is saying without becoming as defensive. Such a comment conveys hope. It indicates that she *can* be more open, and makes the examination of when or why she is sometimes (or even frequently) uncommunicative one that can be faced with greater courage and confidence. We are usually far better able to face difficult issues at moments when we feel stronger than when we are fearfully hiding. Yet that is often just when the therapist is calling attention to such matters. In the version suggested here, the therapist can address a delicate issue without hitting the patient when she is down.

Building on strengths is illustrated in a different way in the work of a student therapist whose supervision had been focusing on precisely this issue. The patient, Jill, was someone who at times could seem quite manipulative and who frequently kept her therapist on her toes. The patient had called her earlier in the week and had asked if she could have her session moved up. The therapist, after attempting to assess just how upset the patient was and whether there was a real emergency, decided that there was not, that this was just one more instance of the patient's trying to pull her out of role, to get her to do things she didn't do for her other patients. So the therapist said over the phone something like: *I know you're feeling upset, but we'll have to talk about it on Thursday.*

As Thursday approached, the therapist was feeling rather apprehensive. She was anticipating being told how cold and insensitive she was, and even hearing about some acting out on the patient's part in order to demonstrate how much she (the patient) had needed to be seen for an extra session and to make the therapist feel guilty. The patient began the session by indicating that the reason she had called was that she had been depressed and upset over some tension in her marriage. She had felt on the verge of a big fight with her husband. Then she said, "It turned out I didn't have a fight with him that night, but I did the next day."

A central problem of this patient's was her tendency to present herself, and to view herself, as totally passive and helpless in her life. The "help me" call had seemed to the therapist just one more instance of this. In her account in this session, the patient initially brushed over the fact that she didn't fight with her husband that night. That she did fight with him the next day was clearly the moral of the story for her. Her therapist, however, did not begin by inquiring about the fight. Instead, she asked, *What helped you not to fight with him on Monday night?*

Now certainly that would not always be the correct focus. Indeed, with a patient who tended to minimize difficulties and conflicts, such a course might be quite counterproductive. But Jill was anything but a minimizer. Her entire relational style (and style of experiencing herself as well) was one of focusing constantly on how things were not going well, how they were out of control. In this instance, consequently, the therapist wanted to interrupt that familiar, and maladaptive, pattern. Having discussed with me in the supervision some of the issues that are the focus of this chapter, Jill's therapist was alerted to the importance of building on the patient's strengths, and she intervened by directing attention not to Jill's later lapse but to her having been able, at least for a while, to delay and control herself.

In response to her therapist's question, Jill said that "thinking about talking to you helped." This was in a sense a transitional response. Jill did not initially attribute her capacity to delay to any thoughts that were truly her own. It was thinking about someone else with whom she was in a dependent relationship that mattered. Yet at the same time, she *was* able to recognize that she had controlled herself and that she had done so when the therapist was not there. She had in one sense borrowed from her therapist the strength to delay, but in another sense she had found it in herself. The therapist's choice about what to comment on and inquire into, and the subsequent exploration it sparked, enabled Jill to sense more clearly the capacities she had to build on. In a small but important way, it contributed to her finding and developing an alternative, and more adaptive, life strategy.

In another case, that of Anna, the patient was distraught because her lover no longer seemed interested in going to bed with her. She had taken up with the lover in part because her *husband* wasn't going to bed with her. Not surprisingly, she felt very humiliated by this turn of affairs (no pun intended).

Anna's therapist, a supervisee of mine, wanted to discuss with me how he could inquire tactfully into what Anna did that turned men off. He sensed that Anna was extremely vulnerable, and he wanted to avoid further damaging her self-esteem. My suggestion was that he not approach the question from that angle at this point. Certainly at some point understanding of what she did to turn men off would be essential. But given her present state of fragility and vulnerability, it seemed to me preferable to address the same set of issues from the standpoint of her strengths, to help create a more solid foundation for her self-esteem even while pursuing the question that was of concern. I thus suggested asking instead something such as: *Tell me, what's your sense of how you got Bob to go to bed with you in the first place?*

There was, we suspected (and later found confirmed) a pattern to these occurrences in the patient's life. There were indeed things she did, both with her husband and with her lover (and with other men in her life over the years) that were consistent and obviously important for her to understand. But finding a pattern, although important, is not enough. If it is done in a way that the patient finds demoralizing, it will be counterproductive. The therapist's aim is to look for clues to *break* the pattern and to look for those clues within the patient's current re-pertoire. By first examining how she *has* been able to achieve her aims, the therapist is in a better position to enable the patient to look at how she has failed. And, importantly, she is also in a better position to enable her to sense her *conflict*, since she can see clearly that it is not a simple matter of men not being interested in her.

NOTICING SMALL STEPS IN THE RIGHT DIRECTION

Somewhat similar considerations are illustrated in the case of Martha, a successful lawyer who encountered frequent difficulties with men, both in her professional life and socially. When therapy began, Martha attrib-uted these difficulties almost exclusively to men being unable to deal with smart and accomplished women. Her therapist, herself a smart and accomplished woman, was able to communicate her understanding of this as a real problem faced by women in our culture, but she hoped to interest Martha in examining whether there were other issues involved in her problems as well.

Early in the work, these efforts proved rather frustrating. Martha stayed on the level of ideological pronouncements about relations be-tween men and women that her therapist experienced as largely de-fensive (notwithstanding the elements of truth in her position). At sev-eral points the therapist raised with Martha whether there was any purpose in her being in therapy: if her problems really were solely a result of men's inability to tolerate strong women and had nothing to do with any personal difficulties of Martha's—even with difficulties Martha had in dealing as effectively as she might with the atitudes of the men she encountered—then what contribution could therapy make?

Martha's therapist felt that Martha's anger at men was as much a *cause* of her difficulties with them as a result of these problems. She could be quite disparaging and seemed likely to bring out the worst in the men she encountered. She had grown up in a home in which her mother was exaggeratedly "feminine" in a passive and self-derogating way. Martha's father seemed to ride roughshod over her mother, paying little attention to her needs and expecting to be waited on hand and foot. Mother seemed to Martha a model of exactly what she did not want to see happen in her own life, and Martha vowed to herself that no man would ever treat *her* that way.

The convergence between, on the one hand, Martha's personal experiences and their impact on her life, and on the other, an ideological position about male–female relations that was rooted in a number of valid observations but was being used defensively by Martha to keep her on a determined but frustrating course, presented a substantial challenge to her therapist. The difficulty was exaggerated, however, because the seemingly implacable wall of ideology led the therapist to feel that nothing she said was getting through to Martha. Through the filter of her discouragement, the therapist could hear only that side of what Martha was saying that reflected Martha's persisting commitment to the view of her life with which she had entered therapy. In order to break the impasse, I suggested that she listen carefully for any indications at all that she was getting through to Martha and that she be supportive of any slight leaning in a new direction. I added that in paying attention to where Martha had succeeded in changing her approach even a little bit, she would make it more likely that Martha would eventually be able to hear what she had to say about the patterns that had not yet changed.

The first opportunity to apply this perspective came when Martha was describing a first date with a man, Bill, to whom a friend had introduced her. Earlier in the session, Martha had made a point of saying that she anticipated he would be defensive with her, since she was a lawyer and he was "only a podiatrist" and earned less money than she did. In discussing what happened when the question came up of who should pay the bill, Martha noted that he had wanted to pay but she had said, "I earn a good living. Why shouldn't I pay my share?"

The therapist, thinking in terms of our previous discussions, said to her: "I notice you didn't say to him that you earned more than he did, only that you earned a good living. I think that's important to notice, because it's an instance of where you communicated clearly, directly, and yet without threatening him or being excessively competitive."

In this way, the therapist was able to introduce the question of Martha's way of communicating with men, including—at least implicitly—the ways she challenged and provoked them, in a manner that built upon whatever capacity she had mustered to communicate a bit more effectively.

A related example, from a later period in the same case illustrates how the perspective offered here can be applied in looking at the behavior of other people in the patient's life as well as in looking at the patient's own behavior. Martha had begun to date Bill more regularly and her therapist began to focus on a pattern that was rooted in the same set of issues addressed above: Martha could offer support to Bill when he was feeling shaky but very rarely asked for any kind of support from him. She was implacably self-reliant and self-sufficient, and there were clear indications that her unwillingness to turn to Bill in any way, to convey to him that he was important to her in the way that she had become important to him, was leading to some rethinking of the relationship on his part. Indeed, in the process of examining this, it became apparent that Martha's exaggerated independence and absence of need for others was one of the key characteristics that was generally responsible for the stormy and unsuccessful nature of her relationships with men.

When this was first raised with Martha, her response was to say repeatedly that men only wanted bubble-headed, incompetent women, and she'd be damned if she'd be like that just to please them. Her therapist attempted to point out to her the caricature nature of this perception, the overly dichotomous thinking that led her to see fierce and unyielding independence as the only alternative to being bubble-headed and incompetent (as she had perceived her mother to be). She tried to help Martha to see how this stance made it impossible for her to gratify, or even to acknowledge, her own perfectly normal and healthy needs for nurturance and caring, as it also prevented any man she was involved with to feel at all needed.

There were some indications that Martha was beginning to let herself hear these comments by the therapist, but progress was slow and halting. Not infrequently Martha would resort to comments such as "Why should I have to fuck up just to make him feel good?" and a different aspect of her tendency to caricature and falsely dichotomize had to be addressed. Greater progress was made when the therapist began, in a slight variation of what she had been doing previously, to ask Martha if there had ever been any times when she *could* turn to Bill for support. On one occasion, she began to talk about how Bill had held her and comforted her when her mother had died. Her eyes moistened when she related this, and she started to tell in considerable detail, and with real affect, how Bill had been steady and sensitive and understanding. Then, rather suddenly, she caught herself and said stiffly and harshly, "Men always like that, they like it when you're weak," and she launched into an extended diatribe that took her far away from the experience she had just been describing.

Her therapist reported in the supervision session that she had thought at first about interpreting the defensive nature of Martha's changing the subject but had decided not to because all the ways she thought of broaching the subject seemed likely just to lead to an argument or further fuel for an ideological smokescreen. Instead, thinking of the general strategy we had discussed for approaching Martha, she simply said after a time, "Let's come back to Bill's holding you and being sensitive to what you were feeling when your mother died. I'd like to hear more about that." Without rubbing Martha's nose in the fact that she had had difficulty staying with that topic, her therapist gently led her back to the experience she had warded off.

THE PATIENT'S OWN SELF-CRITICALNESS

For various reasons, certain patients will seem to go out of their way to make it difficult for the therapist to see progress in the work. Their defensive style can drive them to be relentlessly negative about themselves, and it is often not easy for the therapist to avoid getting caught up in the spiral of negativity. Particularly will this be the case for such patients when they have begun to take a genuinely useful step in the direction of change.

What can be most confusing, and even intimidating, for the therapist is when, after some real and considerable progress, the patient begins to introduce what appear to be "deeper" complaints and experiences that suggest that the previous progress was temporary and superficial. Clearly the therapist must be alert to the possibility that in fact deeper concerns *are* emerging and that attention will have to be paid to some more serious troubles than had yet become apparent. But not infrequently it is the very tendency on the patient's part to present himself as more troubled and damaged than he really is that lies at the heart of his difficulties. In such instances, the therapist's choice to follow the new material to its seemingly more pathological conclusions can lead to the unraveling of the good work done and to a confirmation of the patient's sense of himself as deeply damaged. If, on the other hand, despite the feelings of discouragement and chagrin that such a sequence of events can create in the therapist, she can manage to keep clearly in mind the previous period of significant movement, she will find not infrequently that the apparently greater depth now being reached is in fact a defensive retreat from the threat posed by the prospect of change.

For any change in a long-standing pattern of behaving and of experiencing oneself can be threatening, even if that pattern has been a source of considerable pain.

Sometimes all that is required in such instances is simply a comment pointing the patient back in the direction of her prior progress—for example, *I'm aware that a number of new and frightening feelings have emerged for you recently, but I'm still struck by how much more able you've been to say to people what you're really feeling.* Along with this, it is useful to explore as well what is frightening about the new material that is emerging, what unnamed terrors and anticipations have led the patient to retreat from the progress that had been made. But unless the therapist is careful not to let that progress itself slip out of focus—not to be seduced by the intriguing "deeper" material away from the less exciting, but often therapeutically more significant, steps by the patient to make changes in some aspect of his daily living—a more serious retrogression may follow, and the patient's self-presentation that implies that the earlier progress was superficial and temporary may become a self-fulfilling prophecy.

Weiss and Sampson (e.g., 1986) have written extensively about the patient's posing of "tests" for the therapist and the importance of the therapist passing such tests if the therapy is to be successful. From their perspective, such tests occur whether the therapist is aware of them or not, and therapists operating from therapeutic perspectives other than their "control–mastery theory" can pass the test if they successfully avoid playing into the pattern that originated in relation to the patient's parents and that has been maintained since then by the failure of others to respond differently to the patient's tests. In effect, what I have just described can be conceived of in a somewhat similar manner. From the vantage point of hindsight, on occasions when I have successfully managed to keep the focus on the patient's previous progress, it has appeared that the emergence of the new, seemingly more regressive material was in essence an implicit test of the sincerity of my interest in the patient's really living differently and that I had been presented with a crucial choice point in the work. Because such tests and such choice points are usually presented without fanfare or signal, it is unfortunately the case that often the patient has his fears confirmed (the therapist "fails" the test) without either party even being aware that such an event has occurred.

Put differently, as painful as the patient's neurotic ways of living may have been, they have nonetheless been the route to much of the safety or gratification the patient has obtained in his life (even as they have also been the reason those gratifications have been so limited). They have felt as well (and here we are close to the nub of the problem) like the only way to gain whatever degree of acceptance and warmth from others the patient has been able to wrest and like the only way of creating any sense of contact or connection, however limited or unsatisfactory such connection might be. Consequently, these neurotic ways of living—at once deadly enemies and old and familiar friends—cannot be given up lightly. From the vantage point of the neurosis, it cannot be taken for granted that the therapist will continue to maintain interest and contact with the patient once he relinquishes the neurotic ways of interacting that his skewed life experience has suggested to him are the only way such contact can be maintained.

If the therapeutic work is directed at changing fundamental aspects of the patient's way of living (if it is an intensive, or "deep" or characterological therapy), it is highly likely that such testing-by-regression will occur at one or more points in the work. If the therapist is not alert to this likelihood, there is a reasonable probability that the patient's unconscious pessimism will be "confirmed" by the therapist's interest in his less adaptive modes of functioning as well as by the therapist's apparent readiness to be deflected from the positive steps the patient has taken.

Adding a cognitive perspective to the considerations advanced thus far, Tenzer (1984) has pointed out, in a way that bears interestingly on the above discussion, parallels between the results of some of Piaget's experiments and the process of change in psychotherapy. As she notes, Piaget's subjects often went through a stage in which they were able to change their behavior to successfully master the problem they were addressing, yet they were unable to conceptualize or articulate the change that had taken place. "With remarkable obduracy, they persisted in saying they were doing one thing when in fact they were doing something else. . . . Furthermore, what could be recognized at one moment . . . was often lost at the next" (Tenzer, 1984, p. 428). In similar fashion, she suggests, changes in patients in psychotherapy often occur without the patient at first recognizing them; they may be apparent to the therapist, but not yet to the patient.

Arguing from a position derived from both psychoanalysis and Piagetian theory, Tenzer suggests that patients may actively resist noticing positive changes not just for emotional reasons but because of a basic feature of cognition—the tendency "to organize along familiar dimensions and to discount what does not fit in with prior expectations" (Tenzer, 1984). Such efforts on the part of the patient to maintain old ways of seeing things, though a potential obstacle to therapeutic change, do not in Tenzer's view carry the critical implications sometimes associated with the term resistance. Working through resistances, she suggests, is for all people "an integral part of acquiring knowledge. In this sense, resistance no longer can be used as a term of opprobrium with which to label a recalcitrant patient. It is, rather, a way of maintaining continuity in a world that is subject to constant change" (Tenzer, 1984, p. 422).

Without such a cognitive gyroscope providing direction to our adaptive efforts, we would be in constant danger of being drawn off course by each new stimulus. But there can be a price to pay for this otherwise adaptive conservatism in our vision of the world. The patient's old patterns of behavior, and old ways of perceiving those patterns, feel like reality itself, and even if they have been unsatisfactory, they are not easily relinquished. As Tenzer puts it,

> The fleeting, ephemeral nature of some "insights" in analysis can be attributed in part to resistance to "seeing" whatever does not conform to prior ways of "looking." A new image or impression, a different Gestalt, is likely to vanish unless it is consolidated and repeated attempts are made to "re-view" it, preferably within different contexts or configurations . . . . If contradictions and inconsistencies are to be useful as vehicles of working through toward insight and change, then they must be *noticed*. (Tenzer, 1984, pp. 430–431)

How the therapist might faciliate that process of noticing, in order to assure that changes that have occurred in the patient do not begin to evaporate, is interestingly hinted at by Tenzer in her descriptions of the interaction between subject and experimenter in the Piagetian experiment:

> One moment the child could "see"; the next moment the seeming insight was lost. Pseudo-necessity, what cannot be, over-rode contradictory perceptual and proprioceptive evidence. In the meantime, it was as though a light were flickering on and off outside the subject's control, yet sometimes tantalizingly within his grasp. . . . They were gradually accommodating to the contradictory evidence. *However, it took a concerted collaborative effort—on the part of child and experimenter—for the child to seize hold of these elusive moments of awareness of cognitive gaps and hold on to them.* (Tenzer, 1984, p. 432; italics added)

The therapist too must collaborate actively to help the patient hold on to the elusive changes emerging in the therapeutic work and to help the patient notice and affirm them. The "pseudo-necessity" to which Tenzer refers, the rigidly held conviction that the world (or the self) is a certain way, channeling and organizing perception in a way that prevents the individual from noticing that it is different, must be actively confronted as a countertherapeutic force. Steps in the right direction must be underlined if they are not to be erased.

SEARCHING FOR THE FEELING

One of the situations in which finding and building on whatever assets the patient has is most challenging—but also most important—occurs when the patient claims not to be feeling anything at all. One is confronted with such a state of affairs most often with obsessional and schizoid patients, and not infrequently the patient's report of no feelings is conveyed with a tone of considerable discouragement and even despair.[3]

An approach to this situation that I have found useful is to say to the patient something like *I think that you have some idea of what you should be feeling, and because you're not feeling that, you register it as not feeling anything.*

Then, depending on the exact nature of the case (that is, depending on just what I did think the patient was experiencing), I might say something like: *Indifference is a feeling too. It's not that you're not feeling anything. You're feeling indifference. In fact, you're feeling a great deal of indifference.*

Several patients have reported that this emphasis on there being something that they are feeling (albeit not what they think they are supposed to be feeling) has enabled them to avoid the discouragement and the battles that had occurred in previous therapies, where they felt the therapist was criticizing them for holding back or that he was telling them that they were less than human. (One patient said he felt "like a reptile, cold-blooded and scaly," when his former therapist kept hammering away at how he ran from his feelings. "I didn't know what to do, how to satisfy him. I just kept feeling more and more inadequate, unworthy, inhuman.")

In one instance, a patient reported that his father died, and said he had no feelings. He felt we should talk about his father's death, but didn't know how to because he didn't feel anything about him. From clues in the session and from what I already knew about him, I suggested that it wasn't true that he didn't have feelings about the death. He just wasn't feeling *grief* at the moment. Instead, he was feeling a sense of relief at his father's being gone and a defiant feeling of "I don't care." The patient broke into a nervous laugh and said, "Yes, that's right! But is that a feeling?" He began to reflect that maybe he wasn't "good," but he was a "real person" after all. A variety of meaningful and affect-laden associations began to occur to him and, interestingly, later

---

[3]The apparent contradiction between the claim of "no feelings" and the evident affect that a despairing state implies will be addressed shortly. It is indeed at the heart of how to approach this situation.

in the session he did directly experience feelings of grief and loss. It seems likely to me that had I focused on his defensive pattern of warding off feelings (however "accurate" my interpretations), he would have had considerably more difficulty getting in touch with the range of feelings that the death stirred in him.[4]

An interesting variation on this theme came up with a patient who was frequently silent. At one point, he said, "I just don't have anything to say. I'm afraid whatever I say will be boring." The response to this comment by the patient was: *You know, actually what you're saying* right now *(about fearing being boring) is the furthest thing from boring. You're sharing with me what you're feeling right at the moment.* Here again, the therapist's finding the kernel of something real and valuable in what the patient experiences as just another indication of his worthlessness contributes to reversing the neurotic circle in which the patient is caught. In essence, the patient is helped to see that by *addressing* his feeling of being boring he is actually transcending it. The therapist's readiness to find and to encourage the step that the patient has taken sows the seed for further change.

ATTENDING TO POSITIVE MOVEMENT AND NOT JUST DEFENSIVENESS

One place where countertherapeutic focus on the negative—on the weak, the resistant, the defensive and avoidant side of the patient's personality—can potentially arise is in the carrying out of the frequently cited clinical rule of thumb that defenses should be interpreted before the impulse they are defending against (e.g., Fenichel, 1941). There is much in this recommendation that makes great sense. But as it is frequently applied, it can end up impeding the patient's progress toward health and greater self-esteem and can even impede the deeper understanding of conflict it was designed to promote.

In its historical context, the focus directed to resistance by Fenichel,

---

[4]Contrast the way of responding to the patient described here to that described by Liebowitz, Stone, and Turkat (1986): "With the compulsive we adapt in an opposite way, often expressing in a rather dramatic way ('You mean to say your father died last Saturday, and you didn't even mention it till now!') what the patient may characteristically report in a perfunctory and affectless manner." Although there may be circumstances in which such an approach might be called for, by and large it seems to me both cruel and counterproductive.

Reich, and other analysts of that era was a significant advance. It introduced into psychoanalytic practice a more complex understanding of the personality and pointed toward both a more effective and a more humane treatment. It signified, moreover, an appreciation that merely "knowing about" an unconscious wish or fantasy is insufficient to enable the patient to change. If the patient's defensive efforts are not addressed, if the persisting style of perceiving and thinking that has previously kept certain thoughts out of awareness or out of genuinely lived experience is not modified, then any change will be very temporary. The patient will acknowledge the therapist's interpretation only to have forgotten it by the next session or equally inimical to clinical progress, he will recall it in such a way that the affect or the further implications for his life will be surgically excised.

"Interpreting the defense first" is a strategy designed to prevent this undermining of the clinical process. The aim of interpreting a defense is not just to make the patient aware of the defense; it is, through such awareness, to *disrupt* the defense's operation, to interrupt its automatic and ego-syntonic mode of action. Only if a path is thus cleared for the assimilation of the thought or inclination being defended against is an interpretation of that thought likely to be of value to the patient.

In working, for example, with patients characterized by strong obsessional defenses, interpretations of warded off experiences are likely to have little clinical value until one has first worked on how the patient makes *any* interpretation simply an idea, to be considered logically and intellectually, but not really experienced as truly his. Such a patient's careful, measured manner, his excruciatingly balanced examinations of anything and everything, even, for some patients, the persistent tendency to accompany any acknowledgment of the interpretation with words such as "perhaps" or "possibly," can deadeningly hedge or temper the patient's experience of what is being examined. These characterological operations need to be addressed in their own right if the patient is to profit from interpretations directed toward the inclinations or experiences they are keeping from fully experienced awareness.

But as useful as this perspective on defenses is, it needs to be complemented by a concern with acknowledging and recognizing the patient's strengths and especially with acknowledging the patient's movement in a therapeutic direction. Not infrequently, even when the patient is evidencing considerable defensiveness, we may also note that he is manifesting considerably *less* defensiveness than was evident previously. If this progress is not acknowledged, the effect of focusing on the defense can be not to open up the possibility for effective assimilation of the warded off material, but rather a counterproductive discouragement of the patient.

No one leaps from defensiveness to openness in one fell swoop. The gap is too wide. Consequently, even as the patient is taking important steps in the right direction, it will be possible for the perceptive clinician to see ways in which this movement is being denied, blurred, or limited by intellectualizing. If the clinical maxim that the defense should be interpreted first is applied too strictly or mechanically, the therapist is likely to focus rather exclusively on how the patient is continuing to ward off the impact of what he is discovering, even as the discovery process itself is proceeding. Perhaps, for example, the therapist will point out that the patient's tone of voice did not seem consonant with the feeling he was expressing; or that whereas he acknowledged being hurt by something his wife said, he said he was "sort of" hurt; or that his saying he was "less than pleased" at what his best friend did was a way of reducing the impact of beginning to notice he was angry. As far as it goes, this might well be correct and perceptive. Yet not infrequently it will also be the wrong thing to say.

One useful criterion for evaluating where to place one's interpretive emphasis is a directional or vector approach to change. From this perspective, one asks oneself what the basic direction is in which the patient is moving, both in the overall thrust of the therapeutic work and in the recent events one is addressing. It is one thing to comment on the patient's hedging when it is a persistent obstacle to the work or when it seems to be an instance of backsliding that it might be useful to call attention to before it becomes a trend. If the patient had been talking more openly and genuinely about difficult matters and then began to manifest the defensive operations that had significantly impeded the work earlier, an interpretation of this might well be in order.[5]

It is quite another matter, however, to direct one's comments to the patient's hedging when, despite its persistence, the trend has clearly been toward greater expressiveness and a *reduction* in the defensiveness. This might be the case, for example, when a very vulnerable patient,

[5]Even here, it is important not to be nit-picking or relentless. One should certainly not pick up on every instance of retreat but only on those in which there is reason to think there is either a danger of substantial erasure of the progress that had begun to be evident or the initiation of a trend that may be problematic for the therapy. And when one does comment on the reappearance of defensive hedging, it can be useful to note explicitly that this occurrence contrasts with the overall thrust of the patient's participation in the therapy. See Chapters 8 and 9 for an elaboration of this latter point.

who has relied a good deal on bluff and bravado, begins to acknowledge some fearfulness or anxiety but does so by referring to himself as "a bit concerned," or when a patient who has persistently obscured for himself his impact on other people "sort of sees" how his wife might have experienced what he said as critical. To comment on the manifestations of defense in these instances can be very counterproductive. For many patients, such interpretations can be experienced as a message that their efforts to move beyond their longstanding defensive way of communicating are not appreciated, that the struggle to be more open and expressive has failed, even that the restrictions and inhibitions that have limited their lives are simply too strong to overcome. Rather than promoting the goals of the therapy, the comment induces discouragement or even self-laceration.

An example initially described in *Psychoanalysis and Behavior Therapy* further illustrates the point being made here. A supervisee had been working with a teenage patient who was quite unable to acknowledge that she played any role in what happened to her and who tended to maintain a very passive stance toward the events of her life. This tendency, as well as a rather self-pitying attitude that accompanied it, made it difficult for her to have much success with boys. In the session of interest here, however, the patient reported that boys had been nicer to her recently. From a variety of indications, it was clear to the therapist that this changed behavior on the part of the boys was a response to some changes that the patient had made in how she acted with them. In her characteristic fashion, however, the patient described the changes in the boys' attitudes as if she had had nothing to do with bringing them about.

The therapist was alert to this dimension of the patient's character and, focusing on the patient's continuing defensive hedging of her responsibility, even for something good, said to the patient, "You say it as if you had nothing to do with it." The patient in reponse said "It doesn't matter what I do, you don't think it's good enough." This was a quite characteristic response by the patient, but nonetheless it suggested that the therapist's comment had been counterproductive.

In discussing the comment with my supervisee, I suggested that she could have conveyed her point to the patient in a way that built upon and encouraged the step that the patient had taken by saying for example: *Well, I guess you must have been doing something right to get that response from the boys.* That comment, like the one the therapist did make, focuses on the question of whether she was actually *doing* something. But it does so in a way that highlights the steps the patient has taken rather than the defensiveness that hedges it in.

Another case that illustrates a somewhat similar point was seen by me some years ago. The patient was a very self-deprecating woman who had great difficulty in accepting praise or stating openly that she had done anything well. One day she described being in a car that broke down on a deserted highway, and, because she had recently read a book on auto repairs for women, she knew what the trouble was. She clearly enjoyed this experience of competence and enjoyed as well both demonstrating it to her companion in the car and telling it to me in the session. This display of competence and of taking pleasure in it was rather new for her and of considerable therapeutic import.

Consistent with her general defensive tendencies, and her anxiety about open displays of pleasure or proficiency, the patient made a point, after telling me the story, of adding that the thing that was wrong was the only thing she knew about cars, that she had not really learned anything else from the book and was basically rather ignorant.

I was in no position to evaluate how true that self-evaluation might have been, but in its timing and context it seemed clearly to be an anxiety-provoked, almost automatic effort to retreat, at least momentarily, to her earlier mode of experiencing and presenting herself. Had I followed strictly the rule of first interpreting the defense, I would have commented on her taking back or hedging her expression of pride and achievement before making any comment about that feeling itself. And at certain points in the work (consistent with the guidelines offered above) that is likely what I would have done. In this instance, however, it seemed much more important to affirm a beginning movement in a therapeutic direction. To call attention instead to where it fell short risked driving the still emerging tendency back underground, leaving the patient feeling once more a failure. Indeed, in this particular case, such an interpretation would have colluded in a particularly ironic way with the defense: my commenting on her being defensive would have paralleled her own commenting on how little she really knew. In both instances the message would have been that even if it looked like she had accomplished something, the more basic truth was that really she fell short.

I therefore did not comment at that point about her hedging and instead simply said that I could see she took pleasure in her competence on this occasion and was glad to see that she was now allowing herself this pleasure. My comment on her pleasure was itself an interpretation, since she had not been fully explicit about enjoying this. But it was an interpretation directed toward the emerging trend rather than toward the defense that attempted to constrain that trend. Either focus could have yielded a comment that was in some sense accurate. The choice was made on the basis of which of two accurate, but partial, descriptions were judged more likely to facilitate therapeutic progress.[6]

With another patient, Elizabeth, I did draw explicit attention to her defensively disparaging the progress she had made, but I did so in a way that was specifically formulated to affirm the change she had made and to avoid colluding in her self-disparagement. Elizabeth was a writer whose productivity had been severely limited by strong self-critical tendencies that inhibited her from completing or submitting what she had written. On one occasion, she did manage to complete a piece, and, after first predicting that no one would like it, she received quite a bit of praise for her work. In her characteristic fashion, she then averred that the people who had praised it didn't really know how to judge, that their standards were too low, and on and on.

I wanted to call Elizabeth's attention to how she undid and undermined her progress but was concerned not to fall into the trap I have been discussing above. I therefore decided to call Elizabeth's attention to her defensiveness in the following way. I said to her: *Do you think there's any part of your reaction that is a residue of your old tendency not to give yourself credit?*

In this way, I was able to alert her to how she was undermining her experience, but in a way that did not further contribute to that undermining by seeing only what she was doing wrong. By describing her defensive attitude as a "residue," the comment acknowledged that she has changed and that her general direction was *away* from the old defensive pattern. Calling attention to maladaptive behavior in this particular way can be helpful as a way of at once alerting the patient to problematic tendencies and helping her to maintain her confidence and sense of movement.

It is, of course, essential that such a description have some truth to it, or it will ring hollow and be experienced as evidence that the therapist really is not in touch with the patient's experience. If no change has been apparent, it will be counterproductive to pretend that it has. But

---

[6]With some patients who belittle themselves and present themselves as incompetent, what has proved useful is simply the straightforward strategy of inquiring, whenever they act more competently than usual: *Something enabled you to be more competent there. What made it possible?* By focusing on what made it possible in those instances, a less defense-strewn path is created toward exploring what gets in the way on other occasions and what keeps the patient so often in the stance of the incompetent one. (In further exploring such an issue, Karen Horney's [1945] concept of the "moving-toward" neurotic trend, and the conceptions of anxiety and conflict associated with it, often prove helpful.)

very often—especially after the therapy has proceeded for a while—it is possible to formulate comments of the sort just described that do have some resonance. When this is the case, such comments have the further virtue of suggesting a general direction or pattern to the patient's life—one of movement toward openness and away from defensiveness. Suggestion has been a much misunderstood feature of the psychotherapeutic process, and its potential role in facilitating change has been greatly underestimated. Further discussion of the role of suggestion, and a closer examination of why it is disdained by many therapists and of when and how this disdain can be ill founded, will be found in Chapter 9.

The Interweaving of Content and Defense Interpretations

The above remarks should not be taken as suggesting one should never interpret a defense or call the patient's attention to evasions that keep him from achieving self-understanding. Rather, my point is that it is essential to keep in mind the basic direction of the patient's activities, to consider whether what one is observing (however minimal or hedged it might be) is essentially a move forward into greater acceptance by the patient of her genuine experience or is rather a retreat from whatever degree of insight or expanded self-acceptance had previously been attained. The basic thrust of the patient's communication or mode of expression cannot be understood adequately in cross section alone. Whatever mixture of productive self-exploration and fearful evasion is evident at any moment, it must be understood as part of a continually changing series of mental states in which the degree of defensiveness or expressiveness will vary depending on a host of influences. Effective clinical response to what the patient is saying requires that the direction of change be taken into account, that the complex product of competing inclinations evident at any moment be understood in relation to what has come before and to whether it represents an increase or a decrease in the patient's tendency to give voice to conflicted feelings and wishes.

It is likely that in the early stages of exploring any particular issue, the operation of the patient's defenses will play a predominant role in her experience of herself and others. At that stage the therapist's comments can fruitfully be directed toward calling the patient's attention to this dimension. If these efforts by the therapist are successful, however, there will be a shift in the balance between defensiveness and expressiveness, and it is important for the therapist's efforts to reflect that shift and to acknowledge, implicitly or explicitly, the progress the patient has made. If, for example, the patient had been denying how hurt she felt at her son's failures to call on Mother's Day or her birthday, and now she was acknowledging the hurt a bit but still hedging it with comments such as "But on the other hand, he has a right to independence" or "But I can understand—actually I'm kind of busy myself," the therapist, rather than commenting on the hedging, would be more likely to say something like *I'm getting a sense today of the hurt you feel when he doesn't call. It's not easy to talk about that, and I'm pleased you've found a way to get to it.*

Usually, the course of the work will be characterized by a continuing back and forth. At certain points the patient will clearly be moving forward; at others a resurgence of anxiety may lead her to retreat to a defensive position previously overcome, or to cling to a compromise that earlier represented hard-won new ground but now reflects a certain stasis in the work.[7] If such stasis persists for a while, the therapist can return temporarily to the focus, more prevalent earlier in the therapy, on interpreting the defenses that are impeding the patient's reappropriation of crucial parts of her own experience. The aim is to help the patient regain momentum toward overcoming her anxieties and self-imposed restrictions. Once she has again begun to move forward, the therapist can return the focus of the work to interpreting, acknowledging, and encouraging the steps toward fuller self-expression and self-understanding that the patient has taken. Her attention will shift to the new material emerging or to the fact of change itself.

Defense interpretations never entirely disappear from the therapeutic work, though the relative emphasis is likely to change. Even in the late stages of the work there will continue to be times when the primary vector is one of retreat, when old fears and modes of self-protection gain the upper hand. Although the balance between defense interpretations and interpretations of the feelings and inclinations the defense is designed to ward off is likely to shift as the therapeutic work proceeds, the two sides of the interpretive process must always be kept in mind. The decision as to when to interpret "content" and when to interpret the defense will largely depend on whether in the recent work the patient has been moving toward fuller expression of conflicted inclinations, has been resting on a plateau with little forward movement,

---

[7]There are many reasons why the patient might stand back or retreat. One of the most important to appreciate is that considerable research has demonstrated that after anxiety is diminished there is usually a "spontaneous recovery" in the level of anxiety when the individual is exposed to the frightening situation at a later time. This will temporarily alter the balance between expressive and defensive inclinations, yielding a compromise formation similar to the therapeutic material seen earlier in the work. If the therapist handles this occurrence properly, its effects will be only transient, but if the phenomenon is not properly understood, more serious arrest of therapeutic progress can ensue. For a fuller discussion of the therapeutic implications of this and related phenomena, see Dollard & Miller, 1950; Wachtel, 1977, Chap. 6; Wachtel, 1987, Chap. 5.

or has pulled back from a degree of openness and clarity that had been attained at an earlier point.

In practice, it is often not possible to distinguish very sharply between defense interpretations and interpretations of content. Not only do the two interweave considerably throughout the course of the therapeutic work, but even the very same comment can often be viewed from both vantage points. Greenson, in an important exploration of this dimension of psychoanalytic technique, states that "We analyze resistance before content or ego before id so that when we interpret the warded-off content to the patient, he will deal with it more appropriately and not merely repeat his past neurotic patterns" (Greenson, 1967, p. 138). But he then goes on to add,

> The rule that we analyze resistance before content must *not* be understood to mean that we analyze the resistance alone or approach it first and that we avoid the content completely until the resistance is resolved. Actually, there is not always a sharp dichotomy between resistance and content. . . . [R]esistance [can become] the content and then a given content comes to be used as a resistance. (p. 143; italics in original)[8]

Greenson also notes that it is inappropriate for the analyst to call attention to each and every resistance or manifestation of defensiveness. When the resistance is small or seems temporary, he recommends simply waiting for the patient to move ahead or, if the patient is silent or hesitant, helping out with a simple prompt ("Yes?" "What were you saying?") to help the patient get started again. The pursuit of every small resistance, he adds, "turns the analyst into a nag and the analysis into a harassment. Part of the tact of doing analytic work is knowing how to discriminate between resistances requiring analysis and those which do not" (Greenson, 1967, p. 147).

The tact shown by the skilled therapist or analyst is evident as well in precisely how the interpretation is offered, as I have argued throughout this book. In illustrating concretely the application of the principle of interpreting resistance first, Greenson implicitly illustrates as well a number of the other considerations that have been of concern to us thus far. The patient had related a dream to him with rather provocative sexual content but in a manner Greenson viewed as stilted and defen-

---

[8]In this latter point, Greenson is actually building on an idea first introduced by Wilhelm Reich (1949). As Reich pointed out, resistance can often take the form of presenting enticing content that is seductive to the analyst but has little real impact on the patient or the therapeutic process. Apfelbaum and Gill (1989) suggest that what is "content" and what is "defense" is not a matter of a fixed structure, dam, or armor, but rather a matter of what, at any given moment, is more ego syntonic.

sive. Greenson felt "it would be pointless to proceed to the warded-off content until I had first analyzed and partially worked through some of the patient's resistances." He therefore said to the patient, "You seem to be embarrassed today when you try to tell me about your sexual experiences. Even your language seems stilted" (Greenson, 1967, p. 139).

In some ways, this comment seems like one that could be experienced by the patient as critical. In order fully to evaluate it we would need to know the tone in which it was said, the nature of the relationship Greenson had already established with the patient, and (apropos the preceding discussion) to what degree the patient's report of the dream represented a step in the direction of more open expression or a retreat to greater defensiveness. Two aspects of the way Greenson worded the comment, however, are worth noting. To begin with, he refers to the patient's being embarrassed *today*, and he states quite explicitly that he did so "because there were occasions when he was able to be more direct about sexual matters and in this way I am reminding him of that" (Greenson, 1967). Thus, Greenson is here attending to considerations of variability in the patient's functioning similar to those discussed earlier in this chapter.

Secondly, and less explicitly noted by Greenson, the comment calls attention to the patient's feeling *embarrassed* rather than stating that he was being *defensive* or *resistant*, or that he was *avoiding* or *hiding* anything. Consistent with the considerations advanced thus far, we may see that such a way of putting it is both more respectful and more likely to be experienced by the patient as an empathic appreciation of how he is feeling.

We may further note that the two sentences of Greenson's comment have somewhat different slants. The second sentence ("Even your language seems stilted") is more likely to feel critical (and indeed, the patient's first response to it is defensive: "Well, there is no use in being crude. . . . I don't know what kind of language to use here") Perhaps a better version of the second sentence—given that the patient is sometimes able to be more direct about sexual matters—might have been: *Your language seems* uncharacteristically *stilted*. That not only presents the patient in a more positive light; it also is likely to arouse his curiosity: Why is it that he is behaving uncharacteristically in this instance?[9]

In this chapter I have stressed the importance of attending to the patient's strengths. The temptations our field presents to pathologize and to assume that the sicker the patient appears the more profound

---

[9]If this latter way of putting it seemed to Greenson implicitly to overstate the patient's ease on other occasions, he could have at least said something like: *Your language seems more stilted here than it usually is. I wonder what that's about.*

and acute must be the therapist's perception create a need for continuing reminders on this score. Clearly, however, the patient has come to us because there is something wrong in his life, and it does him no good to wrap him in a warm blanket of good will and reassurance that does not address the patterns of living that cause him trouble. An essential task for the therapist is to meet the challenge of attending at once to the twin poles of affirmation of what is good and strong in the patient and promotion of the changes required if those strengths are to be fully realized. It is to this topic that we now turn.

CHAPTER 8

Affirmation and Change

One of the central challenges facing the psychotherapist is to reconcile the conflicting poles of affirmation and change. On the one hand, the therapist must be able to empathize with her patient, to see the world through the patient's eyes and understand and appreciate his perspective. She must grasp the sense in which the way of life the patient has chosen felt necessary and must comprehend its validity. At the same time, she needs to keep clearly in mind that she is an agent of change, that the patient has come to her because something is *wrong*. She must not become so appreciative of the patient's way of seeing things that she cannot help him to reflect on it and transcend it. Navigating these tricky cross-currents is a far from easy task.

The seeming tensions between these two perspectives can at times lead therapists to bury the contradictions and identify almost completely with one or the other pole of the process. Some therapists, for example, attempt to steer the entire course of the therapy hewing strictly to the standpoint of empathy. Their assumption is that if one attends fully and wholeheartedly to the patient's point of view and the patient's experience, whatever change is needed will follow almost automatically.

Such empathic immersion in the patient's experience is, I believe, indeed a crucial requirement for therapeutic progess. People need to feel understood and appreciated for who they really are before they are ready to relinquish patterns of thought and relationship which, however problematic, have been the basis of whatever security they have been able to achieve in this world. But as important as empathic immersion is, it is not sufficient. The view that once true understanding is achieved, everything else takes care of itself oversimplifies and short-circuits the therapeutic process.

The fears that underlie neurosis are so potent, and the self-deceptions and rationalizations they breed so easy to mistake for reality, that without the therapist acting in certain respects as an agent for an alternative point of view, without her challenges—usually gentle, but necessarily persistent—to the patient's familiar, if not always comfortable, assumptions, change will at best be slow and precarious and may well be deterred altogether.

Moreover, the choices people make in the course of their lives are consequential. We deal as therapists not just with the illusions of the past, or even just with the illusions of the present, but with the accumulated *consequences* of those illusions, with the added burden that a life structure built on a foundation of skewed experiences and exaggerated fears places on the patient's ability to see any other way. Unless the therapist is willing to help the patient overcome those burdens, to help him initiate new patterns in the face of a lifetime of reasons for not doing so, the therapy faces a difficult uphill struggle.

But although an active, and at times even challenging, complement to empathic appreciation is usually essential, equally essential is the maintenance throughout of an empathic bond. Some therapists avoid the tensions between empathic immersion in the patient's point of view and the task of working to change that point of view in important respects by defining their role almost exclusively in terms of being change agents. Attention to the subtleties of the patient's experience gets short shrift, and therapy becomes a technology, a melange of techniques or, even worse, an arena for manipulation.

Most of us, however, whatever our orientations, struggle to reconcile the two poles of the therapeutic process. Sometimes we may lean a bit too much one way, sometimes too much the other, but throughout we attempt, whether implicitly or with full awareness, to steer a course that is not too reductive in either direction. My focus in this chapter is on this necessary tension in the work of the psychotherapist and on how the ways we communicate to patients, the kinds of things we say, can aid in or obstruct the reconciliation of those tensions in a therapeutically useful way.

A DIALECTICAL APPROACH TO THE PROBLEM

Marsha Linehan (e.g., Linehan, 1987; Linehan & Wagner, 1990) has placed particular emphasis on the dynamic tension between affirmation and promoting change and has conceptualized its resolution as requiring a dialectical approach. As she puts it, "a fundamental dialectic in any psychotherapy . . . is that change can only occur in the context of acceptance of reality as it is. And acceptance is fundamentally linked to the possiblity of change" (Linehan & Wagner, 1990, p. 10).

Linehan's work has been particularly focused on patients diagnosed as borderline personality disorder, a population that presents special problems to the therapist. These severely ill, and often dangerously suicidal, patients can place great stress upon the therapist, and it is not uncommon for therapists working with them to experience considerable resentment or temptation to withdraw. Linehan notes that the research literature suggests that borderline patients whose therapists like them tend to do better in treatment, and an important subsidiary aim of her treatment approach is to "create a theory that will enhance therapists' compassion and liking for their borderline clients." (Linehan & Wagner, 1990, p. 10)

In approaching this goal, she centers on two observations: (1) that the therapist cannot like or feel for the patient, and certainly cannot convey such feelings to the patient in a therapeutically effective way, unless she is able to accept the patient as he is; and (2) that the therapist cannot like and accept the patient as he is unless she can see some prospect for change. The patient's present way of life is too chaotic, demanding, and destructive for such acceptance to be sincere without it pointing simultaneously toward change.

Further exacerbating the dilemmas that therapists of such patients face, according to Linehan, is that central to the origins of these patients' difficulties is the repeated experience of invalidation. Significant others in the patient's life have, for their own reasons, been unable to tolerate any negative affective experiences on the part of the patient and have dismissed or trivialized those experiences. They have, as a consequence, also deprived the patient of the opportunity to learn to cope with those experiences. The patient grows up unable to label, control, or trust his emotional reactions. Only extreme displays of emotion seem to get any response, but these extreme displays also further his invalidation. Others recoil or feel blackmailed, and the patient himself feels humiliated, damaged, and tempted once again to block all experiences of negative affect until they once again explode in an outburst or crisis.

The therapist's task, from this perspective, is to help the patient to accept and learn to cope with distressing emotional experiences. But in teaching the patient effective means of dealing with such feelings, the therapist must take care not to convey that what she is trying to do is to make the feelings "go away." That, of course, would simply replicate the pathogenic conditions that got the patient into his dilemma in the first place. Thus, the "dialectic" in this approach is that genuine change can only be brought about through real acceptance of the patient's experience of helplessness and rage, yet that acceptance is likely to be impossible for the therapist if she is so immersed in the patient's experience that she too sees no way out. Only by being able to ride both horses—acceptance and change—at the same time is the therapist able to bring the journey to a successful conclusion.

THE CENTRALITY OF CONFLICT

Linehan's work with borderline patients originally was undertaken from a primarily behavioral perspective, but it turned out to converge in interesting ways with psychodynamic approaches to borderline disorders (Swenson, 1989). Linehan views a dialectical perspective as important not just in working with borderline patients but in all clinical work. Indeed, the approach to the problem of affirmation and change discussed in this chapter, which is largely guided by a broadly conceived psychodynamic point of view, might also be described as dialectical. From the present point of view, a central element in effectively reconciling the stance of empathic resonance and the role of agent of change is attending to the dimension of conflict in the patient's experience. In attempting to embrace the way the patient sees the world now, and at the same time help him to see it otherwise, a key is simultaneously to empathize with his wish for change. That wish, after all, is what has brought him to a therapist's office, and it is as real and valid a part of his experiential world as any other dimension the therapist may address.

It is the almost universal presence of a wish to change, alongside the wish to somehow keep on going just as one has, that gives poignancy to the phenomenon of resistance and that makes it possible to attend to it without abandoning a commitment to empathic appreciation of the patient's experience of the world. It is because the patient is in *conflict* that he at once enlists your aid in changing his life and acts to impede that change. If one keeps the conflict in mind, it is often possible to find an opening wedge into change through the very process of empathizing.

Recognizing the patient's simultaneous wish for change alters the attitude with which one looks at those aspects of his stance in life that can be seen as regressive, maladaptive, or embodying retreat. Behavior which, from one perspective, can be seen as an instance of resistance, can from another be recognized simply as a sign of conflict. The patient is not intransigent, stubborn, or uncooperative; he is afraid, uncertain, and torn between competing visions and inclinations.

When the patient is viewed in this way, it is much easier to see the world through his eyes even as one is committed to helping him *change* how he sees the world. Though it is often true, as some therapists are fond of saying, that there is a sense in which the patient wants to *get better* without really *changing*—that is, without modifying the neurotic assumptions that underlie his life, without giving up the defensive operations that buy him short-term comfort at the cost of long-term adaptation—it is also true that the patient *does* want to get better. The crucial therapeutic task is to help him see how his troubles stem from *competing* wishes and how significant changes in his outlook are already rooted in his present way of experiencing things.

Appreciating the dimension of conflict can enable the therapist to push into forbidden territory while addressing quite sympathetically the organization of experience that makes such a push necessary (that is, that is responsible for the territory *being* forbidden in the first place). Consider, for example, working with a patient who has trouble acknowledging strong anger toward a parent. The therapist's effort to focus on either the anger or the denial of it runs up against considerable resistance, and the experience is one of grinding one's gears, of pushing against rough sand. If instead the therapist says something like, *It's a real bind to be in such a rage toward someone you also love,* she is much more likely to be effective and to be heard. Having experienced attentiveness to both sides of his conflict in this way, the patient can more readily accept the anger and acknowledge it both to himself and to the therapist.

The principle of focusing on conflict in order to address the twin poles of affirmation and challenge was central in the case of Walter. Walter was a very argumentative man who continually chided his therapist for not going deeply enough, but launched into elaborate intellectual arguments or changed the subject whenever the therapist tried to address aspects of his experiences that were not fully manifest. Walter's therapist, when he addressed this issue, tended to say things like: *You say you want to go more deeply, but when I try to do it with you, you don't want to.*

In supervision, I suggested he try instead the following alternative the next time the opportunity came up: *You want to go deeper into your experiences, but it's frightening; so you hesitate and change the subject even though you also want to stay with it.* Such a way of putting it highlights the patient's anxiety and conflict rather than simply his resistance. It acknowledges that the patient's desire to go deeper is also real, and it sides with the patient in a way that the early version tried by Walter's therapist did not.

In the course of generating this alternative, we discussed as well a number of other possible phrasings that also, by highlighting the conflict, would enable the therapist to confront the evasion while sympathetically aligning herself on the side of the patient's experience; for example: *You want to change and yet at the same time you find yourself doing things that make it very difficult to change.* This comment acknowledges and affirms the reality of the patient's wish to change at the same time as it points to his doing things that interfere. As in some of the examples in earlier chapters, the phrase *you find yourself* serves as a means, with this difficult and vulnerable patient, of easing him into an examination of his countertherapeutic behaviors without requiring him to take too much responsibility for them at first.[1]

Another variant went a bit further in extending sympathetic appreciation while calling attention to the problematic pattern: *It must be frustrating for you. You say you want to go deeper, and I can tell that you do; and yet you keep changing the subject or getting very abstract. What do you make of that?*

The effort to combine affirmation and the push for change via the medium of attending to the patient's conflict is illustrated in a different way in the following example. The patient, José, was a late adolescent of Puerto Rican extraction, who had seemed until recently to be on the fast track out of the Barrio. His parents were very ambitious for him and had managed to get him into a prestigious private school on a scholarship. José was very bright and had been doing quite well in the school, more than holding his own with his better-prepared, upper-middle-class peers. When it came time to apply to colleges, however, it turned out that José had so thoroughly alienated and worried his teachers that despite good grades and a desire on the part of the colleges to recruit talented minority students, he did not get into any of the colleges he had applied to. The teachers' letters of reference conveyed a picture of a troubled, rebellious, alienated young man who would be a considerable risk for any college admissions committee to accept.

José struck his therapist not as rebellious but as depressed, frightened, and torn by conflict. Indeed, in many respects his difficulties stemmed not from a rebellious nature but from being excessively obedient. José's parents, who had had to scrape by on menial, low-paying jobs, were very ambitious for their son but not really very trusting of his capacity to think for himself or to make his own choices. They recognized his intelligence but were so suspicious of the outside world that they viewed him as dangerously naive and, essentially, in need of micromanagement of his life by them.

---

[1]Such diminishing of the patient's responsibility might, on first blush, seem to clash radically with Schafer's (1976) emphasis on "action language." Schafer, however, focuses his discussion primarily on the language of theoretical discourse rather than the language used to speak to the patient. He does stress the importance of the patient taking responsibility for disavowed intentions and actions, but he recognizes that the clinical application of this principle must be flexible and attuned to what the patient is capable of assimilating at any given point. What is crucial in phrasings such as "yet you find yourself" is that when employed properly, as part of a sequential strategy of interpretation, their value lies in their utility in furthering the very aim of helping the patient take greater responsibility for his own actions and inclinations.

Their suspicion and hostility toward the outside world were in one sense well-grounded. They themselves were individuals who had suffered considerably from discrimination and found themselves in a station in life quite incommensurate with their own talents. But their negativity was also paralyzing and damaging to José in several ways.

First, the degree to which they took over for José left him with diminished confidence in his own capacity to run his life and, as a defensive reaction to his consequent insecurity, a tendency at times to reject advice or to act impulsively and maladaptively in order (unconsciously) to demonstrate to himself that he was his own man. This tendency contributed directly to his alienating his teachers. Desperately striving to get out from under the obedient, good-boy self-image that had developed in response to his parents' hovering attention, José would act in ways that left his teachers feeling angry, hurt, and rejected, and that led them to see him as troubled, unreliable, and unworthy of trust despite his good grades on exams and papers.

His parents' attitudes also left José suspicious and frightened of the outside world. His intense need to make it in the world of the upwardly mobile middle class was severely hampered by his lack of confidence or sense of safety in that world, which felt to him alien and dangerous. This lack of trust further exacerbated his difficulties with his teachers. Their experience was that they were making sincere efforts to reach out to him and to provide encouragement and support, and José's suspiciousness and even hostility made no sense to them and signified only that he was an ingrate or that there was something wrong with him.

Addressing this complex of feelings, attitudes, and mutual misunderstandings with José was made difficult by the fact that the therapist was, after all, part of that outside world José so mistrusted. The fact that she was herself a member of a minority group helped some in this regard, but it was far from sufficient to allay his suspicions. It was thus particularly important for the therapist to communicate her understanding in a manner that did not dismiss José's own way of seeing things. Although it was important for the therapist to stand for change, to represent the possibilities residing in the world outside, those possibilities had to be conveyed in a way that simultaneously gave real credence to José's quite different experience. The key to doing this lay in addressing the *conflict* that José was in. Based on our discussions in supervision, José's therapist said to him the following[2]:

"My understanding of what you've been doing, and it makes perfect sense given how you were brought up, is that for 17 years you were

---

[2]The comment is quoted verbatim from a tape recording she brought to a supervision session.

told "don't trust that world out there," and I can understand that you want to do whatever you can not to go out there. But I think another part of you recognizes that that doesn't really make sense, that it will be much too limiting. So one part of you really wishes you could be out there, but the reality is that you're very afraid and you're mistrustful, and it's going to take a lot of effort to persuade yourself that it's safe. Part of what we can do together is to work out ways for you to test out this fear and suspicion, work out ways for you little by little to feel safe in that world that your parents say they want you in but that they certainly haven't made it easy for you to go into."

Here the therapist actually takes a rather strong stand with regard to José's mistrust of the larger world from which he is tempted to retreat. Regarding this boy as at a crucial choice point in his life, a turning point that will have an enormous impact on the range of choices subsequently available to him, she wishes to help him grab hold of the possibilities still within reach before he lapses into the confining and frequently self-destructive world of many of his peers. But she plants the seeds for José's reexamination of his mistrustful stance in a way that conveys an appreciation of why he sees things as he presently does. The message is not that José is wrong or mistaken. Rather, his attitudes are perfectly understandable given his life experiences, *but* it may be worth reexamining those experiences to see if they admit of other possibilities.

In stating that "another part of you" has a different view, she is highlighting the experience of conflict. She is also making it clear that it is José too who wishes to move past his troubled orientation to the world and that it is not just the therapist entering his world as a missionary.

AFFIRMATION AND CHANGE IN THE THERAPEUTIC SESSION

The principles that enable the therapist to raise questions in an empathic manner about the patient's behavior in his daily life can be useful as well in addressing problematic behavior within the sessions. Once again it is essential on the one hand to communicate that one understands the patient's experience and sees a validity in his way of perceiving things and, on the other hand, to help the patient, where appropriate, to find a new way of responding to the situation he faces.

A student in a practicum seminar, for example, described feeling continually frustrated by the behavior of his patient, Frederick. Frederick would frequently come late to sessions and miss sessions without calling, and he had not paid his bill at the clinic since entering therapy 5 months before. The therapist clearly liked Frederick a good deal but felt increasingly that he was unable to address Frederick's behavior in relation to him without feeling very critical. As a consequence, he had been avoiding addressing these important issues.

Frederick was a very bright young man from Jamaica, who had recently graduated from an excellent New England college and come to New York to live. He was quite depressed when he came to the clinic, precipitated by the break-up of a relationship with a woman. He couldn't concentrate, slept a good deal, and had generally low moods. As we looked at Frederick's history, some themes became apparent that bore directly on his behavior in the therapy. Although Frederick had a long history of considerable success in school, in every other aspect of his life he had little sense of efficacy and control. His parents had emigrated to the United States when Frederick was 3 years old, leaving him in Jamaica in the care of his grandparents. Then, after 6 years of living with his grandparents, he had been kidnapped and brought to the United States by his mother, who had in the interim divorced his father. His mother had remarried, and his stepfather was cruel and abusive.

Throughout Frederick's life story, from his parents leaving when he was very little, to the kidnapping, to the abuse by his stepfather, to a variety of experiences with friends and girl friends, themes of powerlessness were paramount. Given this understanding, Frederick's behavior in the therapy took on a new meaning. It became clear that his "difficult" and "resistant" behavior in the therapy could be understood as part of an effort at self-healing, at attempting to regain a sense of efficacy and control. At the same time, of course, it was also a disruption of the therapy, the one experience and relationship that might enable him to achieve a fuller and more genuine sense of mastery in his life. Coming late, missing sessions, and not paying his bills all put the therapy greatly at risk.

I suggested to the therapist that he say to Frederick something like the following:

Given your life experiences, I can see how it's important to you not to submit once again to the circumstances other people have set up for you. When you come late, or miss a session, or don't pay your bill, I think it's your way of saying "I'll do things my way, according to my program, at my own pace." It's part of the fighting spirit that even all the blows you've had to endure haven't been able to knock out of you. I think at some point you may want to question whether this is the best way to gain such a sense of efficacy, whether there might be other ways that don't have as high a cost to you, but for now this feels like a way to at least begin to take control.

Clearly the comment contains a message about the need to change this behavior. But it makes its point in a way that is appreciative of the positive thrust to the behavior as well and that comprehends this behavior pattern as making sense, not just as something that must be changed.

Moreover, it functions to oppose a potential vicious circle that could bring the therapy to a grinding halt. If Frederick continues to see the behavior being addressed here (missing sessions, coming late, and so forth) as simply reflecting his not being able to "get his act together" (which is how he had regarded it up until then), he is absolved of a certain amount of responsibility for it, but his sense of inefficacy, of not being master of his own life, is increased. He continues to experience himself as a piece of driftwood carried in one direction or another rather than as an active agent; and this then requires still more of the same passive resistance to combat that sense of inefficacy. In contrast, if his behavior is construed as deriving from his own *agency*, if it feels to him as if he is actively structuring his mode of participation in the therapy (even where it includes behavior that is problematic), this contributes to his sense of being in control, and the resultant sense of empowerment can reduce the necessity to find ways of "sneaking in" little pockets of assertion or mastery.

To be sure, Frederick's behavior could also be understood in other ways as well. It seemed, for example, to be an instance of what in Chapter 6 was called "identificatory transference." Frederick was, one could say, treating the therapist without regard, as he had been treated by his parents. It is likely that behavior of this sort on Frederick's part is implicated in a wide range of his difficulties. Examining how it gets him in trouble in his life, both through the transference relationship and in direct examinations of his daily interactions with others (as well as through the parallels between the two) was a significant part of the overall course of the therapy. At this point in the work, however, when the therapist was looking for some opening into a matter that Frederick was extremely reluctant to address, and that the therapist too was finding it difficult to raise in a therapeutically helpful manner, it proved useful to focus on a different—though not entirely unrelated—dimension of the behavior's meaning and to highlight its implications from a quite different angle.

Obviously a single comment such as the one described in this vignette does not in itself resolve the potential impasse presented by the pattern of behavior it addresses. But it does illustrate how the work can be carried along by a framing that casts the behavior in an appreciative, understanding light even as one is engaged in an effort to participate in changing it.

In another case, the behavior that needed to be addressed involved the patient's complaining constantly about how the therapist conducted sessions. Everything had to be done just so, and the therapist's way was always wrong. It felt to the therapist that the patient was preoccupied with getting her to do various things she didn't want to do or to do things the patient's way; consequently she was very irritated at the patient and thought of him as excessively "manipulative." She felt stymied about how to address this pattern, since she was aware that to say what she was thinking—that the patient was being manipulative—would in truth be more an accusation than an interpretation.

I suggested that she say to the patient simply, *You're afraid I won't do things right.* This construction addressed directly the patient's complaining, but it did so in a much more sympathetic way than any of the comments that had occurred to the therapist. It looked at the experience *along with* the patient, rather than putting the patient down. Once again, the aim was simultaneously to acknowledge and affirm the patient's experience and to point him toward the possibility of change. Calling attention to the pattern and empathizing with it were not alternative courses of action but were combined in the one comment.

A somewhat similar challenge came up regarding a child presented in a case seminar I was conducting. The young patient wanted her therapist to give her food in the sessions, which for various reasons the therapist didn't want to do. The child seemed angry at the therapist's refusal and was largely silent. Here too the therapist was tempted to see this in terms of "manipulation," a category all too prevalent in our clinical thinking. I suggested that she say instead: *I guess it feels only fair that if I don't give you anything, you won't give me anything either.*

This comment addresses itself to the patient's anger, stubbornness, even vengefulness, yet it does so in a way that conveys understanding rather than criticism. It opens up the exploration of the issue without first requiring that the patient see herself as having been wrong.

The general form *I guess it feels only fair that* is a form that can prove useful in a variety of contexts; it encourages the patient to elaborate his feelings or experience rather than to retreat to a defensive stance in the face of a perceived attack.

At a slightly later point in the work with this same child, the therapist wanted to convey to the child her understanding of the symbolic meaning of her asking the therapist for food. As the therapist saw it, the request for food had several overlapping meanings: she felt that in asking for food the child was asking to be nurtured and taken care of, to be paid attention to, to have her requests taken seriously, to have the rules broken for her as a sign she was special, and to have some indication that in the therapy she would not be bound by rigid rules as she was at home. But although the therapist had articulated these meanings to herself quite clearly, she was puzzled by her inability to find a way to convey this to the child that felt comfortable.

As we explored this, it became clear that an important aspect of the problem was that the therapist had put it to herself that "the issue isn't really food but being taken care of, paid attention to, and so forth." As a consequence, the phrasings that came to mind most naturally were ones such as *What you really want is....* Perhaps as a result of being sensitized to nuances of phrasing in the seminar, she (quite properly, I believe) felt uncomfortable with the phrasings that came to mind, but (perhaps because of the way she continued to think about the issue) she could not find an alternative that felt suitable.

The fairly simple and straightforward phrasing that did the trick was: *I guess if I give you food, you feel better taken care of.* Once again, it addresses the same content, but it does so from a point of view that stands beside the patient rather than one that challenges or criticizes. And it does so without relinquishing any of the opportunities for exploration opened up by the more critical *What you really want* comments. Indeed, this is one of the relatively few places I would offer close to an absolute in my recommendations: just about every time you are tempted to say *What you really want* or *What you really feel,* substitute instead a comment of the form offered here.[3]

A somewhat similar recommendation seems to me to be in order when something the patient is saying about someone else is experienced by the therapist as an indirect reference to her or to the therapeutic relationship. It is not uncommon in such circumstances for the therapist to say something like "Perhaps you're really feeling that toward me."

The problem with such a comment again lies in the word "really." It implicitly dismisses the patient's own experience, treating the report of the outside relationship or experience as only chaff, to be discarded in the process of harvesting the transferential wheat.

The seemingly slight variation of substituting "also" for "really"—

---

[3]This same child also worried a great deal about the plants in her therapist's office and whether the therapist was taking care of them properly. Apropos the discussion above, a useful supplementary comment might be: *Maybe you need to be taken care of better, just like the plants do;* but clearly not *What you're really worried about is whether you're being taken care of properly.*

Perhaps you're also feeling that toward me—is a significant improvement. Using "also" instead of "really" is more respectful toward the patient's experience. It doesn't invalidate the patient's way of construing what has transpired; it simply *adds* to it. It doesn't presume that the feelings toward the therapist are more "real" or even that they "underlie" the other feelings the patient has reported. It doesn't imply that the feelings that the patient *thinks* he is having are illusory or superficial. Rather, it points the inquiry in a direction the therapist thinks may be fruitful, while remaining respectful of the patient's own perceptions. In that sense, it too is a way of affirming the patient's experience while simultaneously pointing the way toward a modification or expansion of that experience.

A related, but somewhat different approach turned out to be useful in a case presented to me by a supervisee. The patient was a Hispanic woman who was extremely angry at the staff of the school her child was attending, staff she felt were racist and incompetent. As it turned out, this situation was complicated by the fact that the student therapist had himself been working part time in that school and felt very uncomfortable dealing with this anger toward an institution with which he felt somewhat identified. He sensed that some of the anger at the school was displaced and reflected the mother's frustration at her own difficulties in disciplining her child. But in trying to find a way to convey his perceptions, and to turn the therapy away from what seemed like constant and fruitless complaining about the school, his way of broaching it was quite accusatory: *I guess it's much easier for you to blame the school than to look at what you're doing with your child.*

Not surprisingly, the woman felt criticized and blamed. Having just taken a sociology course in which the concept of blaming the victim had been introduced, she was fully prepared to make her therapist feel absolutely awful. The therapist, to his credit, recognized immediately that his comment was an error, and in the supervisory sessions, we discussed some of what might have been going on. He was able to appreciate his own anger at his patient, both for the way she was treating her child (which had some painful resonances with his own childhood) and for her accusations about the school, which put the therapist into a difficult loyalty conflict.[4] After some discussion both of the countertransference issues and of just what it was that he wanted to get across, he came up with a much more satisfactory alternative to use the next time the opportunity came up: *I can understand why you'd be angry*

---

[4]By the time the therapist realized that his patient's child attended the school he worked in, he had already been working with her for a while. Had this been clear at the time of intake, it is unlikely the case would have been assigned to him.

at the school, and it's important to see if anything can be done about that situation. But I wonder if there are other parts of your life that are also making you angry, and if that's kind of adding to your anger at the school.

This comment had several interesting features. To begin with, like several of the comments described earlier, it was an "also" comment rather than an "instead" comment. It doesn't invalidate the mother's anger at the school but, rather, invites consideration of whether something else might *also* be bothering her. It thus contributes to helping her move away from a pattern of complaining in a ritualistic and rather unproductive way, but it does so much more respectfully than did the earlier comment. It also helps to open up discussion of other sources of frustration in this woman's quite difficult life, helping to point toward topics that needed to be addressed but were being crowded out, as it were, by her complaints about the school.

Even in the way it addresses the anger at the school itself, the comment usefully structures the patient's approach to the issue. *I can understand why you'd be angry* provides acknowledgment of the validity of her feelings, whereas *it's important to see if anything can be done about that situation* both further takes her concerns seriously and moves discussion of them away from repetitive complaining and toward consideration of possible changes or solutions. Not surprisingly perhaps, the patient turned out to be much more receptive to this way of approaching the sources of her anger.

WHEN EMPATHY IS AVERSIVE

In most of the examples discussed thus far, empathic resonance with the patient's experience is a key element in resolving the dilemma the therapist faces. Occasionally, however, the therapist's empathy itself may be a source of distress to the patient. In those instances, if the therapist is to follow the principle of respecting the patient's way of organizing and interpreting his experience, while simultaneously questioning what must be questioned, expressions of empathy with regard to certain experiences must be carefully titrated.

Some patients, for example, seem to be in considerable psychological pain, but feel humiliated if that pain is noticed. The therapist's empathic appreciation of his pain feels to the patient like an attack, like a perception that cuts rather than heals. In such a situation, where the patient's fear of being seen as soft or vulnerable makes empathy itself feel like the enemy, it is useful to consider how the expression of empathy itself can be incorporated into a strategy that at once accepts and works toward changing the patient's view of the world.

One begins by empathizing, in essence, with the resistance, with the patient's insistence on *not* being told about pain, with his *irritation* at having pain addressed. The comment might be simply *You don't like to be told you're feeling pain.*

Such a comment, although directly resonating with and accepting the patient's experience and intention, also implicitly calls attention to both the pain itself and the patient's hypersensitive avoidant stance toward it. Indeed, it is *intended* to do this. But although strategic, it is also genuine. It directs itself to a particular aspect of the patient's experience and conveys an understanding and appreciation of that experience; the patient *doesn't* like being told he's in pain.

The next stage in the interpretive process, the fruit as it were of the workings of the first comment, might be to say: *You feel uncomfortable with the idea of pain.* Here one is still not saying the person *is* in pain. Rather than challenging the patient's experience, one is approaching change from *within* the patient's experience, making comments the patient can accept and affirm.

This second comment might not have been acceptable at the outset. It is bolder, goes further than "you don't like" to be told. It points to the patient's discomfort, broaches the notion that the idea of being in pain, of being the sort of person who feels pain (perhaps of feeling like someone with so much pain to deal with that it must be kept at bay altogether) makes him *anxious.* This is why the comment comes second, only after the "you don't like" comment has had a chance to bring the patient's dislike of talk of pain to his consciousness.[5]

Only then, when this preliminary work has been done, when one has resonated strategically with a *part* of the patient's experience in order to open a door to resonating with the rest, is it likely to be fruitful to comment on the pain itself. One has seen the pain all along, but to communicate about it in a way that will be therapeutic, one must see other things as well. In particular, one must appreciate that the patient's aversion to having his pain seen and commented on by the therapist is not simply a "resistance" to be overcome but another part *of his experience,* of who he is. As such, it requires both respectful empathy in its

---

[5]The "you don't like" comment serves a double function in easing the patient into an area he fears. On the one hand, it reassures: it conveys to the patient that the therapist understands his aversion to such talk, that he is willing to honor it and not bring up something the patient fears hearing. On the other, it also is itself a beginning broaching of the topic. The very sense of safety created by the therapist's appreciation of the patient's distaste for such discourse also makes it a little easier *to* engage in it. It permits the beginning of a desensitization to the idea, so that, in a safe and gradual context, it can become increasingly possible to approach it.

own right *and* an understanding of its position in the overall hierarchy of the patient's goals.

WHAT DOES IT MEAN TO BE "SUPPORTIVE"?

It is possible to conceive of many of the recommendations in this chapter as falling under the rubric of what is usually called "support" in the psychotherapy literature. Support is a key element in all psychotherapy, but it is a highly controversial element, often utilized only covertly for fear that the therapy will seem "superficial." In fact, properly understood, support is in no way antithetical to deep exploration; indeed, the absence of appropriate support is one of the most common *impediments* to the effective exploration of issues that are frightening and conflictual for the patient.

Recent contributions, both conceptual and empirical, have challenged the sharply dichotomous distinction between exploratory and supportive approaches to therapy that had long dominated clinical thinking and have highlighted the critical importance of support for the exploratory process itself. Schlesinger (1969) offered a particularly clear and incisive critique of the way the term "support" is used in clinical discussions and pointed toward a much more differentiated understanding of the meanings and applications of support. Noting that the term supportive has often been used to refer strictly to therapies that are severely limited in their aims and methods, Schlesinger argued that

> by arrogating the name "supportive" for a polar example of psychotherapy in which the purpose of supporting a patient is pursued in a particular way with particular techniques and with limited aspirations, we debase the term "supportive." We tend to obscure the fact that support is one of the essential purposes of all psychotherapy, and we use it to imply a specific *kind* of psychotherapy—which it is not. (Schlesinger, 1969, p. 271)

Schlesinger questions sharply the assumption that therapy that is "supportive" is precluded from utilizing interpretations and exploring unconscious contents. Support is manifested in a variety of ways in all therapies and is a blanket term that refers in fact to many different aspects of the therapeutic process. Schlesinger points us to ask not simply if the therapy is "supportive" or "expressive" (a distinction he believes fails to capture with any degree of adequacy the complexity of the therapy relationship and the mix of techniques and attitudes that all therapies include). Rather, he suggests we guide our inquiry into the issue of support with questions such as the following:

In what sense (areas, instances, etc.) does this patient need support: (1) his sense of reality against the temptations of dereistic preoccupations, (2) his conscience against the temptations of corruption, (3) his frightened ego against the anxiety-inspired wish to banish all derivatives of a troublesome instinctual impulse or even against intense feelings of any kind? Or is it a fragile and remote impulse-derivative that needs support (*e.g.*, a tender, affectionate feeling against defenses that would stifle it), or perhaps it is the shaken patient who needs support against momentarily overwhelming outside pressures, or does his flagging motivation need support in order to continue treatment during a phase of uncomfortable resistance? Or is it the patient's self-esteem that needs support against the painful discovery of the infantile core of certain strivings?

The term "supportive" applies to each of these different situations though the manner in which the support would be offered, if indeed it would have to be explicitly offered by the psychotherapist at all, is likely to be quite different in each. (Schlesinger, 1969, p. 272)

Rockland (1989), building on earlier insights of Gill (1951) and Knight (1954), reached somewhat similar conclusions to those just described, although he differed from Schlesinger in continuing to advocate for a particular category of therapy to be labeled "supportive therapy." According to Rockland,

All psychotherapies contain significant supportive aspects. Even psychoanalysis, the quintessential exploratory or nonsupportive psychotherapy, furnishes the patient significant support via such elements as the frequency of meetings, the structured way of proceeding, and the acceptance of the analyst. . . . A psychotherapy without any supportive elements built into it cannot be an effective psychotherapy, and probably would not be viable. (Rockland, 1989, p. 9)

Particularly strong indication of the pervasiveness and crucial importance of supportive elements in all psychotherapies comes from a major study of psychotherapy process and outcome conducted over many years at the Menninger Foundation. Robert Wallerstein, a leading figure in psychoanalysis for several decades and a central participant in the Menninger study, has been especially clear and forthright about the ways in which the study's findings require modification of key psychoanalytic assumptions about the role of support in psychoanalysis and psychotherapy (e.g., Wallerstein, 1986, 1988, 1989a, 1989b). Although he notes that the implications of the Menninger study must be considered in the light of the particular patient population from which the findings derive, he makes it clear that the results differed dramatically from what was expected by the project's planners, a group that was not only thoroughly familiar with the patient population on which the study was based, but that also included some of the most prestigious and sophisticated individuals in the psychoanalytic movement. As Wallerstein reports,

> an overall finding from our project—and almost an overriding one—has been the repeated demonstration that a substantial range of changes, in symptoms, in character traits, in personality functioning, and in life-style rooted in lifelong and repressed intrapsychic conflicts, have been brought about via the more supportive psychotherapeutic modes and techniques, cutting across the gamut of declared supportive *and* expressive (even analytic) therapies, and that in terms of the usual criteria—stability, durability, and capacity to withstand external or internal disruptive pressures—these changes can be (in many instances) quite indistinguishable from the changes brought about by typically expressive–analytic (interpretive, insight-producing) means. (Wallerstein, 1988, p. 146)

Wallerstein adds that from the vantage point of the standard psychoanalytic assumptions about the relative roles of exploration and support and their relationship to each other—assumptions which guided the planning and implementation of the Menninger Foundation project and which continue to be highly influential in psychoanalytic circles to this day—there is "considerable real surprise" in many of the findings of the project: for example,

> that these distinctive therapeutic modalities of psychoanalysis, expressive psychotherapy, supportive psychotherapy, etc., hardly exist in anywhere near ideal or pure form in the real world of actual practice; that real treatments in actual practice are inextricably intermingled blends of more or less expressive–interpretive and more-or-less supportive–stabilizing elements; that almost all treatments (including even presumably pure psychoanalyses) carry many more supportive components than are usually credited to them; that the overall outcomes achieved by those treatments that are more "analytic" as against those that are more "supportive" are less apart than our usual expectations for those differing modalities would portend; and that the kinds of changes achieved in treatments from the two ends of this spectrum are less different in nature and in permanence than again is usually expected, and indeed can often not be easily distinguished. None of this is where, three decades ago, we expected to be today. (Wallerstein, 1988, pp. 149–150)

Understanding of why these findings were so surprising, and of the largely unrecognized and unarticulated assumptions that have shaped therapists' views of support and its relation to exploration, is quite germane to the central themes of this entire book. On close inspection, one can see that in fact much confusion has been introduced into discussions of support in the psychotherapy literature by a failure to distinguish between two rather different meanings of the term support, rooted in quite different ways of thinking about the therapeutic process. On the one hand, many discussions of support are implicitly grounded in an essentially adversarial view of the therapeutic enterprise. Exploratory therapy is conceptualized as *tearing down* defenses, and support is understood as shoring them up, and *therefore* as antithetical to exploration. This conception is closely related to the view of resistance, examined critically at several points in this book, in which resistance, too, is implicitly conceived of in adversarial terms, with the patient trying to manipulate, avoid, or wrest inappropriate gratifications, and the therapist attempting to overcome the resistance through firmness, persistence, refusal to gratify or be seduced, and interpretations directed against the patient's efforts to cover up.

Newer models of therapy, however, tend to stress not the *tearing down* of defenses so much as the *building up* of a curative relationship. These models are likely to generate a quite different tone, not only in theoretical discourse on the therapeutic process but in how one interacts with patients as well. In contrast to the view of support that equates it with "shoring up" defenses or with "covering over" unconscious material, support from this framework is an essential part of the process of exploration itself, the basic grounding of the relationship that makes such exploration possible.

The implications of this alternative conception of support are further clarified in terms of the revised understanding of anxiety discussed in Chapter 3. If the patient feels threatened by what the therapist says (or, for that matter, by what she *doesn't* say; that is, by the stance and attitude of the therapist vis-à-vis the patient), his defenses are likely to intensify. Far from promoting the patient's access to unconscious material, the absence of sufficient support is likely to impede that access.

The importance of the patient's feeling secure if exploration of unconscious material is to proceed effectively has increasingly been recognized by psychoanalytic writers—for example, in Schafer's (1983) discussions of the "atmosphere of safety." But the persistence of certain theoretical confusions (examined at various points in this book) and ties to certain formal features of the therapist's stance that are closely related to some therapists' professional identities, have prevented this newer understanding from being fully assimilated into common therapeutic practice. It is one of the aims of this book to facilitate that assimilation.

The dichotomy between support and insight is a false one, which has hampered considerably the development of a more fully effective—

and more fully empathic—psychotherapy. Support—especially as it is embodied in the therapeutic interactions described here—is perfectly consistent with, indeed is an essential component of, the exploratory process. The approach advocated here, although it contains many supportive elements (in the sense described by Schlesinger, Wallerstein, and others as facilitating the exploratory process), clearly is not "supportive therapy" as that term is typically used.[6]

In much of the literature on support in psychotherapy, it is commonly assumed that when one is supportive one places limits on the depth of change that can be achieved and that, therefore, it is only patients who are not "fit" for the rigors of more demanding therapeutic approaches who by default are assigned to "supportive therapy." Werman, for example, states that

> insight-oriented psychotherapy is based on the assumption that the patient possesses psychological equipment of adequate quality, but that the function of this mental apparatus has to be freed up from those influences and conflicts that inhibit its fullest utilization. *In contrast, supportive psychotherapy assumes that the patient's psychological equipment is fundamentally inadequate.* (Werman, 1984, p. 13; italics in original)[7]

This attitude seems to me highly problematic for two reasons. First, it is difficult to see how one can be genuinely supportive toward anyone one regards as "fundamentally inadequate." Much of the discussion in this and the preceding chapter is directed toward helping the therapist overcome precisely such attitudes both in her thinking and in her communications with the patient. Second, the sharp distinction between insight and support contributes to a pervasive tendency to offer less support than is optimal for those patients who do get referred for more

---

[6]Rockland (1989), for example, states that "exploratory psychotherapy seeks to uncover unconscious mental contents, whereas supportive therapy covers them over" (p. 16), and that supportive therapy "does not include interpretation among its techniques, nor is making unconscious content conscious a goal" (p. 243). The approach described in this book, no matter how supportive, bears little resemblance to such a "supportive therapy."

[7]The literature on supportive therapy, like the literature comparing the indications for psychoanalytically oriented psychotherapy in contrast to psychoanalysis, often claims that no value judgments are implied, that it is simply a matter of finding the most appropriate therapy for the particular patient. Writers who make this claim may even bolster it by declaring they regard supportive therapy as "better" for the patients assigned to it since they are people who would not be helped by more fully exploratory therapies. The hidden value judgments that lie behind this seemingly egalitarian position are discussed in Wachtel (1987, Chap. 12).

avowedly exploratory therapies. Wallerstein (1989a), referring to the commonly made distinction between supportive and expressive psychotherapies, describes the maxim that typically guides psychoanalytically oriented clinical work as "Be as expressive as you can be and as supportive as you have to be." The position taken here, in contrast, might be stated as "Be as supportive as you can be *so that you can be* as expressive [as exploratory] as you will need to be."

Support and Autonomy

A further source of confusion about support, and of the hesitancy of some therapists to think of what they do as supportive, is a function of the (negative) link between the concept of support and those of neutrality and autonomy. It is sometimes assumed that, in contrast to a supportive stance, the therapist with more ambitious goals and with a stronger patient (see above) assumes a stance of neutrality and that such a stance, permits the patient to find the authority for his actions within himself rather than turning to others. In the process, according to this view, he is able to achieve a measure of automony and a depth of change that is otherwise unattainable.

To be sure, it is very important that the therapist not simply take over for the patient in such a way that he temporarily feels better but without having achieved the ability to later master things himself. The concern of many analysts that "structural change" be achieved is, in that sense, appropriate and important. But the observations made by Wallerstein in his analyses of the Menninger study data, and the considerations advanced in this chapter and elsewhere in this book suggest that change of this sort is not necessarily best accomplished by seeking to minimize the therapist's role as giver of directions, permission, or encouragement.

Sometimes the argument against being too supportive is made via the metaphor that the therapy should not serve as a "crutch." If we take that metaphor seriously, however, we may notice that crutches are not always meant to be permanent; often crutches are used as a temporary way of enabling a healing process to proceed so that crutches will no longer be necessary. And the *failure* to provide a crutch, requiring the person to stand on his own two feet prematurely, can render appropriate healing—and the achieving of a more enduring capacity to stand unaided—virtually impossible. It is in this spirit that I advocate the therapist's bearing more of the burden of change than has been traditional in therapies that seek to promote insight.

The therapist temporarily does some of the things the patient must eventually do for himself in order to help the patient gain sufficient strength to be able to do well without him. The dependent tie to the therapist is "resolved" not so much through insight into its childhood roots as by the patient's developing effective and gratifying patterns of living—through the skillful and supportive ministrations of the therapist—that make further dependency unnecessary.

CHAPTER 9

Attribution and Suggestion

Truth is not static. The therapist must help the patient grasp the truth about his life, but the nature of that truth is continually changing. If the therapy is going well, the patient is, almost by definition, a person in transition. In this chapter I wish to discuss a number of strategies of therapeutic communication that are centrally rooted in this perspective. They further have in common that in one way or another they are designed to facilitate the process of change by predicting it or describing it as already having progressed. They are thus future-oriented redescriptions of the patient and his life circumstances.

We have already encountered a number of such comments in the course of discussions of other topics in earlier chapters. The reader may recall, for example, the case of Tina discussed in Chapter 6. Following what seemed to be the family rules, Tina was compulsively flip and bouncy and avoided discussion of anything that bothered her. Building on only the tiniest indication of change in this pattern, the therapist was advised to say to the patient, *I'm amazed you've been able to do it all these years, and I'm not surprised that you're now finding it a bit exhausting.* This is an example of what I will call an *attributional* comment. A feeling is attributed to the patient that she has not reported having. (Put differently, it is a feeling that she has not *yet* reported having. I am reminded here of Picasso's remark when told his portrait of Gertrude Stein did not look like her. Reportedly, his comment was "It will.")

An attributional comment will be useful, of course, only if it addresses a tendency that is at least potential in the patient, if it has some ring of truth or familiarity to it. In a sense such a comment makes something that is not yet true, or is *potentially* true, truer than it otherwise might have been had the comment not been made.

From a different vantage point, one could view the comment just described—as many of the others discussed in this chapter—as a suggestion. The suggestive element in psychotherapy has been much misunderstood over the years and has been a source of considerable conceptual confusion. The difficulties can be traced back to Freud, who actually had a more complex, less thoroughly rejecting attitude toward suggestion than many contemporary therapists, but whose struggles with the implications of suggestion for his theoretical endeavors fatefully shaped the course of later developments. Later in this chapter, after offering the reader a picture of the range of ways in which attributional comments can be employed to further the progress of therapeutic work, I will take up the potential objections in some detail, explicating some of Freud's views on the matter in a way that sheds new light on our understanding of suggestion in psychoanalysis and in other therapeutic approaches.

An attributional perspective similarly underlay a comment made to another patient, Barbara, who was extremely submissive and permitted her parents and her husband to examine every minor detail of her behavior for potential misdeeds, failures, or slips of propriety. At one point I said to her, "I have a sense that you're getting sick and tired of being scrutinized all the time," and hoped that in the saying a path would be cleared for her to be able in fact to feel more of a right to be irritated.

Once again, for such a comment to be helpful it must make contact with a real emergent (though not yet clearly overt) trend in the patient. Otherwise it can be an unrecognized attempt to impose the *therapist's* irritation, or the therapist's values or predispositions on the patient. Moreover, (reflecting a danger not inconsistent with the one just stated) it can be experienced by the patient as an implicit criticism of her: "What's wrong with you that you're not sick and tired of this?"[1]

CONFLICT AS A KEY TO ATTRIBUTIONAL COMMENTS

As with so many other aspects of therapeutic work, understanding of and attention to conflict is often central to an effective use of attributional comments. Part of why the trends addressed by such comments have not yet emerged as clear and unambiguous, part of why they must be helped along, is that they have been submerged in conflict. And part of why they are important, and have the potential to play a larger role

---

[1]As the reader will no doubt suspect, the issue of feeling scrutinized eventually came up in relation to the therapy as well. Ways of employing the principles adduced here to address the patient's feelings about the therapist and the relationship are discussed later in this chapter and elsewhere in the book.

in the patient's psychic life, is that they do represent genuine inclinations of the patient which, though now largely buried, would readily gain expression if the conflict were resolved.

Christine, for example, was a young woman entangled in an enmeshed family who had to struggle considerably to achieve even a minimum sense of independence. Having a right to pursue her own inclinations or to exercise her independent judgment was not something that had any place in her family system. Even during those periods when Christine had a boy friend, her family and her boyfriend's family would go together to shop in a nearby suburban mall.

The formulation that I suggested her therapist present to her was centrally rooted in the idea of conflict. I suggested she say to Christine something like the following: *I can see that you're in a lot of conflict. Part of you feels you don't have the right to go your own way and part of you realizes you do.* Several things are worth noting about this comment. First of all, we may see that it subtly promotes the patient's independence by using the word "realizes" in describing her right to go her own way rather than "feels." Secondly, it attributes that realization to the patient. It is described not as something the therapist is telling her but rather as something that *she* realizes.

This way of communicating, it should be noted, *blurs boundaries*. What is the therapist's viewpoint and what is the patient's is for the moment partially obscured. And of course, this is precisely its point: it is *designed*, in essence, to insert a new idea into the patient's inner dialogue, to encourage the patient to adopt a perspective from the therapist, to identify with a different point of view that, it is hoped, will be liberating. Interestingly, formulations in psychoanalytic circles of how therapeutic change occurs have increasingly centered on the crucial role of some kind of identification with the therapist or analyst. Terms such as "transmuting internalization" and "benign introject" have become important parts of the theoretical vocabulary. Implicit in such formulations is that change *requires* that some blurring occur, that the patient take in something from the therapist. If the boundary between patient and therapist is kept too hard and fast, if the sole means of taking in an idea is confined to conscious, rational appraisal, the therapy operates under a severe handicap, indeed one it is unlikely to be able to overcome.

To those used to thinking in more traditional terms of neutrality, of the total "resolution" of the transference, and so on, this description may sound troubling. What is to guard against the insidious injection of the therapist's own values into the patient's life? This is a question that must indeed be taken seriously (see in this regard Wachtel, 1977, Chap.

12, and Wachtel, 1987, Chaps. 10 and 11). But one safeguard that should be kept in mind—and it should as well be a safeguard in relation to the therapist's grandiosity—is that the therapist's comments are far from omnipotent. Apropos the discussion in Chapter 1, they are less like an injection than a tissue transplant: they can easily be rejected if they are read as alien. And they are likely to be experienced as alien if they do not in fact resonate with some aspect of the patient's own aspirations, values, or vision of what is possible in his life. Here then, in a different way, is another place where accurate empathy is a crucial element in the therapeutic process. It enters in, invisibly but powerfully, as a safeguard. The therapist who does not properly understand her patient will be ineffective.

LABELING MALADAPTIVE TENDENCIES AS "RESIDUALS"

My emphasis here on turning a predictive, magnifying lens on the tiny buds of change, nurturing them, and helping them to grow more prominent, should not be taken to imply that one turns a blind eye toward those aspects of the patient's behavior that are maladaptive. Such behavior, after all, is likely to constitute the bulk of what the therapist is required to attend to in the course of the therapy. Often these problematic behaviors (in therapy or in the rest of the patient's life) are readily addressable using the familiar constructions and forms of speech that are the therapist's stock in trade. Not infrequently, however, situations arise in which the therapist may sense, either quite explicitly or perhaps only dimly, that the very act of addressing the patient's problematic behavior, although crucial, is also a danger to the patient's progress. This can particularly be the case with patients who are very prone to hear other people's comments as critical and to feel hurt by them, and with patients who are overly and harshly *self*-critical and who are likely to seize on any description of their persisting maladaptive behavior as one more sign that they are bad, or a failure, or hopeless.

An interesting example of this occurred at an important juncture in the case of Eva, who was being seen by a therapist I was supervising. Eva's parents had made it very difficult for her to separate from them. They would rarely be completely open about their opposition to her going off on her own, but they would manage to convey their disapproval through questions that undermined her resolve and highlighted the negative in whatever step she was taking. In addition, they somehow always managed to create disasters whenever Eva did go off. When mother didn't have the flu or father a backache, father would lose a job, mother would have a bad fall, father would smash up the car, mother would start a fire in the house by leaving some paper near the stove, and so forth. All these things happened with extraordinary regularity only when Eva had recently gone off on her own (for example, to summer camp, to college, to graduate school, or to take her first job).

At the time of the session to be discussed here, Eva had decided to take on a job that would be a quite significant advance for her, but one which required her to be out of town for several days a week. As a consequence, she had suggested to her therapist that perhaps they should cut back from twice a week to once a week.

When Eva broached the idea, her therapist attempted not to take a stand one way or the other but, rather, to explore with Eva how *she* felt about the decision. Eventually Eva did decide to take the job, and in many ways it seemed to have been a very good decision. But she became increasingly anxious in the sessions, feeling (incorrectly) that her therapist disapproved of her decision, that she resented Eva's cutting back to once a week and felt hurt by it. There were clear but unacknowledged signs that Eva felt angry at what she felt was an attempt by the therapist to hold on to her at the expense of Eva's freedom and best interests, and there were signs as well that Eva felt guilty about this unacknowledged anger.

Eva's therapist saw Eva's concerns about the therapist feeling hurt, and her fear that the therapist would reject her if she persisted in her successful move toward greater autonomy, as a continuation of Eva's old way of experiencing the world. She felt it important to help Eva see this connection in order to aid her in breaking the pattern that had so dominated and limited her. She was concerned, however, that Eva would experience her pointing out the parallels between what she experienced with her therapist and what she had earlier experienced with her parents as a further attempt to keep Eva in her place, to show her that nothing had really changed. She worried as well that a message that conveyed to Eva "You're still doing the same old thing" would feel discouraging and undermine the sense of growth Eva had experienced when she took the new job.

I suggested to the therapist that she could address the parallel in the following way: *You've taken a big step in accepting the new job, and you've confronted what you used to fear. So of course you're bound to still have some residual anxiety and to feel with me some of what you used to feel much more with your parents.* Such a comment addresses directly the parallel between Eva's experience with her therapist and her longstanding pattern with her parents. It does—as it needs to—point out to her how she's "still doing the same old thing." But it does so in a way that has a very different meta-message. By describing the anxiety as *residual*, one is in effect making a prediction. One *hopes* it is residual, and one is trying to create the circumstances under which it will in fact *become* merely residual. By highlighting the distinction between the past and present circumstances, even as one is also pointing out the consanguinity, one hopes to further the process of that distinction.

Other details of the way in which the comment was designed also were chosen to facilitate its function as pointing toward change and to diminish Eva's experience of guilt and self-criticism. The comment begins by pointing to the step she has taken and pointing out that it entails her confronting what she once fearfully avoided. It then states that "*of course*" she's "*bound to*" still have anxiety, thus presenting the anxiety not only as residual but as perfectly normal and understandable, something anyone in her circumstances would experience. It ends, again with a change-amplifying implication, by describing her as feeling now "*some of*" what she used to feel with her parents, but characterizing what she used to feel with her parents as "*much more*" than what she now feels with the therapist.

Thus, even as a parallel or continuity between past and present is being focused upon, so too does the comment point to the overcoming or reduction of that continuity, to the possibility of change, and the amplification of a progressive view of Eva and her life course.

A similar kind of therapeutic challenge arose in the work with Stanley, an extremely self-critical patient who, as one manifestation of his self-criticalness, berated himself for not making progress in therapy fast enough. It was important for him to understand that this self-judgment and impatience was itself part of the very pattern he needed to notice and understand, but there was also a danger in pointing it out that it would become still further fuel for his self-flagellations, one more thing for him to criticize himself about.

The persistence of this pattern was addressed without further fueling his critical side by pointing it out in the following way: *A little bit of the old pattern of self-criticism is still around, in the impatience you're feeling regarding your progress. That's to be expected. You can't, after all, get rid of it all at once.*

In such a comment, the primary vector is pointing to change. The pattern that the comment points out is presented as not so much a part of the present, of the thrust of his life's course, but as "a little bit of the old," an anomaly slowly but steadily in the process of disappearing. Thus, the message is essentially equivalent to the earlier locution in which the patient's anxiety is referred to as "residual anxiety."[2]

[2]It should also be noted that the comment serves as well to challenge the self-criticalness, to alienate or distance the patient from it. By addressing it as an anomoly, as something from the past inappropriately intruding into the present, room is cleared for less critical self-perceptions, and support is given to them.

In the case of Kathleen, a similar approach was useful at a later stage of the work. Kathleen, a very self-critical woman with a rather harsh superego, had made considerable progress in therapy and had changed her life quite substantially. At one point she began to talk about being less self-critical recently, and added "I guess I've lowered my standards."

I wanted to call attention to the recurrence of self-criticalness in that comment and work on the anxiety that stirred it. But as in the cases just cited, I was concerned not to feed her self-criticism further in pointing it out. I therefore said to her, *Talking about lowering your standards sounds like a piece of the old way of thinking creeping up for a moment, putting it in a self-critical way. As I hear what you're saying, you haven't lowered your standards; you've let yourself recognize better when you've met them.*

Here again the self-criticalness is labeled as "old," as *not* part of the newly dominant, emergent pattern in her life. Moreover, describing it as "creeping up for a moment" both treats it as temporary ("for a moment") and furthers the process of alienation from it ("creeping"). Beginning the next sentence with *As I hear what you're saying*, contributes a further attributional dimension to the comment. It makes that sentence quite different from just stating, "You haven't lowered your standards," or even from beginning the sentence, "It seems to me" you haven't lowered your standards. The latter two ways of putting it have at least implicitly an adversarial or corrective aspect: the therapist is telling the patient what's really happening. In contrast, "As I hear what you're saying"—that is, "As I hear what *you're* saying"—largely attributes the understanding to the patient. In effect, the therapist merely overhears; it is the patient who has made the point. Thus, as discussed below, the patient's *ownership* of the insight is enhanced.

At another point in this same stage of the work with Kathleen, I commented on her renewed nervousness as follows: *The nervousness you're feeling now is different from the nervousness you used to feel. That came from the jangled feeling of being stuck. The nervousness now is the anxiety that is always associated with entering new territory, with daring to approach what you had previously felt was forbidden.*

The reader will readily see that this comment is in a similar spirit to many of those discussed in this chapter. It distinguishes between past and present, attributes a certain momentum of change to the patient's activities, and redescribes her experience in a way that magnifies the change-oriented dimension.

Finally, a variant on the preceding strategy is illustrated in the case of Anthony. There were a number of steps Anthony had hesitatingly begun to take, but at a very halting pace, and I found myself about to say "Now it's time for you to start to. . . . " As that phrase came to mind, however, so too did a better one: *You've already started moving in this direction implicitly. Now it seems we're at a point where you're ready to start consolidating those intial steps and taking some new ones.*

Here again, a certain momentum is attributed to the patient, and it is hoped that that attribution will itself provide a bit of further momentum. It may also be noted that the construction used was not *Now it's time to start consolidating . . .* , which would still have a bit of the tone of coaxing and recalcitrance, but rather, *Now we're at a point where you're ready to start consolidating.* The use of the word *consolidate* here further adds to the same tone: one can only consolidate something that, at least to some degree, has already begun.

DESCRIBING BEHAVIOR AS TEMPORARY OR TRANSITIONAL

Still another way to convey your understanding in a way that structures it toward forward movement is to describe a source of distress or a problematic pattern of behavior as *transitional* or *temporary*. One might say, for example, *Yes, I can see you are temporarily more distressed [or, in other cases, more reluctant to reach out, more inhibited, more self-doubting, etc.], but it seems to me that that's a transitional response to the new situations you're encountering as you change.*

In a related vein, one might comment that the patient has "entered a stage of the work" in which greater anxiety is to be expected. Here there are *two* elements helping to frame the patient's experience constructively. Not only is this described as a "stage" and hence, temporary. The anxiety is also described as expectable, and it can therefore be taken as a reassuring indication that the process is on course rather than as a sign of trouble.

In a variation of this last sort of phrasing, I said to one patient, who was in acute conflict over competitive feelings toward his father and experienced any step in a direction his father had not taken as a betrayal: *It's not easy to pass through a stage in which you surpass your father.*[3]

One might note in this comment both the phrase *pass through,* which further emphasizes the temporary nature of his present state of distress, and the opening phrase *It's not easy to . . .* , which conveys an

---

[3]In casting his surpassing of his father as a stage to be passed through, the comment contains a certain ambiguity. Certainly I was not trying to convey that he would later revert to being inferior to his father, though at some level that may well have been part of what, from the perspective of his guilt, he found reassuring in the message. At another level, a more complicated notion of stage was being suggested: his present anxiety over

empathic appreciation, a sympathetic understanding of his distress.

In these various comments, as in those discussed earlier in the chapter, there is again a suggestive or predictive element. It might well be that without such a comment the patient's response might *not* be transitional or temporary, that it might be a real setback that could presage the unravelling of the therapy. The aim of the comment, however, is for the direction and encouragement that the comment provides to enable its implicit prediction to come true.

Once again, of course, such comments are only appropriate (and only likely to be effective) if they have a significant element of truth to them. As Freud found a century ago, suggestions that are just magic amulets have at best just a temporary effect. But as I've argued throughout this book, truth in human affairs is more ambiguous and dynamic than we are sometimes accustomed to imagining it. The way we articulate the truth will inevitably change it in some way. Knowing how to articulate it so as to facilitate movement in a progressive direction is a central feature of the good therapist's skills.

Along similar lines, when I wish to address some more resistive behavior or some more regressive portion of the personality without labeling the patient as such-and-such kind of person, or pinning him down in a discouraging and static picture, I will say something like: *You're beginning to rethink a lot of how you approach things, but the old ways are still very strong and we need to keep being alert to their appearance.* Consistent with the general line of argument in this chapter, such a way of communicating conveys *movement.* By labeling the maladaptive pattern as "the old way," one helps the patient to disidentify, to become alienated from it, and as a consequence such a comment can aid him in examining it and changing it.

HELPING THE PATIENT OWN HIS INSIGHTS

The attributional dimension can also be employed fruitfully in helping the patient to own and embrace the insights that are attained in the course of the therapeutic work. One potential problem with the standard interpretive stance is that it can convey to the patient the message that the therapist sees him more clearly than he sees himself. This can

---

surpassing his father was a stage in that it was expected that over time he would stop construing every achievement as a betrayal; indeed, that he would reach a point where he would simply not be categorizing experiences in this way, would not be measuring every step he took for whether it surpassed his father's equivalent steps.

lead both to passivity on the patient's part and to the strengthening of inclinations toward self-deprecation.

Thus it can often be useful, rather than saying some variant of *you feel such-and-such* or *you seem to be feeling such-and-such* (with their implication that the therapist is talking about something the patient has not yet grasped), instead to frame one's comments in a form such as *With all that has been going on in your life, I can understand how you'd feel such-and-such [angry/rejected/etc.].* Such a way of putting it has several advantages:

First, it implies that we are talking about something *both* of us know about; by, in effect, *assuming* the patient feels angry/rejected/etc. (and assuming too that the patient knows this), it puts the feeling out there for both of us to examine and gives the patient credit for already knowing at least something about it instead of it being an insight *offered* by therapist to patient.[4]

Second, it has a *normalizing* dimension to it. The therapist is conveying not only that he sees such-and-such a trend in the patient. He is conveying as well that such a trend is *understandable*, and thus, at least implicitly, that it is *acceptable*.[5] Thus, taking the trouble to phrase one's comment in the manner just suggested also contributes to a more *empathic* stance toward the patient rather than (a potentially demeaning) objectivity.

A number of variant forms of attributional comments also can be used to help the therapist convey to the patient a sense of owning the insight being addressed and of being an active participant in the process. Again they entail the therapist's foregoing the (inappropriate) pleasure of being smarter than the patient, of knowing something the patient doesn't, and substituting for it the more mature pleasure of being therapeutically helpful by enabling the patient to feel he has discovered something himself. In one way or another, these comments entail standing beside the patient, seeing something along with him, *assuming* he already knows and therefore that one is addressing something of *common* knowledge between them. These include such phrases as *As we've both seen . . . , As I know you're aware of . . .* , and *If I'm understanding you properly, what you're saying is. . . .*

---

[4]Here again, two elements are important to keep in mind. First, we are once again operating in an implicitly *predictive* realm; the patient may not *yet* be clear, but by our very efforts we make it more likely he *will* be. Second, it is once again crucial to recognize that, on grounds of both ethics and efficacy, the tendencies we are identifying in the patient must be tendencies that we genuinely see and that he can genuinely experience.

[5]It should be clear that this does not imply that all *actions* are acceptable. It is one thing to *feel* enormous anger at someone close to one and obviously quite another to act in a violent manner toward that person.

An interesting variation on this theme—again involving a kind of standing beside the patient and assuming something is understood—entails casting the patient's and the therapist's understanding in relief in relation to *others* who don't fully understand. In this variation, one raises with the patient the question: *Is there any way to make him/her/them understand?*

In the case of Jo Ann, for example, a patient prone to severe headaches, there were numerous indications that her headaches developed most often after her mother had behaved in a critical and intrusive way. Cowed by guilt, Jo Ann had had a difficult time realizing how angry this behavior of her mother's made her and, indeed, even in registering her mother's behavior as critical or intrusive. We had begun to make some progress in clarifying these dynamics, but Jo Ann still largely extended to me the pattern she had learned in relation to her mother: she implicitly took my comments as rebukes and experienced any comments about her being angry at her mother or experiencing her mother as intrusive as occasions for further self-criticism or self-abnegation.

In the context of one effort to address these issues, I said to Jo Ann, "Is there any way you could make your mother see how angry her intrusiveness makes you?" As she later discussed this comment, there was something in the matter-of-factness of it, in its taking as a *given* that mother was intrusive and (implicitly) that *of course* she'd be angry about it, that enabled her to hear and accept the message in a way that she hadn't previously. By standing side-by-side with the patient, and together looking at the *other* who doesn't understand what patient and therapist already do, the therapist can clear a path for the patient to assimilate an understanding that she would otherwise still find unacceptable.

THE SEQUENCING OF ATTRIBUTIONAL COMMENTS

The next example amplifies on several themes already introduced, but it indicates how a *series* of attributional comments can help the therapist guide the patient step by step toward understanding and dealing with difficult issues in her life. To begin with, it again illustrates empathetically standing side by side with the patient as she attempts to come to grips with the behavior of a significant other—in this case particularly severe and disturbing behavior. It also aims to help the patient assume *ownership* of the insights and perceptions that develop as a result of the therapeutic work, and again it does so in part through comments that attribute to the patient a degree of understanding that she had not yet attained prior to the comments themselves. In this example, however, the reader can gain greater understanding of how attributional comments can be put together in a sequence or set that is designed to promote new understanding and a new perspective in a stepwise fashion.

The patient, an 18-year-old named Vicki, was being seen by a student in our psychological clinic. Her mother was a quite disturbed woman who was using her daughter, and her fantasies and projections with regard to her, to keep herself together. In numerous ways, Vicki's mother would convey the conflicting, but powerful, messages that (1) Vicki was crazy and (2) she (the mother) would fall apart if Vicki were not there holding her together. In response to much of Vicki's behavior (including a good deal that was typical of most teenagers), she would say to Vicki that "You're killing me." And in response to anything Vicki did that she disapproved of, she would label Vicki as "subhuman," something there was good reason to think Vicki's mother actually felt about *herself*. By and large, the message that Vicki was damaged or crazy was generally quite explicit; the message about the mother's own terrors, and her desperate need for Vicki was usually covert and, indeed, implicitly forbidden to be noticed or commented upon by Vicki.

At one point in the treatment, Vicki began to insist that the therapist prescribe medication for her. It became apparent that this was in response to her mother's telling her she was crazy and needed medication. It also became apparent (to the therapist, but not yet to the patient) that it was in fact *the mother* who needed medication and that Vicki's mother seemed, in effect, to be seeking medication vicariously through her insistence that her daughter take it. The therapist was reluctant to refer Vicki for medication under the circumstances but was having difficulty dealing with Vicki's own increasing insistence.

Among the key issues that needed to be addressed with Vicki were her difficulty in acknowledging how seriously disturbed her mother was and the corollary imperative to play out the sick role, to take on the role of the crazy one, in order to help mother deny her own disturbance. Several strategies for opening up this set of issues were devised that bear on the central theme of this chapter. To begin with, the therapist told Vicki that medication was always potentially available, and that they could consider it together at any point, but that she felt that part of Vicki's wanting medication was to shut herself up because it was hard for her to believe that her therapist wanted to hear about her experiences. She then added *I can understand how you'd feel that way since your mother clearly doesn't want to hear much about your experiences, and immediately calls them crazy.* Thus the issue of her mother's role in Vicki's difficulties, and the inappropriateness of describing Vicki as crazy, was introduced in the context of an *I can understand* communication.

The aim of the therapeutic strategy described here was eventually to be able to address both Vicki's mother's craziness and the prohibition Vicki experienced regarding openly seeing it. But a number of preliminary lines of intervention were necessary before Vicki could hear this. One involved helping Vicki see how desperately she tried to please her mother and how impossible that was to do.

One phrasing that proved helpful was the following: *It must be hard to know that no matter what you do you can't please her.* Interestingly, earlier efforts by the therapist to point out to Vicki that her mother was impossible to please had had little impact. Their structure was such that they seemed to convey that the therapist was *arguing* with Vicki. The therapist would say something along the lines of: *There's no pleasing your mother,* or *Whatever you do she finds fault with,* and Vicki would then feel compelled to defend her mother. The structure of the communication was subtly adversarial, with the therapist trying to *persuade* Vicki that her perception was incorrect. In contrast, the slight (but significant) change in the phrasing just noted placed the therapist *side-by-side* with Vicki. "*It must be hard* to know" is sympathetic rather than adversarial, and "It must be hard *to know*" gives credit to Vicki for *already* knowing (and places therapist and patient side by side in examining a kind of objective reality) rather than having the quality of a *challenge* to Vicki's way of seeing things. As with many of the examples I have cited, it enables messages to come in freely through the side door while the front door is being heavily guarded.

Having achieved some success with an *It must be hard to know* message, we attempted to extend this strategy further. I suggested Vicki's therapist next find an opening to say to her: *It must be hard to have to pretend that you can please her, knowing that that's really impossible.* The necessity of pretending was a crucial element to address, since it contributed significantly to Vicki's terrible feelings about herself. Believing that it was possible to please her mother played a significant role in Vicki's feeling that if her mother were *not* pleased, it must be Vicki's fault. Once again, though, we were addressing a perception that was taboo for Vicki, and she seemed able to hear it only when we made an end run around the taboo by treating a more accurate perception in essence as a *fait accompli* ("knowing that that's really impossible").

Preliminary work of this sort eventually made it possible for her therapist, further utilizing this communicative structure, to successfully say to Vicki *It must be very hard to know your mother is crazy.* This was followed by a tearful acknowledgment by Vicki that "I kind of knew that all along, but I couldn't really admit it to myself."[6]

POINTING THE PATIENT TOWARD ACTION

Attributional comments may be employed not just to promote the patient's assimilation of new understanding and perspective but also to help the patient initiate new, more adaptive actions. As discussed in Chapters 2, 3, and 4, the operative causes of the patient's difficulties are not solely internal, and their solutions cannot be achieved solely in the patient's head. Because of the circular nature of maladaptive patterns and the critical role of "accomplices" and of the feedback the patient receives from his transactions with others, effective efforts at change must enable the patient to take steps in daily living that complement intrapsychic reorganization and further promote and consolidate whatever insights have been attained.

One of the circumstances where attention to the attributional dimension may be particularly useful in promoting such steps is in instances where processes of modeling and identification are brought into play. Such processes figure prominently in the patient's move toward more adaptive action, whether utilized as part of an intentional therapeutic intervention or occurring implicitly and without specific intention or awareness on the therapist's part. Their therapeutic value, however, will depend considerably on how much the patient experiences the new behavior as "his own" rather than as simply imitating or copying the behavior of another. In nurturing this sense of ownership of the new behavior, an attributional perspective is once again helpful.

Particularly useful are comments of the form: *It sounds like what you'd like to say [do] is. . . .* Such a comment, rather than being couched in the form of advice or direction from the therapist, attributes both the inclination and the particular shape it might take to the patient. In its manifest form, it is not about what the *therapist* suggests the patient might say or do but about what the therapist perceives the *patient* as already having come up with.

---

[6]Once again it is important to be clear that the form of the comment is not in itself determinitive. If the therapist says the "wrong" thing in the "right" way, she is not likely to be successful; although (as therapists are realizing) there is no *one* right content to an interpretation, what one says must resonate with the patient's experience. Nonetheless, although the medium is by no means the entire message, the central point of this book is that it is a highly significant part. Indeed, without the right form to the message, the content—however "correct" it might be—will not get through.

Such comments are, of course, only ethical (and only effective) if they in fact address something the patient really *is* inclined to do. But like many comments made by psychotherapists, they are likely to be addressing feelings and inclinations that the patient has not yet articulated very clearly. In effect, what they do is both to help the patient bring to awareness feelings and inclinations that have not gained full access to consciousness and to help link those feelings and inclinations, from the outset, to possibilities for effective action. The therapist, in effect, lends her ego to the patient at the moment of birth of the emerging idea, and thus she helps to give it a shape more likely to fit with the most forward-reaching structures of the patient's psychological organization. By helping to structure the emerging ideas and images not just as inner states to be observed, but as precursors of, or even first steps toward, effective action, such comments assist in the patient's growth and his developing sense of competence in dealing with the world.[7]

Both the therapeutic effectiveness and the ethical soundness of this sort of attributional comment can be further enhanced by addressing the comment to the *conflict* that the patient is facing, thus more fully encompassing his implicit experience. One might, for example, extend the paradigmatic comment depicted above by adding a further element: *It sounds like what you'd like to say [do] is such-and-such, but you feel that if you do, it will be selfish/mean/dangerous/etc.* Such a comment has the advantage both of addressing in advance the resistance (you feel it would be selfish/mean/dangerous/etc.) and of conveying to the patient a fuller appreciation of the extent and dimensions of his experienced dilemma.

A further safeguard against the therapist merely pawning off on the patient her own preferred way of dealing with life situations is rooted in an experience familiar to all therapists. When the therapist says *It sounds like you're feeling like you want to do X,* the patient will almost inevitably hear it in his own fashion, and say "Yes, you're right, I do want to do X-prime [or even Y or Z]." Even when not attending to the attributional dimension in the fashion described here, but simply in offering an interpretation from a traditional framework, therapists are aware of how often this kind of reinterpreting by the patient occurs. It is not at all uncommon for therapists who think they give no advice whatsoever to hear patients coming in and saying "I did what you said

---

[7]It is the way in which the comment is framed as "here is what I perceive *you* as wanting to do," when the patient, although able to embrace the comment, could not have generated it unaided, that gives it its attributional dimension.

I should," and then to be further flabbergasted to hear what it was the patient interpreted her as saying in the last session.

Thus, even if we attempt quite consciously to guide the patient in a particular direction—and it must always be in a direction that is our best guess as to what *the patient* would do if he were free of irrational anxiety or conflict, not what the therapist might prefer to do—we can be confident that the human tendency constantly and actively to organize and reinterpret material will assure that what follows will not be simple parroting of our message. The strongest likelihood, indeed, is that the suggestion the therapist makes will lead the patient in quite unanticipated directions.

A different kind of attributional pointing toward action was evident in the case of Edward. Edward was a young writer who came into therapy because he had been severely blocked for some time in work on his novel. In exploring the issues associated with Edward's writer's block, it became clear that part of the problem was that Edward never experienced the writing as really his. His father, a cold and dominating man, had also been a writer, and his shadow loomed over everything that Edward wrote. A central theme in Edward's life was that of powerlessness, and in following in his father's footsteps, that sense of powerlessness was magnified for him. On the one hand, he felt he would never measure up to his father as a writer (or that he "didn't have the balls" to bear his father's rage if he did). On the other hand, even the not inconsiderable success he had already achieved as a young man played into his dilemma, because it felt not completely his. He worried if his short stories were published only because he was his father's son and, beyond that, worried that becoming a writer altogether was not really his idea but just going along with the powerful force field emitted by his father.

His writer's block seemed to be a way of going on strike, of gaining what he came to call "negative power." He did this in a number of ways in his life, but a key one was in "not being able" to write.

After a while, he reached a point in the therapy where he began to talk spontaneously and explicitly about wanting to say "I will" instead of "I can't." As we discussed this, and started to put it together with what we had discovered about his feelings toward his father, I said to him,

> So one thing seems important at this point, when you're beginning to say "I will" and "I can," and when you're thinking along with this about whether writing is going to be the work you'll do or whether you want to do something else: it seems very important that if you do decide you want to continue to be a writer, you make sure you're doing it for *you* this time around and not doing it for him.

This comment had several aims. To begin with, it implied clearly that it is *possible* for him to write, that it's within his power. By emphasizing that he should only do it if he feels that it's for him, by talking about whether he *decides* to continue to write, the comment implies that it's not a matter of whether he *can* write but of whether he *wants* to. Similarly, by placing the discussion of the writing in the context of his earlier comments about "I will" instead of "I can't," his *activity* is also being stressed. The comment, in effect, *clears a space* for his writing. By distinguishing writing that is *his* from writing that is for his father, the comment conveys that there *is* writing that is his. It in effect *protects* or shields the writing from the conflict it had previously been caught up in. Finally, the phrase "this time around" implies that this is a fresh start, a new round, in which, potentially, the old assumptions no longer need hold sway.

THE CHALLENGE OF SUGGESTION

Common to many of the constructions I have labeled as attributional in the preceding discussion is an element of suggestion. The patient, in effect, is given a running start by already attributing to him an inclination or a capacity that it is one aim of the therapy more fully to develop. Suggestion is a concept that makes some therapists uneasy, raising concerns about the patient's autonomy and the danger of the therapist imposing her values on the patient. It is these questions and concerns I wish to take up here.

An ambivalent, if not outright negative, attitude toward suggestion is particularly strong in the psychoanalytic tradition, and this skepticism can in large measure be traced back to Freud and to the roots of his development of psychoanalysis. Psychoanalysis, it might be said, was the child of suggestion[8]; and like the Oedipal child so central in psychoanalytic narratives, it showed noteworthy hostility toward the parent from whose loins it sprang. Differentiating the "pure gold" of psycho-

---

[8]The psychoanalytic method evolved out of Freud's efforts to utilize, and then to modify, the suggestive therapies that were the dominant therapeutic approach when Freud began his practice. Influenced first by the theories of suggestion of Liebeault and Bernheim, and then by the results of Breuer's (and Anna O's) experiments with hypnosis, Freud began as a practitioner of suggestion. Over time he progressively modified his use of suggestive methods until, eventually, the psychoanalytic method he developed seemed to bear little resemblance to the approach from which it evolved. As the discussion below indicates, however, the role of suggestive influences in psychoanalysis was never as minimal as is sometimes supposed.

analysis from the supposedly inferior ministrations of the practioners of suggestion was a lifelong aim of Freud's.

As is often the case, however, Freud's own views on the matter were more open, more complex, and more honest than those of many of his followers. Although Freud could at times be quite thoroughly dismissive regarding the role of suggestion in analysis or regarding its therapeutic value more generally (see below), there were numerous instances when he acknowledged the pervasive influence of suggestion in all psychotherapy and even the necessity of explicitly and thoughtfully utilizing it if one is to obtain the best possible results. In "On Psychotherapy," for example (Freud, 1904/1959), an early paper that is of note because the question of suggestion is a particularly central concern, he states that "an element dependent on the psychical disposition of the patient enters as an accompanying factor" in all therapeutic efforts and notes that

> We have learned to use the word 'suggestion' for this phenomenon . . . . All physicians. . . are continually practising psychotherapy even when you have no intention of doing so and are not aware of it; it is disadvantageous, however, to leave entirely in the hands of the patient what the mental factor in your treatment of him shall be. In this way it is uncontrollable; it can neither be measured nor intensified. Is it not then a justifiable endeavour on the part of a physician to seek to control this factor [suggestion], to use it with a purpose, and to direct and strengthen it? *This and nothing else* is what scientific psychotherapy proposes. (Freud, 1904/1959, p. 251; italics added)

This last statement in particular ("this and nothing else") is certainly a rather striking endorsement of the central importance of suggestive influences. Other passages in the paper as well indicate Freud's appreciation of the importance and appropriateness of suggestive influences, while conveying to us as well an interesting perspective on why on other occasions he treated them less than enthusiastically. For example:

> There are many ways and means of practising psychotherapy. *All that lead to recovery are good.* Our usual word of comfort, which we dispense very liberally to our patients—"Never fear, you will soon be all right again"—corresponds to one of these psychotherapeutic methods; only, now that deeper insight has been won into the neuroses, we are no longer forced to confine ourselves to the word of comfort. We have developed the technique of hypnotic suggestion, and psychotherapy by diversion of attention, by exercise, and by eliciting suitable affects. *I despise none of these methods and would use them all under proper conditions.* If I have actually come to confine myself to one form of treatment, to the method that Breuer

called *"cathartic"* [italics in original], which I myself prefer to call "analytic," it is because I have allowed myself to be influenced by purely subjective motives. Because of the part I have played in founding this therapy, I feel a personal obligation to devote myself to closer investigation of it and to the development of its technique. (Freud, 1904/1959, p. 252; italics added)

A number of features of this passage are noteworthy. Certainly not the least of them is Freud's forthright indication of his personal motives in confining himself to what might be called the "pure form" of psychoanalysis, one in which suggestive influences are largely ruled out. In effect, he is acknowledging that the determining factor in the way he approached therapy was not necessarily what provided maximum benefit to the patient in his office; his approach reflected as well his own interests in pursuing his research and his destiny.[9]

It could be argued that Freud's less than thorough repudiation of suggestion here (at least in terms of its therapeutic value, rather than whether it accorded with his personal agenda) is reflective of this being an early paper, and that once psychoanalytic technique evolved to the point of incorporating more modern and sophisticated techniques of resistance and transference analysis, the suggestive methods lost their last measure of justification. In fact, however, roughly equivalent passages can be found throughout Freud's writings, right up to the very end.

In "The Future Prospects of Psycho-Analytic Therapy," for example (Freud, 1910/1959), he suggests that as the prestige of psychoanalysis increases, the results should improve. "I need hardly say much to you about the importance of authority. . . . The extraordinary increase in the neuroses since the power of religion has waned may give you some indication of [man's craving for authority]" (p. 290). He even declares that it is "surprising that any success was to be had at all" without reliance on the therapeutic power of suggestion.

To be sure, Freud takes these successes as a sign that there is indeed something valid above and beyond suggestion in psychoanalytic ideas. But his argument clearly implies something quite akin to what I am arguing here—that to attempt to achieve therapeutic results without at

---

[9]Freud only reluctantly, and under financial pressure, turned from a career in research to one as a practitioner. He acknowledged on a number of occasions that he was "lacking in therapeutic zeal" and that his interest in the psychoanalytic enterprise was above all an interest in the research possibilities it afforded. He argued, of course, that there was a necessary convergence between his interests as a researcher and the patient's interest in being cured. There is reason to think, however, that this fortunate harmony was considerably exaggerated (see Wachtel, 1987, Chap. 12).

all trying to harness the power of suggestion is like trying to work with one hand tied behind one's back.

Freud makes a related point in his *General Introduction to Psychoanalysis*:

> When the patient has to fight out the normal conflict with the resistances which we have discovered in him by analysis, he requires a powerful propelling force to influence him towards the decision we aim at, leading to recovery.... The outcome in this struggle is not decided by his intellectual insight—it is neither strong enough nor free enough to accomplish such a thing—but *solely* by his relationship to the physician. In so far as his transference bears the positive sign, it *clothes the physician with authority, transforms itself into faith in his findings and in his views*. Without this kind of transference or with a negative one, the physician and his arguments would never even be listened to. (Freud. 1916/1943, p. 387, italics added)

He goes on to note that this phenomenon is a universal one in human beings and is identical to that which Bernheim had earlier called suggestion. "What [Bernheim] called suggestibility is nothing else but the tendency to transference.... And we have to admit that we have only abandoned hypnosis in our methods in order to discover suggestion again in the shape of transference" (pp. 387–388).

Later in that same work, Freud further acknowledges that the analyst makes it possible for the patient to overcome his resistances "by suggestions which are in the nature of an *education*. It has been truly said therefore, that psycho-analytic treatment is a kind of *re-education*" (italics in the original). He goes on to say that by "manipulating" the transference, "it becomes possible for us to derive entirely new benefits from the power of suggestion; we are able to control it; the patient alone no longer manages his suggestibility according to his own liking, but in so far as he is amenable to its influence at all, we guide his suggestibility" (p. 392).

In these passages we see not only an open acknowledgment that suggestion, when properly used, constitutes one of the most powerful tools available to the psychotherapist, but we also have a tying of the issue of suggestion to that of transference. Increasingly for Freud these two themes were linked. In his final summation of his thoughts in *An Outline of Psychoanalysis* (Freud, 1940/1949), he puts it quite clearly. The transference relationship, he says, has the advantage that

> If the patient puts the analyst in the place of his father (or mother), he is also giving him the power which his superego exercises over his ego, since his parents were, as we know, the origin of his superego. The new super-

ego now has an opportunity for a sort of *after-education* of the neurotic; it can correct blunders for which his parental education was to blame. (Freud, 1940/1949, p. 67; italics in original)

Freud does go on to warn of the dangers of crushing the patient's independence in the process or of trying to create the patient in one's own image, and he emphasizes the importance of respecting the patient's individuality. He argues for limiting the amount of influence exerted to the minimum required by the patient's inhibitions. He adds, however, that "Many neurotics have remained so infantile that in analysis too they can only be treated as children" (Freud, 1940/1949). Freud thus not only points to the indispensibility of suggestive efforts on the analyst's part; he also, without intending to, alerts us to a factor that may be much more potent in determining whether the patient is "treated like a child" than is the willingness to acknowledge and openly employ suggestion—namely, the view that the patient somehow remains "infantile."

All this is not to say that Freud was sanguine about the role of suggestion. Indeed, determining the proper role of suggestion, both in therapeutic technique and in theorizing about what occurs in the therapeutic process, was one of the most vexing of all issues for him, an issue to which he continually returned and about which he demonstrated noteworthy inconsistency. Throughout Freud's writings one can find a tendency, often in the very same paper, on the one hand to acknowledge in surprisingly straightforward fashion the importance that suggestive influences retained even after the development of psychoanalysis, and on the other, either to sharply contrast psychoanalytic methods with suggestive ones or to hedge the role of suggestion so severely that one wonders what to make of those passages in which he treated suggestive influences as so significant.

In the 1904 paper noted above, for example, notwithstanding the passages already quoted acknowledging the centrality of suggestion in all scientific psychotherapy, Freud claims that there is "the greatest possible antithesis" between suggestive and analytic technique. The technique of suggestion, he states,

> is not concerned with the origin, strength and meaning of the morbid symptoms, but instead it superimposes something—a suggestion—and expects this to be strong enough to restrain the pathogenic idea from coming to expression. Analytic therapy, on the other hand, does not seek to add or to introduce anything new, but to take away something, to bring out something; and to this end concerns itself with the genesis of the morbid symptoms and the psychical context of the pathogenic idea which it seeks to remove. (Freud, 1904/1959, p. 254)

A similar distinction is offered in the *General Introduction*, designed in like fashion to temper the implications of his acknowledgment in that work that "we have only abandoned hypnosis in our methods in order to discover suggestion again in the shape of transference." He describes the ways in which suggestion was used at the time by those therapists who were primarily hypnotic and suggestive in their orientation and differentiates it from the use of suggestion in psychoanalysis:

> The hypnotic therapy endeavours to cover up and as it were to whitewash something going on in the mind, the analytic to lay bare and to remove something. The first works cosmetically, the second surgically. The first employs suggestion to interdict the symptoms; it reinforces the repressions, but otherwise it leaves unchanged all the processes that have led to symptom-formation. Analytic therapy takes hold deeper down nearer the roots of the disease, among the conflicts from which the symptoms proceed; it employs suggestion to change the outcome of these conflicts. (Freud, 1904/1959, p. 392)

Perhaps the clearest statement of this general approach to the problem of suggestion appears in an encyclopedia article Freud wrote in 1922. His argument in that article enables us as well to discern more clearly Freud's strategy for reconciling his wish to minimize the role of suggestion in psychoanalysis and his recognition that in fact suggestion plays a key role in *all* therapies, *including* psychoanalysis. "Psycho-analytic procedure," he wrote there,

> differs from all methods making use of suggestion, persuasion, etc., in that it does not seek to suppress by means of authority any mental phenomenon that may occur in the patient. It endeavors to trace the causation of the phenomenon and to remove it by bringing about a permanent modification in the conditions that led to it. *In psycho-analysis the suggestive influence which is inevitably exercised by the physician is diverted on to the task assigned to the patient of overcoming his resistances, that is, of carrying forward the curative process.* (Freud, 1922/1959, p. 126; italics added)

This last statement points us toward at least a partial resolution of the seemingly contradictory views about suggestion that Freud presented at different times. It indicates that it was not suggestion per se that was ruled out of psychoanalytic practice, but a *particular kind* of suggestion—that form of suggestion that it was the destiny of psychoanalysis to replace. Prior to Freud's discoveries, suggestion was primarily employed in a manner both unsophisticated and rather authoritarian. The therapist would state quite explicitly, and without any understanding of how the symptoms had come about, that they would now disappear. Sometimes, perhaps surprisingly, that would be perfectly sufficient, and the symptoms in fact would disappear. On many other occasions, however, this technique either failed to bring about the desired results or the results were only temporary. In many respects, it was this rather primitive utilization of suggestion that Freud had in mind when he distinguished psychoanalysis so sharply from suggestion and which he rightly argued psychoanalysis had replaced. In contrast, when the aim of suggestion was the pursuit of uncovering the hidden recesses of the mind and encouraging the patient to give up his defenses and resistances, Freud welcomed this powerful force as an indispensible ally.

Such a distinction would seem to offer an acceptable, and quite logical, reconciliation of the differing evaluations of the role of suggestion cited above. Indeed, in its light, the statements are not even so sharply contradictory. Suggestion is indeed an important element in any therapy, and the requirement is only to use it in a sophisticated fashion that furthers the deeper and more extensive aims of the patient and the therapy rather than the short-sighted aim of achieving merely temporary relief. From this perspective, the suggestive elements in the attributional comments described earlier in this chapter would be relatively uncontroversial. Those examples, though employing suggestive influences in a way that differs in important respects from traditional psychoanalytic practice, are also aimed at furthering the patient's efforts to come to grips with warded off experiences and inclinations, not at bolstering the repression of those tendencies.

This seeming reconciliation, however, is not quite sufficient. For Freud had still another requirement. "In every other suggestive treatment,"[10] he said, "the transference is carefully preserved and left intact; in analysis it is itself the object of the treatment and is continually being dissected in all its various forms. At the conclusion of the analysis the transference itself must be dissolved" (Freud, 1916/1943, p. 394). Something akin to this idea is influential as well among many therapists who do not think of themselves as psychoanalysts but who practice some form of interpretive or exploratory psychotherapy.

In part this requirement of dissolving the transference reflects ethical and value concerns, concerns centering on the importance of fostering the patient's autonomy, on enabling him to emerge from the therapy as a free person who makes his own decisions rather than living out an orientation to life in which irrational attachments to others

---

[10]Note here once again that the phrase "in every *other* suggestive treatment" clearly implies that psychoanalysis too is a suggestive treatment.

determine his views and choices. I have addressed this set of concerns in some detail elsewhere (Wachtel, 1977, especially Chap. 12; Wachtel, 1987, especially Chaps. 10–12). Suffice it to say for now that I believe that the formulation Freud puts forth here is neither as feasible nor as desirable as he implies. The idea of "dissolving" the transference is one of those initially appealing rhetorical tropes of which Freud was such a master. Its empirical substance, however, much less any reliable evidence for its occurrence, is not so close at hand. Moreover, if one examines carefully the basis for preferring such an outcome, it turns out to rely on a set of ideas, rooted in the highly individualistic ethos of our social and economic structure, that are far more problematic than they first appear to be (Lukes, 1973; Lux, 1990; Rieff, 1966; Schwartz, 1986; Wachtel, 1989).

Freud's Epistemological Anxieties

I wish now to turn to another, less commonly remarked upon reason for Freud's effort to present psychoanalysis as a therapy in which the role of suggestion was somehow transcended. Perhaps the most weighty factor in Freud's opposition to openly embracing the role of suggestion was epistemological—indeed, one would not be exaggerating very much to refer to his concerns in this regard as *epistemological anxieties*. In the very paragraph in which he ends up arguing that the transference is "dissolved" at the end of the analysis, Freud takes up quite explicitly the challenge that "regardless of whether the driving force behind the analysis is called transference or suggestion, the danger still remains that our influence upon the patient may bring the objective certainty of our discoveries into doubt; and that what is an advantage in therapy is harmful in research."[11] He notes further that if this claim were justified, "psycho-analysis, after all would be nothing else but a specially well-disguised and particularly effective kind of suggestive treatment; and all its conclusions about the experiences of the patient's past life, mental dynamics, the unconscious, and so on, could be taken very lightly" (Freud, 1916/1943). This, clearly, is Freud's real nightmare.

The apparent inconsistencies in Freud's view of suggestion and the evident struggles discernible in his efforts to come to grips with it can be best understood, I believe, if we recognize that Freud was struggling with two quite different implications of suggestion, one therapeutic and

---

[11]Note here again the implicit acknowledgment that the employment of suggestion *is* indeed an advantage in the therapy.

one essentially epistemological. As the passages cited earlier indicate, Freud was too honest and perceptive an observer to deny the highly significant role of suggestion in psychotherapeutic change. Though he endeavored to develop a therapeutic method that was more than *mere* suggestion (and succeeded in this endeavor quite considerably, I believe), he could not—as much as he wished to—consistently argue that he had *replaced* or *eliminated* suggestion as a therapeutic force. The most he could do was to claim that he had *harnessed* it, that he had turned it to the purposes of analysis: to uncover the hidden and rejected portions of the psyche and overcome the resistances, rather than to bolster those resistances and achieve relief at the price of once again burying what was struggling to come to light.

From the perspective of the *therapeutic* function of psychoanalysis, such a recasting of the role of suggestion in analysis was quite enough for Freud; as we have seen, on those occasions when he was directing his attention to the therapeutic process, he was inclined to give suggestion its due. But being a psychotherapist was never the central core of Freud's professional identity. As numerous observers (including Freud himself) have noted, Freud's commitment to psychoanalysis as a method of *research* was much stronger than his therapeutic zeal. It was most of all as a researcher and as a theorist, as a discoverer of new facts about the mind, that Freud hoped for immortality, and it was on these grounds that he experienced suggestion as a specially dangerous and alien presence.

If we can appreciate how strong a threat suggestion was to the veracity of the data of Freud's new science, how powerful was the motivation on *these* grounds for disavowing the suggestive elements in the method that was simultaneously his therapeutic and research tool, we may be in a position to reassimilate what he himself had recognized (albeit never without considerable discomfort and ambivalence) about the considerable role suggestion plays in the therapeutic effectiveness of his method.

We may then conclude, following Freud, that suggestion is an almost inevitable element in all psychotherapeutic efforts, certainly in those that are successful. But we may further note that the development of psychoanalysis—and later of other modern therapies derived both from psychoanalysis and from other sources—opened up possibilities for incorporating suggestions into an entirely new context, changing their use in ways that made old distinctions anachronistic. Rather than simply suggesting away the symptoms that brought the patient to treatment, the suggestive element in modern psychotherapies (whether implicit or explicit) is employed in a wide range of ways to enable the patient to confront the conflictual issues in his life. As depicted earlier in this chapter, for example, the patient can be helped temporarily to gain the confidence to face what he has fearfully avoided or to take the steps necessary to change a troubling life pattern. The initial pivot of change includes suggestion as a central element; but if the therapy is grounded properly, the processes brought into play by the actions initiated with the aid of suggestion create changed psychic circumstances that are independent of the original suggestive influence. Once the patient starts moving in a direction that furthers his psychological growth, new forces come into play differing from those that led to that movement.

One may see a parallel here to Freud's claim that the suggestive element in the transference is dissolved by the end of treatment, but the parallel is a loose one. It is not through interpreting the suggestive element itself that it is transcended. It is that the changes initiated have further consequences that enable consolidation of the improvement to proceed. In this, the interlocking set of processes that have been addressed throughout this book again must be taken into account.

The psychological import of suggestion is not fully appreciated from within a strictly intrapsychic model. Viewed interpersonally, suggestions can be understood as a way of *initiating* a process that *then* gets maintained by its effectiveness in eliciting new and different responses from other people in the patient's life. This in turn contributes to further intrapsychic changes in the patient or to preserving those changes that have accrued. It is in this sense most of all that the effects of suggestion are transcended, to be replaced by the forces that, in any life, are responsible for sustaining psychological structures and patterns of interaction and relationship. Without an appreciation of this transactional dimension, understanding of the suggestive element in the therapy is limited and distorted.

Predictive Interpretations and Tacit Knowledge

Suggestions can be understood as essentially *predictive interpretations*, interpretations directed toward inclinations or possibilities in the patient that have not yet found adequate expression. Not just any prediction, however, can be effective; the suggestion will only have a chance of being met by a positive response on the patient's part if it is in fact a reasonably accurate interpretation of the patient's potential experience. A suggestion that is not rooted in an understanding of the patient's conflicted inclinations will have little impact. Fears that attending to the suggestive dimension of the therapeutic interaction in the way described earlier in this chapter will somehow rob the patient of his autonomy actually do the patient a disservice; they show insufficient respect for the individual's ability to resist directives that do not accord in some way with his own real, if as yet unrealized, dispositions. Indeed, even in hypnosis, much less in the context of the gentle and empathic suggestions advocated here, there is evidence that suggestions that are not consonant with the individual's own value system are rejected (Orne, 1972; Orne & Evans, 1965).

In some ways, this argument for the legitimacy of attending explicitly to the suggestive dimension in therapeutic practice dovetails with considerations offered by Freud as a further part of his defense of the epistemological foundations of psychoanalytic discoveries. Addressing the possibility that suggestive influences might account for the findings of psychoanalysis, Freud argued that "[a]ny danger of falsifying the products of a patient's memory by suggestion can be avoided by prudent handling of the technique; but in general the arousing of resistances is a guarantee against the misleading effects of suggestive influence" (Freud, 1922/1959, p. 126). In his paper "Constructions in Analysis" (Freud, 1938/1959), he further argues that "the danger of our leading a patient astray by suggestion, by persuading him to accept things which we ourselves believe but which he ought not to, has certainly been enormously exaggerated. An analyst would have had to behave very incorrectly before such a misfortune could overtake him" (pp. 363–364).

Resistance, one might say, has a silver lining. Although it can be a powerful impediment to therapeutic progress, it is also in a sense a guarantor of the legitimacy of the process. Patients are far from putty in the hands of the therapist. And if the therapist's efforts are at cross purposes with those of the patient, her efforts will be ineffective but are unlikely to move the patient very far in a direction he does not wish to go.

Perhaps one of the most useful ways to think of the suggestive dimension of therapists' comments is in terms of the philospher Michael Polanyi's notion of tacit knowledge (Polanyi, 1958, 1966). In offering attributional interpretations, we are helping give shape to an urge or tendency that is *in process*, that is *becoming* something but is as yet still partly inchoate, or as Polanyi might put it, that is as yet tacit. As therapists we help to give voice to those implicit dimensions of the patient's experience, and in doing so we contribute to the shape that they take. But the basic architecture is always supplied by the patient.

Taking this a step further, and consistent with the view guiding the entire approach described in this book, our attempt to give voice to the patient's tacit inclinations is paralleled by an effort to help the patient also find *actions* that can further define and develop his evolving sense of how he wants to be in the world. Thus, the suggestive dimension described in this chapter can be seen as part of a broader attempt to aid the patient in shaping his life in accord with his continually changing and emerging sense of self.

CHAPTER 10

Reframing, Relabeling, and Paradox

The difficulties that bring people to therapy derive in large measure from the ways they interpret and give meaning to the events of their lives. Correspondingly, much of what contributes to the resolution of these difficulties involves helping them to create *new* meanings, to find different ways of making sense of their experiences and, as a result, new possibilities for adaptive action. The therapeutic interventions that fall under the rubric of reframing or relabeling are designed to promote just such creating of new meanings.

The concept of reframing has been especially prominent in the work of therapists operating from a family systems perspective, though it will be apparent as we proceed that important developments in contemporary psychoanalytic practice are rooted in a somewhat similar outlook. In its systemic applications, reframing tends to be based on a pragmatic view of interpersonal reality. Rather than emphasizing the dimension of self-deception (with its implicit corollary that when the self-deception is overcome the patient will be more in touch with the truth of his life), this work stresses the multiple nature of truth itself. That is, it is assumed that at best we can only grasp partial truths about interpersonal reality, and that the primary source of psychological difficulties is not so much that we operate under a false rather than a true picture of psychological events as that the particular partial truth we have constructed is one that perpetuates rather than resolves the dilemmas we face.

Watzlawick, Weakland, and Fisch (1974), for example, argue that our view of reality is never a simple matter of what is "out there"; it depends ultimately on how we define and make sense of what occurs. With homage to Saint-Exupery, they note that truth "is not what we discover, but what we create." This position closely parallels Whorf's in his classic work *Language, Thought, and Reality* (1956): "The categories and types that we isolate from the world of phenomena we do not find there because they stare every observer in the face; on the contrary, the world is presented in a kaleidoscopic flux of impressions which has to be organized by our minds" (p. 213).

Indeed, it is a central feature of intellectual life in the late 20th century—extending well beyond the confines of the therapist's office into literary studies, philosophy, history, and social thought—to point out in one way or another the social *construction* of reality and to challenge the positivist and objectivist notions that are often implicit in accounts of interpretation as a process of "discovery" (see, for example, Berger & Luckman, 1966; Gergen, 1985; Harre, 1986; Heller, Sosna, & Wellbery, 1986; Hoffman, 1991; Messer, Sass, & Woolfolk, 1988; Rabinow & Sullivan, 1979; Rorty, 1979).

In one sense, a reframing of the patient's experience is very much like an interpretation. Both terms refer to efforts to state the facts of experience and their connections in such a way that the patient can see something he did not see before, or see what he has already seen from a different vantage point. In practice, however, the two terms can have significantly different implications. The concept of interpretation, although currently employed in a variety of therapeutic traditions, derives from Freud's efforts to find the hidden meanings behind the manifest actions and communications that the patient presents. Interpretation, as it is usually undertaken, is a *convergent* process. That is, interpretations are thought to become increasingly accurate as the work proceeds, to *converge* toward the true or real meaning that has been disguised by the defenses and resistances. Interpretation tends to be undertaken with the intention of illuminating what is "really" going on.

Reframing, in contrast, tends to be approached from a more constructivist view of reality. Rather than attempting to find the "true" meaning of a pattern of behavior, therapists employing reframing seek the *most useful* way of understanding that pattern. Their epistemological presumptions are *divergent* rather than convergent. That is, there are presumed to be *multiple* meanings to any given pattern, many different ways of construing and understanding.

It is not that the use of reframing reflects a lack of interest in the truth. Both interpretation and reframing may be viewed as truth-seeking processes. But they derive from different epistemologies. Proponents of reframing see truth as multiple and perspectival; one constructs the truth rather than piercing through to it. In some instances, one might think of the use of reframing as similar to what trial lawyers do when they piece together the facts to suit their purpose. One looks at all the evidence and says, in effect, "I know it has looked to you that such and such is the case, but let me show you a different way of putting all this together, one that makes things look rather different."[1]

The above considerations notwithstanding, it is important to be clear that interpreting and reframing are not really sharply distinguishable activities. The preference of some therapists to describe what they are doing as intepreting and others to depict themselves as reframing can reflect semantic preferences or allegiances to different groups and traditions rather than any fundamental difference in strategy or conceptualization. Merton Gill's approach to interpretation, for example, is in large measure a perspectival one, an effort to present "plausible" alternatives to the patient's way of construing his experience (e.g., Gill, 1982, 1983). His explicit acknowledgement of the multiplicity of perspectives from which the patient's experiences can be be understood, indeed his embrace of this multiplicity, has a noteworthy kinship to some of what we will examine here under the rubric of reframing. (It will also be apparent, however, to those familiar with Gill's work, that there are ways in which his approach differs very substantially from much of what is described in this chapter.)

Spence's writings (e.g., Spence, 1982, 1987) similarly illustrate the difficulties in easily distinguishing between interpretation and reframing. Spence too writes from the point of view of the psychoanalytic tradition, with its venerable emphasis on interpretation; but he adopts a view of the process of interpretation in psychoanalysis that accords in large measure with the epistemological perspective shared by leading proponents of the notion of reframing. In Spence's view, when we offer the patient an interpretation,

> we are finding a narrative home for an anomolous happening. We are using language to clothe this event in respectability and take away some of its strangeness and mystery, and by fitting the language into the patient's life story, we are giving it a narrative home. The linguistic and narrative aspects of an interpretation may well have priority over its historical truth. . . . An interpretation satisfies because we are able to contain an unfinished piece of reality in a meaningful sentence. (Spence, 1982, p. 137)

---

[1] I offer this analogy only very tentatively. Despite having a number of very close friends who are lawyers, I have not been persuaded that the efforts of attorneys operating under the adversary system have much to do with truth-seeking. Indeed, in many instances it seems to me more accurate to say that lawyers are paid to *disguise* or *distort* the truth. Therapy, however, is not—or should not be—an adversarial activity, and so the skillful mustering of observations to "make a case," to ask the question *might it not instead be the case that. . . ?* seems to me less suspect in the therapeutic context.

Spence's criteria for judging interpretations are largely aesthetic and pragmatic. If it holds together well, if it conveys a new understanding of the patient's life that is persuasive to the patient and helps him gain a greater feeling of coherence and a revisioning of his life story that opens new possibilities, it is a good interpretation. That it is not the one true story is not a flaw but a necessity. Our lives permit of many narratives. Consequently, according to Spence, "it seems more appropriate to conceive of an interpretation as a *construction*—a creative proposition—rather than as a *reconstruction* that is supposed to correspond to something in the past" (Spence, 1982, p. 35; italics in original). This by no means implies that interpretations are arbitrary or "fictions." Spence is centrally concerned, in fact, with detailing the criteria that distinguish adequate from inadequate interpretations. But in his emphasis on the aesthetic and pragmatic dimension of interpretations, in his view that the interpretation is "first of all, a means to an end," which "may become true for the first time just by being said," he evidences an epistemological position that shares significant commonalities with the stance more customarily associated with proponents of reframing.

Although there is nothing intrinsic about the concept of reframing that requires reframings to be "positive," in practice this is most often the case. Reframings are often an alternative route to the process of building on the patient's strengths described particularly in Chapter 7, but of concern throughout this book. This does not mean that reframings are the voice of Pollyanna, sentimentally offering an unearned optimism closer to the "spin" of the insincere politician than to the unflinching perceptions of the seeker after truth. Rather, positive reframings are paths *back to* reality, illuminated by the therapist for the patient who has wandered in the darkness of self-deceiving or self-limiting negativism. Put differently, reframings are ways of giving meaning to psychological events that point to potential solutions to dilemmas that have been construed in a way that renders solution impossible.

As I have discussed in a number of ways in earlier chapters, it is certainly the case that patients must frequently face unpleasant truths that they have shrunk from for years at a psychic cost that is in total greater than the cost of open eyes. But equally often, it is the very way in which the truths of the patient's life have been subjectively constructed that makes them seem so impossible to face. When reframed, reality often can be more readily braved, and a way of life pursued that requires *less* of the denial and distortion that it is the aim of psychotherapy to counter.

In my own practice, reframing is rarely an isolated intervention, but is rather part of a more extended effort to help the patient come to grips with the conflicts and binds that have been at the root of his problems. The following excerpt illustrates how reframing fits into a larger therapeutic strategy that, in this case, included pointing out to the patient the contradictions and vicious circles associated with his orientation toward pleasing others. The reader may notice as well that it illustrates how a cyclical psychodynamic analysis addresses such concepts as the true and false self in a fashion that emphasizes how true- and false-self experiences are linked to actions and transactions in the real world.

Grant, a 44-year-old corporate executive, had struggled all his life to be successful and, even more, to be appreciated. The event leading up to the therapeutic work described below was Grant's failure to receive a promotion he felt he deserved. He had worked very hard for the company, and the subdivision he headed had outperformed most of the others in recent years. When he inquired as to why he had not received the promotion he anticipated, he got feedback indicating that he had been too self-promoting, that in effect his very effort to be recognized had gotten in the way of his getting the recognition he wanted. He had indeed made an effort to let those above him know how much he had done for the company and how successful his efforts had been, but he felt he had done so in a low-key, "nice" way, and he felt hurt and humiliated not only at being passed over for the promotion but at the perception that he was tooting his own horn too loudly.[2]

Prior to the excerpt described here, Grant had been discussing his feelings about this rebuff and his conflict between, on the one hand, trying simply to be more self-accepting and to let more of himself come through regardless of the impression it might make, and on the other, striving to make people notice him by his sophistication and his achievements. His way of putting it is illustrated in the following sequence, which also includes my response and a portion of the ensuing dialogue:

PATIENT: Of course you'd rather just everyone say "you're a good guy and we all think you're terrific." But if that doesn't happen, or if you can't accept that as enough, then at least you want the recognition. To me it seems that if your parents give you that kind of undemanding

---

[2]Judging from my own experience of Grant, as well as from the descriptions of his interactions with others that came up in the therapy, it seemed to me too that he was not an overtly pushy or aggressive person—indeed, that he was someone who, notwithstanding his efforts to be recognized as a "success," tended even more to strive to please and be well-liked—but apparently, in the context of the culture of this particular corporation, he was perceived as not enough of a team player.

love, unconditional love, then you don't look for it so much later in life; you're able to deal with life as it comes. But if the love is highly conditional, as my parents' was, then you strive for whatever it is that your parents demanded. Partly you strive for it and partly you rebel against it. So some people become the biggest deal maker, and others become totally dysfunctional and rebel like my friend Joe; and I'm kind of some of both. Some days I'm Donald Trump, some days I'm my friend Joe. But the point is that when you're Donald Trump on your Donald Trump days, you want *Time* magazine to do a piece on you and say you're the biggest deal maker in America. Why? Because it was a pretty bad bargain that you had to be a big shot, you had to be an A student to get any recognition as a son, but at least that was the bargain. So if you become an A student, you don't then want to be told that "Well, now it's a different test, today the test is you have to be the best swimmer." So I think that's what it is. But knowing that doesn't seem to help me.

THERAPIST: I think one piece getting in the way is that you're caught in another one of those vicious circles we've talked about. It goes back to the question I asked earlier: If you put aside what will get you the most recognition, what is it that really feels most like you, most like what you really want to do? And you answered, I think very honestly and accurately, that you're not sure, that that's hard to know.

[*Describing Grant's saying he wasn't sure what he wanted to do as "honest and accurate" is, of course, supportive. It also, as will become more apparent shortly, is the first step in the reframing that is the focus of this therapeutic vignette. We may also note that the phrase "one piece" used to introduce the comment breaks up the issues Grant must deal with into manageable chunks. Apropos Chapter 9, we may note an element of attribution or suggestion to it as well. It implies a step-by-step process the the patient will be able to handle.*]

PATIENT: Right

THERAPIST: But what happens is it's hard to know *because* you're looking so much for the cues as to "what will get me approval?" and so on.

PATIENT: Absolutely! That's what ruins these meetings for me.

THERAPIST: And then you're very much at the mercy of other people; and I think it's part of why you're often worried about being jerked around, whether it's in a restaurant or at a meeting or even in a taxi. [*The patient had frequently referred to feeling "jerked around" by people who didn't show him sufficient respect.*] And I think part of what happens is that people can jerk you around without even intending to, because you're looking so much out there, you're so focused on what they think. And then, because you don't have such a clear sense from inside, you have to look out there again, and it further keeps you from knowing what's going on inside, and so the whole pattern keeps itself going.

PATIENT: Right. It always goes back to what you've been saying: "Who's the real Grant?" We can't seem to unravel it enough to know.

THERAPIST: Well maybe the problem is that you don't hear that question as a real question on my part, something I'm interested in knowing. Instead it feels like just one more test. I think what happens is that when you hear that question, you become a little anxious, a little apologetic, because you think you're supposed to know the answer. And so it changes into another test. So let's just try to figure out together [*collaboration*] how we can move into that question *without* it being a test. We both know [*shared attribution*] that you're not sure of the answer to that, you're kind of feeling your way into the answer to that. [*"feeling your way into" restates the situation in a way that depicts him as more active and implies some motion is already being achieved.*] So one answer to the question is that the first step in *being* in touch with the real Grant is that the real Grant is at this moment confused. And that that confusion is real. [*In acknowledging this about his confusion, the main reframing of this vignette begins.*] I think what usually happens is that the confusion feels to you like something shameful, something contemptible, something that needs to be evaded.

PATIENT: That's true.

THERAPIST: If instead you recognize that the confusion itself is at this moment a real part of the real Grant, that's our first contact, our point of contact, with what is truly Grant rather than Grant trying to be for others or be what he's "supposed to be."

This last comment completes the main reframing in this sequence. Grant's confusion, which he had experienced as a failing, as one more reason to get down on himself, is now reframed as something real and genuine about him, and therefore worthy of paying attention to. Previously his shame over the confusion led him quickly to turn away from it, with the consequence that he was further alienated from his own experience and further driven instead to look for cues from others as to what he *should* be feeling and striving for. The result of such efforts was a heightening of his feelings of rudderlessness, as he drifted first toward one external directive, then toward another. Ironically, his retreat from the sense of confusion maintained it, whereas the opportunity the reframing provided to embrace the confusion has the potential to diminish it. In accepting his confusion about what he is experiencing, and even valuing it as itself a genuine expression of who he is, Grant thereby puts himself on the road toward greater clarity and self-integrity.

We may further note that in this comment the confusion is framed as what is true of him "at this moment." Thus there is also an attributional element to the comment: the confusion is real, but temporary; movement toward a less confused state is both possible and likely.

In what followed, Grant spontaneously, and in a manner that seemed genuinely insightful and deeply felt, spoke about how much of what he does in his life seems to be a version of pleasing his mother. He also examined, in much greater detail than he had previously, how, as he put it, "I hide the aggressive me by putting another me over it, and then I hide the *less* aggressive me by putting a *more* aggresive me over it, and all I get is a lot of confusion but very little feeling of accomplishment *or* being liked." Able, at least for the moment, to *look* at his experience of confusion, rather than immediately taking flight into doing something to suppress or cover it, Grant apparently was able to see with greater clarity a central dynamic in his difficulties.

Reframings can also be used to help point the patient toward action and may contain a suggestive element similar to that of the attributional comments discussed in the last chapter. The reader may recall the case of William, discussed in Chapter 6, in which the therapist asked, *What makes it hard to tell your wife you read her diary?* We noted then that the question, by implying that it should not be hard, was implicitly accusatory, and we examined an alternative: *I guess at this point it feels kind of difficult to bring it up.* In the present context, we consider a further variation in that series that is closely related to the central theme of this chapter. The variant I want to consider here is: *It's going to take a lot of courage for you to discuss the diary with your wife.*

Far from implying that the patient's hesitancy to bring the matter up is puzzling (as, subtly, the original question did), this last comment further underlines the therapist's appreciation that it is not at all easy to raise such a matter, especially given the surreptitious nature of what had gone before. The comment reframes the patient's experience to emphasize the courage that would be reflected in his taking action rather than the avoidance he had manifested previously. In this framing, the courage is figure and the avoidance ground. His previous avoidance is acknowledged and accepted (and indeed will later be further explored, when William can approach it from the vantage point of a greater sense of self-worth); it is not, however, taken as a sign of his character or his destiny, both of which are seen as being constructed in the choices he is now in the process of making.

The comment may also be seen as having an attributional dimension of the sort described in Chapter 9. It attributes to the patient an inclination to address matters that he still has not fully given voice to. In saying it is "*going to*" take courage, the comment conveys confidence that the patient *will* take the step, and it frames it in such a way that the patient can feel courageous when he does so.

REFRAMING AND UNDERSTANDING THE OTHER

Perhaps reflecting its close associations with family therapy approaches, reframing is frequently employed to help patients gain a new perspective on the behavior of other people in their lives. It thus is well suited for a therapeutic approach rooted in appreciation of the crucial role of vicious circles and in analysis of the ways in which people mutually maintain patterns of interaction that are problematic for each of them. The changed perspective afforded by effective reframings can contribute to enabling the patient to behave differently toward the other and thereby to disrupt the cyclical pattern in which both are caught.

In the case of a patient I shall call Marie, for example, the reframing focused only indirectly on providing another way of looking at her own experience. The primary focus of the reframing was on the experience of her husband. By reinterpreting what *his* experience might be, the therapist hoped that Marie might be able to begin participating with him in a way that differed from the dance of withdrawal whose steps they both had learned all too well.

Marie entered therapy because of feelings of shyness and insecurity, but as the work proceeded, she complained as well about feeling that she and her husband Charles were not as close as she wished they were. It seemed to Marie that Charles was not that interested in her, and she felt hurt and helpless. Charles indeed did seem to withdraw into his work a good deal, and he tended to spend his free time with his friends rather than with Marie. As I began to hear the story more fully, however, it seemed to me likely that Charles felt as hurt as Marie did, and that from his perspective his distancing was in response to distancing by her.

The first opportunity to introduce this perspective came in the process of exploring what their fights were usually about. Marie mentioned that it was usually Charles who initiated them by complaining that he didn't feel cared for by Marie, that he felt she didn't really need him or that she wasn't really there for him. I pointed out to Marie that she usually thought of Charles as not caring, as not being interested in her since he spent so much time away from her, but that *It sounds like he cares a lot about the relationship but easily feels hurt and not taken care of.*[3] *It's hard for you to see this because he deals with the hurt by withdrawing, and so, understandably, it looks to you like he's not very interested in you.*

A further opportunity to convey something of this perspective arose when Marie described an occasion in which Charles went with his friends to a ballgame instead of accompanying Marie to a party being given by a co-worker at her new job. Here the therapist said: *I certainly understand why you felt hurt and angry at Charles's not accompanying you. But I'm thinking of the picture we're beginning to get of Charles as someone who is easily wounded. I wonder if we might take his withdrawal here not as a sign of his not caring but as a sign that he felt hurt. Can you tell me a bit about what led up to this situation?*

As we inquired into the antecedents of this situation, it turned out that Charles and Marie had had a fight shortly before Charles had gotten the call from his friend inviting him to go to the ballgame, and one of the issues in the fight was, again, that Charles felt that Marie wasn't there for him. Marie hadn't really taken this claim by Charles very seriously because her experience was so strongly that the opposite was the case. But as we discussed it further, she began to see ways in which it might feel quite different to Charles. One of the ways that Marie had developed over the years to cover her feelings of insecurity was to strive very hard to look cool and unflappable. And even with Charles, she rarely felt free to show feelings of hurt or upset. Fearing she would appear too "clingy" and "dependent," she strove to appear self-sufficient, and at times she succeeded all too well: Charles, it began to be clear, experienced her as not needing him very much at all. Moreover, because she didn't want to appear to be a nag, and because she felt humiliated showing feelings of hurt, she tended to respond to Charles's withdrawals by withdrawing herself. (From Charles's perspective, of course, the sequence was reversed: he withdrew in response to *her* withdrawal.)

[3]In saying that Charles "easily" feels hurt and not taken care of, the comment provisionally shifts the responsibility away from Marie and toward Charles's sensitivity to this issue. It contributes to Marie's being able to hear this alternative without having to feel that Charles has good reason to feel hurt and not taken care of. It thus resembles what I called in Chapter 6 "externalization in the service of the therapy." As the work proceeded, we concentrated more on exploring Marie's role in how Charles felt. By explicating the vicious circle in which the two of them were caught, it was possible gradually to enable Marie to see her participation in the pattern without her feeling that it was "her fault."

When, shortly after the fight, Charles got a call from his friend indicating that he had unexpectedly gotten tickets to the ballgame, he said to Marie that he would go to the party "if you really want me to," but that he thought "you'll do fine without me." Marie's response, which she said she made in a cool and aloof tone, was "I'd prefer if you went with me, but if you don't I'll enjoy myself anyway." Her more private thought, however, was "What kind of marriage is this anyway? We're like ships passing in the night." I commented, *I can understand very well your feeling that, and also why you'd feel hurt and angry. But I wonder if there's an irony here. I have a hunch that Charles too feels upset that you're like ships passing in the night. From everything you've described about him, he seems to me to be kind of a sensitive guy who feels hurt pretty easily but doesn't know what to do with it. He seems to deal with feeling hurt in much the same way you do; he withdraws and feels he has to hide how hurt and vulnerable he feels. I think his withdrawal could be a sign that he feels hurt rather than that he's not interested.*

Marie was surprised to find herself feeling more sympathetic to Charles after this discussion and felt that it would be easier for her to reach out to him next time and let him know that she really wanted and needed him to be with her. She realized that when she thought of herself as chasing after him, and of him as reluctant to spend time with her, it felt humiliating to her to expose her neediness. As a consequence of this she had acted aloof and indifferent, thereby maintaining or exacerbating the pattern of mutual withdrawal. With the aid of the reframing, she could feel she was doing something *for him* when she expressed her need for him. She could, in effect, think of *him* as the needy one, even if she were the one who actually was saying "please."[4] As a consequence, conveying more openly her wish to spend time with her husband and acknowledging that she felt better about herself when he accompanied her, didn't seem as humiliating.

This is the sort of shift in perspective one hopes for in response to a reframing. In effect, Marie responded by spontaneously reframing her own behavior, turning it from a sign of neediness and weakness on her part to an attentiveness to *Charles's* needs. As our exploration of this theme proceeded, Marie was also able to see how her not wanting to appear to Charles as nagging or clinging could leave him feeling she really didn't care. She could recognize that indeed he probably did not

---

[4]Clearly this attitude would have to be only a transitional one if the relationship were to prove to be truly satisfactory. A good relationship must be built on mutual respect, not covertly seeing the other as "needy." But the change described here was an important way station on the path toward a more fully satisfying relationship, and for Marie it seemed that that path had to pass through this point.

like to be nagged but that he found her apparent equanimity in the face of their not connecting even more disturbing.

Another case in which a reframing of the other person's behavior proved useful involved Bret, whose wife experienced considerable social anxiety with people she did not know well. As a consequence of the anxiety, Bret's wife was hesitant to go to parties, and when she did, she stuck very close to him in a way that he labeled as "clingy." Bret was quite bothered by this behavior, and it was a source of considerable conflict in their marriage. At the same time, Bret found himself troubled by his attitude toward his wife, whom he loved and enjoyed being with when they were alone together. The reframing that seemed to be very helpful to Bret was: *Your wife seems to feel most relaxed when she's alone with you.*

It is interesting to note that the comment simply restated what Bret had been describing, but from the opposite vantage point. One could equally describe Bret's wife as *less* comfortable with strangers, or as *more* comfortable alone with him. But although the two ways of framing the facts were logical equivalents, they were not at all equivalent psychologically. The second vantage point highlighted a different meaning to the behavior and had different implications for their relationship. Moreover, by interrupting the pattern of bickering that had developed between them about this issue, the reframing created space for a different equilibrium to develop and for them to renegotiate how they would deal with their differing experiences of social occasions.[5]

REFRAMING IN THE THERAPEUTIC RELATIONSHIP

Reframings can be employed not only in reinterpreting the patient's experiences in relation to his spouse, friends, parents, and other such "external" figures; they can readily be incorporated as well into efforts to help the patient gain a new understanding of what is transpiring between patient and therapist. Indeed these are often among the most useful reframings one can employ and can greatly aid the process by which the events in the therapeutic relationship serve as a fulcrum for change.

---

[5]As the reader might speculate, at another point Bret's own conflicts over "clinginess" versus bravely venturing forth became a topic of discussion, and Bret began to recognize ways in which he had dealt with his own conflicts through his feelings about his wife (in psychoanalytic terminology, through projection and projective identification).

Consider, for example, the case of Michael, who engaged in seemingly endless repetitions of the same complaints over and over. The repetitiveness and closed, conclusory quality of Michael's monologues, in which he seemed to have little interest in input from the therapist and little inclination to examine in any way what he was repeating, rendered the therapy lifeless and ineffective. Numerous attempts to invite Michael to explore marginal thoughts or to be alert to unexpected associations met with little success. Michael would announce that what he had just said *was* what came to mind and that nothing else had occurred to him.

The sequence to be described here seemed to be a significant turning point in the work. It began with a fairly traditional transference interpretation. But as the reader will see, the followup to this interpretation included a series of further statements by the therapist that were more in the nature of positive reframings—reframings, however, that were directed toward the events in the room. Michael had been telling the therapist that his boss always wanted things done exactly his way, and he had been indirectly implying that he subtly sabotaged the boss's directives by being overly literal in following them. The therapist commented that perhaps something similar was happening in the therapy. Perhaps, he suggested, Michael felt that the therapist too was imposing his way of doing things in the way the therapy was conducted, and Michael resented the feeling that he had to conform to the therapist's regime.[6]

Michael was very receptive to this interpretation, and his conversational style in the rest of the session showed a greater reflectiveness and openness than had been characteristic of his participation previously. He also saw clearly that he had experienced the therapist's request that he pay attention to marginal thoughts as a demand that he relinquish his own highly logical style and proceed in a fashion that conformed to the therapist's needs and preferences. This felt both like a submission and like a threat to his ability to feel he had control over his own thoughts.

A bit later in the session, Michael stated that something had just

---

[6]The therapist also had in mind that Michael's way of filling the session with a deadening display of diligence, and then explaining that "I'm just doing what you asked; I'm telling you what comes into my mind," was a similar instance of sabotage through seeming compliance with what was requested. He did not comment directly about this pattern and its meaning at this point, however, feeling that it would be experienced by Michael as a criticism. Conveying understanding of Michael's resentment at what he experienced as the imposition of another's style seemed more likely to enable Michael to feel it was safe to take a step forward.

occurred to him, but it was something he didn't want to tell the therapist about. Rather than commenting on the resistance dimension of what had just transpired, the therapist instead offered a comment that reframed what Michael had said in a positive way. He told Michael that he had just done something quite important: Michael had made room for himself in the therapy; he had asserted that he could have some control over how the session proceeded and did not have to conform totally to what the therapist wanted. The therapist also pointed out that by Michael's saying directly that he didn't *want* to tell the therapist what he had thought, he had been able to achieve his aim without paying the price of appearing helpless. This was quite different from what Michael used to say all the time, which was that nothing had occurred to him.

Michael did not, of course, entirely overcome his hesitancy to share his thoughts as a result of this one comment, nor indeed did he henceforth invariably recognize that thoughts were occurring to him. The comment did seem to contribute to improvement in Michael's ability to participate in the therapeutic process, but as is usually the case, it was often a matter of two steps forward and one step back. There were still times when Michael rambled on in a way that allowed no reflection or no new input, and still times when, asked about marginal thoughts, he said he had none. Michael did seem more receptive, however, to comments by the therapist that perhaps a thought had occurred to him that he simply didn't want to talk about.

At one point a few sessions later, Michael commented, in the midst of another obsessively bounded narrative, that the only thought that had popped into his head while telling his story was that he had no marginal thoughts to tell the therapist. He added that he hadn't felt it was worthwhile interrupting what he was saying to report this. The therapist responded that Michael's thought about not having any marginal thoughts was itself a marginal thought and that it was as valuable and useful as any other. He expressed appreciation that Michael indeed *had* told him about having the thought, and wondered aloud if there had been other such thoughts as well in the past that Michael had felt weren't worth relating.

This reframing regarding the value of Michael's thought about not having marginal thoughts led to an important exploration of Michael's fears that his efforts would be regarded as not good enough and to his recollections of having grown up with many exacting demands and few indications that he had satisfied them or had gained any respect for what he had done. He was able to discuss as well, in a fashion that represented a considerable advance in insight and frankness, that he had taken to hiding rather than risk the ridicule he thought would follow if he really opened up to people.[7]

PARADOX

I wish now to turn to the element of paradox that is frequently evident in efforts at reframing. The meanings and formulations of some of them may seem a bit odd, not quite in keeping with the way we usually think about the causes and consequences of human action. That, of course, is precisely their intention. They are ways of looking at things *differently*, ways of reorganizing our view of matters in order that we may be more able to see our way out of the locked-in perceptions that have kept us steadfastly on a self-defeating course.

Paradox is not necessarily limited to reframings, though the two are not infrequently companion perspectives. Paradox has been employed by therapists from a wide variety of orientations, and there are elements of paradox tucked into many fairly common and familiar clinical maneuvers. Greenson (1967), for example, in his text on psychoanalytic technique, discusses instances where the patient declares there is something he cannot and will not tell the analyst. He suggests that the analyst say something like: *Don't tell me what your secret is, but tell me why you can't tell me about it,* or *How would you feel if you did tell me about it?* Such inquiries go around the resistance temporarily and enable the patient to initiate exploration of a topic he has declared he cannot explore.

It is but a short distance from this kind of inquiry to one more frankly paradoxical, such as *What would you tell me if you <u>could</u> tell me?* Remarkably enough, patients who have previously declared their inability and unwillingness to communicate regarding some matter or another sometimes do so in response to such a (seemingly absurd or contradictory) request. The key to the effectiveness of such an inquiry (and, I suspect, the key to most effective paradoxical communications in therapy) is that the patient is in conflict. In this instance, the very fact that the patient has *informed* us that there is something he won't tell suggests that there is also a wish *to* tell. The *What would you tell me if you could?* serves in effect as a kind of releaser, shifting slightly the balance

---

[7]Once again, it must be emphasized that this painfully conflicted and constricted man did not magically change in a trice after this sequence. There were many further advances and regressions. But the exchange described here did seem to be an important moment in the overall process toward change, and I believe that the positive reframing played a significant role.

between the wish to communicate and the wish not to and thereby clears a path for the patient to express what he is ambivalent about expressing.

Also paradoxical is a phrase discussed by Havens (1986) under the rubric "complex empathic statements." When one says to a patient *No one understands how you feel,* one is at once accepting the patient's discouraged sense of not being understood and paradoxically, in doing so, simultaneously conveying that he *is* understood. As Havens puts it,

> Ostensibly, "No one understands" translates a feeling of being misunderstood or abandoned. But the statement contains a systematic ambiguity that allows it to be still more serviceable. It suggests that both "I" and "no one" understands . . . . As a result "no one" statements stand in relation to other empathic statements as scouts do to the main body of soldiers. Both reconnoiter unknown territory. (1986, p. 54)

Other therapists rely on paradox more centrally in their work. Paradoxical interventions have been especially prominent in the practices of family therapists (see, for example, Hoffman, 1981; Selvini Palazzoli, Cecchin, Prata, & Boscolo, 1978; Watzlawick et al., 1974; Weeks & L'Abate, 1982), but they have been pivotal as well in Marie Coleman Nelson's "paradigmatic" approach (Coleman & Nelson, 1957; Coleman, 1956; Nelson, 1962), a variation on psychoanalytic therapy, and in certain applications of behavior therapy (e.g., Ascher, 1989; Chambless & Goldstein, 1980; Fay, 1978; Schotte, Ascher, & Cools, 1989). They are also very much at the heart of Victor Frankl's logotherapy (1960), an existentially oriented therapeutic approach.

A key aim of paradoxical comments is to help the patient relinquish those efforts to solve his problems that in fact end up making the problems worse—efforts at solution, in other words, that themselves have paradoxical consequences. The efforts of insomniacs to fall asleep are a simple and familiar example of this; such efforts almost always end up instead contributing to wakefulness. Similarly, the efforts of sufferers from agoraphobia and panic attacks to battle the anxiety that plagues them often make the anxiety worse, whereas the seemingly contradictory effort to make themselves even more anxious can at times cause their anxiety to recede. The reason for this is probably that in the effort to increase the anxiety, they are thereby exerting at least some measure of control over it. Instead of being passive victims, running constantly from an experience of which they are terrified, they are taking an active stance in relation to it, even if that activity is for now limited to one direction.

In some instances, therapists using paradoxical techniques ask the patient to *increase* the frequency of the behavior that has been disturbing him. In other cases all that seems to be needed is that the patient be asked to *observe* the problematic behavior. He is not explicitly asked to increase its frequency or to intentionally produce it, but just to be alert and keep careful notes about it. Such a request in itself turns the behavior being focused on from an unwanted intruder that must be fearfully avoided to something to be looked for and welcomed. It thus changes the relation of the person to his own behavior. The patient may be asked something such as *Please don't try to reduce this behavior just yet.*[8] *We first need to understand better what it's about and what it's related to, so simply try to keep track of it as it occurs through the week.* Here again, the paradoxical and the straightforward understandings of what is happening proceed side by side. We certainly do want to understand what the behavior means and when it is most likely to occur. At the same time, the request is made with an expectation that it may well lead to a reduction in that behavior.[9]

Another kind of therapeutic message that can be seen either in paradoxical terms or more straightforwardly entails suggesting to the patient that he not attempt to prevent himself altogether from engaging in some problematic behavior, but instead designate a particular time and place for it to occur. Once again this approach is likely to be chosen when the patient has tried many times to control the behavior and has been unsuccessful. From a straightforward perspective, it can be explained to the patient that in so designating the setting for the problematic thought or behavior, its links to other locations and activities in the patient's life can be weakened, helping to restrict it to a particular time and place.

This is akin to the recommendation sometimes successful with smokers that they only smoke in a particular room in the house and that they not do so when they are working or eating or having a conversation. In that way they can continue to smoke if they need to, but the links between smoking and the fabric of their lives are being severed. After a while, smoking becomes dissociated from most of their life activities and the elimination of the now more encapsulated habit is easier (and

---

[8]The phrase "just yet," of course has a suggestive or attributional element (see Chapter 9). It implies that change *will* occur and, indeed, even that a certain effort or restraint must be exercised to prevent it from happening too soon, before we understand it better.

[9]Kenneth Frank, who has made important contributions to the utilization and understanding of active techniques in a psychoanalytic context (e.g., Frank, 1990, 1992), reports: "I have found that monitoring, in itself, is a remarkably effective technique. It is, for example, an introductory element of an anger management program I administer at times, and often the patient's anger will diminish so significantly from the monitoring alone that it is unnecessary to go further." (personal statement)

even if the remaining remnants of the habit are not given up, their smoking has been very substantially diminished). Similar recommendations are often helpful with people trying to lose weight. If they often eat while watching television or doing paperwork, requesting that they get up and do their eating at the dining room table can sometimes enable them to make a dent in their habit, whereas requests that they *not* eat reproduce once again the experience of "I can't."

Depending on the nature of the case, the proclivities of the patient for cooperation or opposition, the urgency of the situation, and a host of other matters, the idea of continuing the problem behavior but in a designated locale or time can be introduced in a relatively straightforward or a relatively paradoxical fashion. The explanation can emphasize how such a strategy can help the patient gradually establish control over his behavior in a way that he previously couldn't; or it can emphasize the importance of "doing it right," doing it "wholeheartedly," so we can really see what the experience is about without the distractions of ordinary daily chores and demands. In either case, this new way of approaching the problem often enables the patient to "save up" the problematic thoughts or compulsive behaviors for their scheduled time, thus freeing him of them in the course of his everyday activities. The patient can be advised that when the thought arises, instead of attempting to oppose it, he can tell himself that this will be "good material" to use in his exercise at worry or self-criticism at the end of the day, but meanwhile he can go about his business. And the message from the therapist that this will provide us with good material to use in understanding what this is all about is not simply part of a structure of paradox; it has contained within it as well a good deal of truth.

Patients often respond to such suggestions with confused laughter—but with a touch of exhilaration as well. At some level they "get it," and see it as a path toward liberation from something they have been terribly stuck in. The liberation is further experienced when the patient approaches the time when he is supposed to think a particular compulsive thought, or engage in a ritualistic worry or self-criticism, and finds that he "fails" at the task—that, for example, when he tries to think self-critical thoughts intentionally, the bottomless well of self-loathing seems to run dry. Patients also sometimes find that the same thought or accusation that seemed deadly serious when they fought against it all day seems rather peculiar when engaged in in this way. They are able to see things in a new perspective and may find themselves laughing at what once almost brought them to tears.

One of the characteristics that makes certain comments by the therapist paradoxical is that in their manifest form they embrace behavior that it is in part the aim of the therapy to diminish. Although it is certainly true that comments of this sort, simply by virtue of this dimension, have a strategic quality, they can at the same time be empathic responses to the patient's actual experience. Indeed, it is often the combination of an empathic message that in some sense resonates with the patient's experience and a simultaneous element of irony and contradiction that gives the comment its impact.

A supervisee of mine, for example, was treating a young woman who quite regularly came half an hour late to sessions. The therapist's efforts to address the lateness had thus far been unsuccessful, and she was growing increasingly frustrated with the truncated sessions that resulted. I sensed that she might begin to fall into an uncharacteristically adversarial stance with the patient over this issue, and suggested she say to the patient something such as the following: *I've been thinking about your coming late to the sessions, and what occurs to me is that you come late because you sense that 15 or 20 minutes is all you can tolerate. I think that's because our work together is reaching down into some of the things that we need to be reaching, and that's hard; it hurts. But it shows us we're on the right track, and maybe now we can figure out together how to make it easier to tolerate what we're dealing with, how to enable you to bear it longer. Got any ideas?*

This way of putting it enabled the therapist to address the lateness in a way that was not scolding, indeed that reframed it as a sign of something positive. The result was a greater readiness on the patient's part to engage in an examination of the lateness, where previously she had responded to the issue's being raised either with irritation or by brushing aside any inquiries on an instance-by-instance basis (the train was delayed, "something came up," and so forth). It certainly remained the therapist's hope that the patient would begin to come to the sessions on time. But by addressing the lateness in this fashion, embracing as a positive sign the very behavior she viewed as a problem, she was able at once to empathize with the patient and to increase the likelihood of change in that very behavior.

Another patient, Robert, also seen by a supervisee, attempted to deal with his anxiety and depression by efforts at maintaining total control over family members. Robert was a man of some wealth, and attempted to deal with his grown daughter by a combination of bribery and demands that everything be done precisely his way or the money he dangled would be cut off. His daughter was increasingly bridling at this control, and there were indications that if Robert did not relent he was in real danger of losing his relationship with his daughter.

The therapist had tried in various ways to point out to Robert what he was doing and what the possible consequences might be, but had had little success. It became apparent that in his frustration the therapist was increasingly engaging the issue in ways that amounted to arguing with Robert. Not surprisingly, this had little impact on Robert's behavior.

Some progress was made as Robert's therapist began to follow my recommendation that he address the *conflict* Robert was experiencing. Robert was able to acknowledge that, yes, he wanted his daughter to do just what he said (because he felt that what he demanded was both reasonable and correct) and at the same time worried that his daughter was pulling away from him. But although this way of communicating with Robert interrupted the problematically adversarial tone that had entered the therapy, it did not seem to enable Robert to relinquish any of the demands on his daughter.

Finally I suggested to Robert's therapist that he say to Robert (mustering as much straightforward and genuine sympathy and empathy as he could muster—in effect, trying sympathetically to see it through Robert's eyes, *but with a twist*): *I can see where holding the beliefs that you do, things would look pretty impossible.* What was helpful about this comment is that it conveyed an appreciation of Robert's experience, but did so in a way that did *not* offer a possibility of change. Its focal message was essentially the same as would be the comment (only slightly different in its wording but very different in its emotional tone): *The way you look at things makes it impossible to see any possibility for a way out of your impasse.* In contrast to this latter comment, the one suggested was not adversarial and thus could not readily be countered. Robert could feel understood, but in a way that left him with a starker sense of the consequences of his demands. It is the element of "going with the resistance" that gives this comment a somewhat paradoxical quality and that gives it a greater likelihood of having a therapeutic impact.

Paradoxical communications generally aim to get a point across that, in principle, could be gotten across in a more direct interpretation, but they attempt to do so in a way that does not generate so much resistance. Their most appropriate application arises when the patient is locked into a self-defeating and self-perpetuating pattern that not only causes him considerable pain but also blocks him from seeing the possibility of alternatives and renders him virtually impervious to more straightforward communications. Central to what enables the paradoxical form of the message to filter through the resistance, and to introduce the potential for new ways of seeing things and new possibilities for solutions, is its element of irony.

That irony, sometimes close to the surface of the communication, and sometimes woven deeply into the helix of the message, casts the patient's psychological situation in a new light; but if not conveyed with considerable skill, it carries the danger of sounding not just ironic but sarcastic. One safeguard against that danger is clear appreciation of the multidimensionality of truth discussed earlier. The therapist who imagines she knows "the" correct way of seeing the situation is much more likely to lapse into countertherapeutic sarcasm when attempting such comments. Even more, it is the element of genuine empathy for the patient's dilemma that counters the potential for sarcasm and renders such comments genuinely therapeutic. In this respect, of course, paradoxical comments are no different from any other aspect of psychotherapy. Empathy is the precondition for all effective psychotherapeutic work, the basic foundation upon which an enormous range of creative and effective interventions can be constructed but without which only a surface resemblance to psychotherapy can be achieved.

CHAPTER 11

Therapist Self-Disclosure
Prospects and Pitfalls

For many therapists, some of the most difficult moments they experience in the course of their work occur when the patient asks them to disclose something about themselves. "How do you feel about what I just said?"; "Do you get frustrated when I talk on and on about the same thing?"; "Do you think about me between sessions?"; "Are you married?"; for some therapists, even, "Where are you going on your vacation?"—depending on the therapist's temperament and theoretical orientation, some or all of these questions may generate considerable conflict and uncertainty. On the one hand, the therapist may feel that the questions are perfectly "reasonable," and even that answering them might be useful to the patient or to the building of rapport. On the other, countervailing that inclination, may be either some fairly explicit theoretical notion of one sort or another or only a vaguely articulated sense that one isn't "supposed to" answer the patient's questions or reveal much about oneself or one's reactions to the patient.

This chapter will consider the question of whether and when to respond to such queries by the patient in the context of the larger question of therapist self-disclosure per se. It is not only when asked a direct question that the therapist must confront this issue. Even apart from the pressures created by direct questions from the patient, most therapists are aware of times when the idea of revealing something about themselves to the patient seems tempting, when it seems that such sharing of their own feelings or experiences might enable the patient to hear what they have to say with less defensiveness, might render their comment less painful or less damaging to the patient's self-esteem, or might convey to the patient a perspective that would enable him better to come to grips with some dilemma he is confronting. Many therapists, however, feel they must resist such a temptation, either on explicit theoretical grounds or on the basis of a vague sense that it "isn't done." In what follows I examine in some detail the question of therapist self-disclosure and consider when it might be appropriate and useful to the therapeutic process and how it might best be undertaken.

Although there are reasons to be cautious about what one reveals to the patient, and although there are certainly times when such communications burden the patient with the therapist's own problems or represent an "acting out" of something that is more for the therapist's benefit than for the patient's, judiciously employed self-disclosures can make an important contribution to the therapeutic process in all its aspects (including the furthering of inquiry into and understanding of the patient's own experience). Indeed, unyieldingly holding to a rule that prohibits all disclosures, and retreating to a reflexive "neutrality" or "anonymity," can be a source of needless pain for the patient and even of therapeutic failure.

In my teaching and supervision of therapists in training, I have found the question of how much to reveal of oneself in the course of the therapy to be one of the most puzzling and difficult questions these therapists face, and it is often not an easy one for experienced therapists as well. The confusion arises from the dual nature of the therapeutic relationship. On the one hand, it is a relationship that is deeply personal and intimate, dealing with matters usually obscured or submerged in everyday conversation. It is in addition, if engaged in properly, a relationship characterized by a deep respect for the patient's capacities and an interest in honest engagement of all aspects of his experience. On the other hand, it is a relationship that is professional and limited, and that is by its very nature asymmetric, focusing on the patient's experience in a way that differs from its attention to the therapist's.

The confusion is further deepened by the view, held by many therapists, that the most effective way to pursue and clarify the patient's experience is to keep the *therapist's* experience out of the picture as much as possible. According to this image of the therapeutic process, the ambiguity introduced by the therapist's stance is a crucial factor in enabling more of the patient's experience to be revealed. In a similar vein, the metaphor is sometimes introduced of the analytic situation as a sterile field in which contaminants are excluded (or at least minimized) in order to afford both analyst and patient the opportunity to observe the patient's unconscious wishes and fantasies in pure culture, as it were.

The classic statement of this general position, of course, was by Freud, though its influence is by no means limited to Freudians. According to Freud,

The young and eager psycho-analyst will certainly be tempted to bring his own individuality freely into the discussion, in order to draw out the patient and help him over the confines of his narrow personality. One would expect it to be entirely permissible, and even desirable, for the overcoming of the patient's resistances, that the physician should afford him a glimpse into his own mental defects and conflicts and lead him to form comparisons by making intimate disclosures from his own life. One confidence repays another, and anyone demanding intimate revelations from another must be prepared to make them himself. (Freud, 1912/1959, p. 330)

Freud contends, however, that such an expectation of therapeutic gain from self-disclosures is based on a superficial psychology of consciousness and that "experience does not bear witness" to the value of such a method, which, he claims,

achieves nothing towards the discovery of the patient's unconscious; it makes him less able than ever to overcome the deeper resistances, and in the more severe cases it invariably fails on account of the insatiability it rouses in the patient, who then tries to reverse the situation, finding the analysis of the physician more interesting than his own. . . . The [analyst] should be impenetrable to the patient, and, like a mirror, reflect nothing but what is shown to him. (Freud, 1912/1959, pp. 330–331)

Gill (1983) has argued that the import of these recommendations by Freud has been seriously misunderstood, and he notes that Freud himself was displeased by how his recommendations were applied by some of his students. Gill quotes in this context from a letter Freud wrote to the theologian Oskar Pfister in which he laments "the human propensity to take precepts literally or exaggerate them" and notes that "in the matter of analytic passivity that is what some of my pupils do" (cited in Gill, 1983, p. 207).

There has been a great deal of debate about the "blank screen" model of therapy in recent years, both among analysts and in a broader circle of psychotherapists, and a number of influential writers have presented arguments highlighting the importance of showing caring toward the patient or pointing toward a more liberal interpretation of the stance of the mirror or blank screen (see, for example, Greenson, 1967; Hoffman, 1983; Schafer, 1983; Stone, 1961; Tansey & Burke, 1989). Nonetheless, the issues of whether, and when, to reveal aspects of one's experience to the patient remain problematic for many therapists. Indeed, within the Freudian community, Gill (1983) suggests that "Despite recent emphasis on the real relationship and the various alliances, there is no doubt that insofar as there is an official Freudian position, it is to advocate a lesser participation by the analyst than Freud did. Freud is frequently criticized by Freudian analysts for having been as interactive with his patients as he was" (p. 208).

Gill's own position is a complex one. On the one hand, he is acutely aware of the obfuscations that analysts engage in to disguise the extent of their interaction with and influence on the patient. Addressing the phenomenon that when there is indication of more severe pathology (and also in work with children) analysts sometimes feel they have an "excuse" for being more real and interactive, Gill notes that "the emphasis on inevitable major participation in treating patients with severe pathology can be used to sidestep the question of the average expectable participation in treating the average expectable neurosis—the patient who meets the ordinary criteria for a classical analysis." He adds pithily that it has occurred to him that "an analyzable patient is a patient with whom the analyst can maintain the illusion of neutrality" (Gill, 1983, p. 213).

As a consequence of these insights, Gill states quite explicitly, "I do not think it is always wrong to report one's own experience" and notes that "often the very inquiry into a particular exchange may be so revealing of something the analyst is experiencing that it would be fatuous to pretend one has not revealed it" (Gill, 1983). His caution about this, that "when one does so one must be especially alert to how the patient experiences such a report," is perfectly consistent with the position taken here. He does, however, end up taking a more conservative position on the question of self-revelation than will be argued in this chapter. Notwithstanding the considerations just advanced, Gill states that "it is best to be quite chary with such revelations," adding,

> I believe they have a tendency to shut off further inquiry into the patient's experience, not least because such inquiry might lead to the exposure of something on the analyst's part which he would rather not know about. (Gill, 1983, p. 228)

As will be apparent below, I too actually regard the potential anxiety of the therapist as one of the important factors placing limits on the therapist's revelations about herself, and for a similar reason—because once that possibility is opened it can constrain the therapist in her pursuit of conflictual, anxiety-laden issues with the patient. It will also be apparent, however, that I advocate dealing with this potential obstacle in a different way than Gill and that I regard the advantages of therapist disclosures in certain circumstances to be substantial enough that we must be wary of imposing so oppressive a burden of proof on this activity that it is de facto excluded from everyday practice.

VARIETIES OF SELF-DISCLOSURES

Part of the confusion in the literature and on the part of practicing therapists regarding the issue of self-disclosure derives from the many different meanings that the term can have. Discussions of whether the therapist should disclose something about herself to the patient often do not distinguish among these various kinds of disclosure nor among the differing ways that information about the therapist can be conveyed. Not all are appropriate in any given clinical situation, and some are more generally useful than others. But as this chapter will illustrate, almost all have their place in some instances.

Confusion about the issue of self-disclosure has been heightened by the hesitancy of a significant segment of the therapeutic community even to acknowledge that the therapist's personality and her own emotional reactions had much to do with the direction the process took. The therapist was viewed as essentially an observer or as a passive object or container for the patient's reactions, and those reactions were regarded as "emerging" or "unfolding" more or less independently of the reactions or characteristics of the therapist (so long as the therapist stayed out of the picture enough not to interfere with their emerging or to "muddy the water.")[1]

As Kantrowitz (1983) has noted, "the analytic literature, while conceding both abstract and specific manifestations of countertransference, rarely considers the impact that the particular qualities of an analyst may have on the treatment process." Instead there is an assumption that the analyst is a "uniform analyzing instrument" and that analysts are "relatively interchangeable." Kantrowitz's own work on the "match" between patient and analyst is a noteworthy exception.

Reflecting this state of affairs, when some writers refer to a greater tendency in recent years to acknowledge the therapist's involvement or participation in the process, they do not have in mind at all actually communicating anything to the patient. Rather, they are referring simply to a greater readiness on the therapist's part to be *aware* that the real qualities and reactions of the therapist have an impact on the process. In the context of a paradigm that was loathe to acknowledge such influences at all—Kantrowitz, for example, describes the psychoanalytic literature as "virtually devoid" of references to the influence of the analyst's characteristics on the material elicited in the analysis—or that relegated them to the realm of countertransference in the narrow sense of reactions by the therapist that reflect neurotic distortions or unresolved childhood

---

[1]For further discussion of the metaphors of emerging and unfolding and their implications, see Wachtel (1982).

issues, such acknowledgment was an advance. If the therapist is in any way made freer to notice her participation and her reactions, understanding of the patient is significantly enhanced (cf. Burke & Tansey, 1991; Gill, 1983; Hoffman, 1983; Racker, 1968; Tansey & Burke, 1989; Wachtel, 1977, 1987). In the present context, however, it should be clear that what I am addressing is the question of the therapist's acknowledging *to the patient* something about her own reality. Our focus will be on when such explicit acknowledgments and disclosures are appropriate and how they should be conveyed when they are.

Disclosures of Within-Session Reactions versus Disclosures about Other Characteristics of the Therapist

Clearly one of the key distinctions in pursuing the question of whether to disclose—a distinction, indeed, that for some therapists virtually defines the boundary between disclosures that are acceptable and those that are not—is that between disclosures about what is transpiring in the session and those about the therapist's life outside. It is my impression that a considerably larger number of therapists are comfortable with the former than with the latter. Basescu, for example, states that "what the analyst says about his or her reactions to what transpires in the relationship between the two people . . . is the predominant arena of analysts' self-disclosure" and notes that it is predominant "in importance, in relevance to the therapeutic work, and in frequency of occurrence. It is also probably the least controversial area of analysts' self-disclosure" (Basescu, 1990, p. 55).[2]

In contrast, revelations about the therapist that are not about what is transpiring at the moment between patient and therapist are much more likely to be regarded as inappropriate. There are a number of reasons for the greater hesitation in this realm. To begin with, many therapists feel that the therapy should be concerned almost exclusively with the *patient's* experience, and that to introduce aspects of the therapist's is not only a distraction but, for some patients, a repetition of one of their earliest and deepest traumas—not having been attended to in a manner that was sufficiently empathic and appreciative of their needs. In effect, the claim is that the parents were unable to be "selfless" in the way that very young children require, and the excessive and premature intrusion of the parents' needs and the parents' reality required the

---

[2]Although Basescu refers here to the "analyst's" self-disclosure, his remarks are equally apt in characterizing the self-disclosures of therapists from most orientations. Basescu himself is not a Freudian but, rather, a leading proponent of the Existential and phenomenological point of view in psychotherapy.

child to *adapt* too early, resulting in the formation of a false self or overconforming exterior. From this vantage point, one of the therapist's chief tasks is to be there *for the patient*, to put aside her own needs in the service of the therapeutic task.

This objection, of course, holds to some degree for the therapist's revealing her own reactions in the therapy as well. In a narrowly literal sense, mentioning such reactions too is a departure from exclusive focus on the patient's experience. Such disclosures, however, are less of a breach in this regard than disclosures about the therapist's life outside the consulting room, because one's reactions *to the patient*, after all, (if they are not rather idiosyncratic "countertransference" reactions in the narrow sense) are further indication that one is paying attention to and emotionally responding to him. (Indeed, one argument *against excluding* such reactions from the therapeutic dialogue is that if one does, the patient can feel that he has no impact on his therapist and can be retraumatized by the experience of insigificance thus engendered.) Moreover—and perhaps the weightiest reason so many therapists who are not comfortable with any other kind of self-disclosure are comfortable with sharing this aspect of their experience with the patient—focus on the therapist's experience in this respect is widely acknowledged to be useful in promoting greater understanding of the *patient's* experience. Put differently, a narrowly rigid interpretation of "attending continually to the patient's experience" can seriously interfere with that very aim, whereas attention to the emotional field between the two participants is the medium for the most sensitive exploration of the subtleties of the patient's emotional makeup.

Even in considering self-disclosures by the therapist that are not directly about her experience of the interaction with the patient,[3] unduly narrow restrictions on the grounds of a presumed need by the patient for *his* experience to be the exclusive focus can be problematic. The conception of the infant and young child as requiring the absolute and selfless attention of the parent is altogether too precious and out of

---

[3]It is worth noting that the particular experience or characteristic the therapist feels moved to disclose is not likely to be unrelated to the events in the room. That is, even if the therapist discloses to the patient something about herself "outside" of the relationship and what is happening in the session, there is a good chance that she was moved to do so, or that it occurred to her at that point, because of something evoked by the interaction with the patient. Thus, if the therapist reflects on why she chose to disclose some particular incident or characteristic, she may find that it sheds light on the patient's experience and the relational matrix in much the same fashion that examining the therapist's more immediate reaction to the patient's productions does. In that sense, disclosures of "outside" material may often be simply a more indirect form of disclosure of one's reactions to what is taking place in the room.

touch with the reality of life as it is lived by flesh and blood human beings. The needs and personal idiosyncracies of the parents enter into the interaction with the child from the very beginning, even in the best of parenting. Indeed, totally selfless child rearing, in which the parents' own needs and feelings are kept out of the picture, is not only impossible but undesirable. Children need to *know* their parents, even as they need to be known by them. The foundations of the capacity both for intimacy and for personal identity require a sense of the parent as another experiencing being and as an active agent with wishes of his or her own. Both essential identifications and the roots of object relatedness cannot flourish if the parent is a blank screen. No matter how attentive the parent is to the moods and qualities of the child, if the light shown on the child is entirely reflected light, if no independent input originating in the parent's views and interests enters the interaction, an essential nutrient for growth will be missing.

Self-Disclosure and the Need for Ambiguity

A second objection sometimes raised to the therapist's revealing anything about her own life is that it interferes with the ambiguity and anonymity necessary to explore the less conscious aspects of the patient's personality. According to this view, the more the therapeutic interaction resembles ordinary social intercourse, the more likely it is to elicit those more stereotyped and surface reactions with which the patient is already familiar. To reach the less accessible layers of the psyche that are causing the patient's difficulties requires removing the guideposts that enable the patient to find the socially appropriate response rather than encountering those feelings and fantasies that are more deeply his own. To the degree that the therapist lets it be known what she is "really" like, according to this view, the patient will be inhibited in revealing his more private and idiosyncratic fantasies and even in letting them take shape. Moreover, if there is evidence that his fantasies are in fact *based on something*—that is, if the therapist's revelations seem to provide a justification for the patient's fantasies—it will be all the harder to persuade the patient that the fantasies are a product of his unconscious rather than a "realistic" appraisal of reality.[4]

---

[4]Closely related to this reservation are the kinds of concerns discussed in Chapter 9 under the rubric of "epistemological anxieties." For those therapists or analysts who wish to believe that what they observe in their patients are spontaneous upwellings revealing the contents of the unconscious independently of any input from the therapist, the stance of nondisclosure is seductive. The therapist holding such a view essentially tries to "get out of the way" and let the patient's "inner world" emerge. My skepticism regarding this conception of the clinical process will be clearly evident to the reader of this book.

Once again, the objection here holds in principle both for revelations about the therapist's outside life *and* revelations of her reactions to the patient in the immediate setting. It leads many therapists to be chary about both but seems to be especially inhibiting of the former, which is in effect regarded as "gratuitous." That is, although there may be reason why one might "have to" reveal something of one's immediate reactions to the patient, and (as noted above) might even *choose* to do so on certain occasions, there seems, to many therapists, almost no reason to go still further and reveal aspects of one's life outside the therapy situation.

Such arguments, it should be understood, are implicitly rooted in a conception of transference that is radically acontextual. The vision that guides them is in essence that discussed in earlier chapters in terms of the transference "emerging," "unfolding," and "bubbling up" (see especially Chapter 4 and Wachtel, 1982). From the vantage point of this image of what transpires in the session, it does indeed seem that the therapist must be extremely cautious about disclosing anything about what she is "really" like, lest she distort or obscure the transference.

The arguments put forward by Gill (1982, 1983), Hoffman (1983, 1991), and others, like those I have presented throughout this book and elsewhere (e.g., Wachtel, 1977, 1981), suggest that such a conception of transference is misleading and limited. Transference, from the perspective of these writers and of cyclical psychodynamic theory alike, must always be understood contextually. There is no one "true" transference, but rather a bounded manifold of reactions and perceptions that is unique to each individual and rooted in his character and his history but always codetermined by the particulars of the person and the situation to whom and to which he is reacting. What the patient must see is not that his reactions are "unrealistic" but, rather, how they reflect his historically and characterologically determined proclivities to experience certain relational configurations in certain ways. In so doing he gains, in fact, a more differentiated understanding of the *multiple* potentials for transferential reactions, as well as of the ways these are related to his vulnerabilities in particular situations. When disclosures by the therapist contribute to the particular shape and direction the transference takes (as they undoubtedly do), that contribution is not a distortion of the transference; it is an extension of the field of observation to be explored, an opportunity to observe still another dimension of the patient's rich store of transference potentials. Moreover, when the patient comes to appreciate not only how he can react to new situations based on experiences in the past, but also how specific transferential reactions are elicited by specific interpersonal situations in the present, that understanding is more complete than when he is persuaded that the true source of the reaction lies completely within him.

Now to be sure, therapists who operate from the view just described do not necessarily advocate the therapist's informing the patient about characteristics of her personality apart from her immediate reactions to the patient; and indeed I too believe that greater hesitation is appropriate in considering whether to reveal information about aspects of the therapist's life outside the interaction with the patient. It is important to recognize, however, that the constructivist view of transference shared, for example, by Gill, Hoffman, and cyclical psychodynamic theory suggests that—regardless of whether such a disclosure is a good idea in any particular instance—when such disclosures *are* made, and become one source of the patient's transference reaction, such reactions are as "analyzable" as any other.

The views and recommendations in this chapter regarding the range of possible disclosures by the therapist are predicated in part on the considerations just advanced. They are predicated as well on a view of the therapeutic process, depicted throughout this book, in which the exploration of the therapeutic relationship is but one aspect of a comprehensive approach to therapeutic change. As will be apparent below, when the crucial role of "accomplices" and vicious circles in maintaining patients' difficulties is taken into account, one is likely to see more instances when reference to some characteristic or experience of the therapist outside the immediate therapeutic context appears to be of therapeutic value.

Self-Disclosure and Idealization

Still another objection, somewhat related to the issue of ambiguity already noted, is that introducing information about the therapist's outside life or personal characteristics interferes with the process of idealization that is an important part of the therapy. The importance of idealization has been particularly stressed by Kohut and his followers, who view idealization as a normal and necessary developmental process that for some patients was not permitted in the course of growing up and who see its occurrence and working through in the therapy relationship as an important mutative experience. But some notion of idealization of the therapist is implicit in the practices of many therapists outside the school of self psychology. Even some cognitive therapists recognize that it is not just the sheer logic of what they say that induces the patient to change. The persuasive power of the therapist, the capacity of the therapist to assume in effect a parental-like role in which, much as the parent of a young child, she serves almost as a kind of interpreter of the world for the patient, as a mediator of reality, is recognized by many therapists to be a powerful factor in the therapy.

Most therapists are ambivalent about this power, recognizing its potential for abuse and wanting to treat their patients with respect, not as children. But most also recognize that, like it or not, this dimension of the therapeutic process is in fact a central one. Whether one talks of it in terms of an "after-education" (Freud, 1940/1949), as a replacement of the archaic and harsh superego with a more accepting and reality-oriented one, as a matter of identifying with the therapist's values or with the therapist's valuing of the patient, or in any of a variety of other related theoretical terms—and whether one sees a need eventually to "resolve" or "dissolve" such an influence or sees it as unrealistic to think such a dissolving possible—most therapists recognize their powerful role in the patient's life, and many are reluctant to interfere with that idealization by revealing themselves, warts and all.

There is indeed some reason to be reluctant to interfere with the patient's perception of us as perhaps more worthy than we are. Our valuing of the patient, even our "absolving" of some of his inappropriate guilt, provides a benefit to the patient whose roots are not wholly rational. For this reason, as well as for many others, our revelations about ourselves to the patient must indeed be judicious. But several countervailing considerations must also be taken into account in formulating an overall approach to the question of disclosure.

To begin with, it should be clear that a balance needs to be maintained regarding our idealization. If we permit ourselves to remain too idealized, an invidious comparison is implicitly set up in which the patient is diminished. Moreover, excessive idealization makes of the therapy an authoritarian rather than a collaborative enterprise. Therapy need not become a confessional or a masochistic orgy by the therapist for the patient's idealizations to be tempered by doses of reality. Indeed, at times such tempering is conveyed simply by asking the sort of pseudoquestions not uncommon in the therapist's discourse (e.g., *You assume I never have any anxieties?*). Since, however, as stressed throughout this book, words alone are not magic, and tone and intent are crucial as well, it is important that the therapist be clear in such instances that she is not *simply* asking a question, not solely engaged in an exploration of what the patient *assumes*, with no element of actual disclosure on the therapist's part. If the statement is truly intended to be ambiguous, if it is *really* just a "question," then the patient is left with the same nagging doubts and uncertainties. If, on the other hand, the therapist does intend to convey a deidealizing point, then it is disingenuous to do so in a way that pretends that all that is transpiring is that the therapist is asking a question that explores the patient's inner world.

A good illustration of a more forthright approach to conveying a version of Sullivan's "we are all much more simply human than otherwise" is offered by Basescu:

> One woman said, "I had a bad weekend. Other people are stable. I'm so up and down. I hide my rockiness." I said, "Don't we all." She: "You too?" I: "Does that surprise you?" She: "Well, I guess not. You're human too." I understood that to mean she also felt human, at least for the moment. (Basescu, 1990, p. 54)

Had Basescu hidden behind the formal structure of his words— had he insisted, to the patient or to himself, that "Don't we all?" and "Does that surprise you?" were simply questions, *not* self-disclosures, the salutary effect of his comments would have been very unlikely. Indeed, a deterioration of both the patient and the therapeutic relationship would have been more probable. The question form that Basescu's comments took was not inappropriate; the overall thrust of his efforts clearly was still exploratory. But by not hiding behind that form, by conveying clearly that he was indeed letting on something about *himself*, he effected one of the many small increments in reappropriated humanity that in their sum constitute a successful therapy.

From the perspective of therapists whose work is guided by Kohut's theories, the matter of dealing with the patient's idealizing of the therapist is approached somewhat differently. Kohut stressed the gradual disillusionment that is an inevitable consequence of the empathic failures that the merely human therapist must evidence at times. If the experience of these disillusionments is gradual enough, and is not intentionally forced on the patient with premature interpretations of his idealizing, self psychologists expect the patient to learn to accept the limits that inevitably characterize human beings, and to gain a more three-dimensional picture of the therapist and, eventually, of himself as well—a picture in which both self and other can be valued for their real qualities rather than for their apparent (and necessarily fragile) similarity to some grandiose imperative.

A second set of considerations countervailing the contention that one should let the patient's idealization of the therapist stand and not interrupt it by revealing too much of oneself—indeed, weighing against the full range of justifications for attempting to eliminate self-disclosure from the therapeutic process—centers on the *impossibility* of hiding nearly as much of ourselves as some of our theories—or our self-protective efforts—imply. The pervasive tendency for the therapist's views and values to come through, even when he believes he is being quite neutral and noncommittal, is well illustrated in a clinical vignette offered by

Ralph Greenson (1967). The patient, a conservative Republican, told Greenson that he had tried to change his political attitudes to bring them into greater agreement with Greenson's liberal Democratic views. Greenson, who had thought he had been successfully anonymous and nonintrusive, asked the patient how he knew what Greenson's views were. As Greenson reports it,

> He then told me that whenever he said anything favorable about a Republican politician, I always asked for associations. On the other hand, whenever he said anything hostile about a Republican, I remained silent, as though in agreement. Whenever he had a kind word for Roosevelt, I said nothing. Whenever he attacked Roosevelt, I would ask who did Roosevelt remind him of, as though I was out to prove that hating Roosevelt was infantile.
>
> I was taken aback because I had been completely unaware of this pattern. Yet, at the moment the patient pointed it out, I had to agree that I had done precisely that, albeit unknowingly. (Greenson, 1967, p. 273)

The point is conveyed in a different, and equally vivid way by Basescu. Therapists, he says,

> show themselves all the time in their dress, in their office surroundings, in their manner of speaking, in the way they establish time and money ground rules, and in the myriad ways of being that are publicly observable. One person knew when my eyeglass prescription changed. Another took me to task for the horrible painting I had on the office wall. . . . Somebody was pleased that I didn't wear a tie. Somebody else assumed I was going to a bar mitzvah when I did wear one. (It was actually a funeral.) My books have been criticized. My plants have been taken to mean that I'm good at making people grow. My cough meant I was getting a cold. My eyes showed I was tired. My car proved I didn't know much about cars, and the loud voice on the other end of the phone indicated I was a henpecked husband. Not all of such conclusions are accurate, but some are, and some are more accurate than I initially gave them credit for being. (Basescu, 1990, pp. 51–52)

Even in the ordinary course of giving interpretations, we reveal more of ourselves than we are used to believing. As Singer has put it, "The more to the point and the more penetrating the interpretation, the more obvious it will be that the therapist is talking and understanding from the depth of his own psychological life. . . . It takes one to know one, and in his correct interpretation the therapist reveals that he is one" (Singer, 1968, p. 369).

Self-Disclosure and the Therapist's Vulnerability

Finally, there is the objection to self-disclosure from the perspective of the *therapist's* anxieties and vulnerabilities. I have briefly alluded to this in my discussion of Gill above. Gill's point is an interesting one, and though not ordinarily discussed in the literature, it is never very far away when I have discussed the issue of self-revelation with students. Indeed, I believe that central to understanding when it is useful to reveal something about oneself to a patient, and when it is not, is an appreciation of the threat *to the therapist* in doing so. Therapy is demanding work, and the therapist must be protected in certain ways if she is to do it effectively. If our most private fears and most shameful traits are in constant danger of being exposed, we will be highly motivated to keep the therapy superficial and "polite," and to avoid topics that are too uncomfortable. If every time we explored a patient's most private sexual fantasies and anxieties our own were to be exposed, if every time we tried to help the patient come to grips with unpretty feelings toward those he loved, or with thoughts and feelings that could seem petty, jealous, or nasty, our own were equally on the table, we would have to be paragons of strength and virtue to do this work. Since few if any of us are in fact such paragons, we need the protection that the structure of the therapy situation provides in order to have the courage to pursue matters wherever they may lead. Such protection for the therapist, indeed, is very much to the *patient's* benefit, since without it we simply could not do the work in the way that is necessary.

One of the unique features of the therapeutic situation is that—in different ways for the two participants—it provides safeguards against certain kinds of threats that ordinarily limit the depth of our inquiries and relationships. On the patient's part, the protection resides in the commitment of the therapist not to judge or criticize, to put away as much as possible those reactions that might well come up in response to the same revelations by the patient if it were an ordinary relationship. This can provide the patient with the sense of safety that enables him to explore previously avoided memories, thoughts, and feelings. Put differently, this is the sensible core of the concept of neutrality, whose efflorescences I have criticized at numerous points in this book and elsewhere (e.g., Wachtel, 1987, Chap. 11).

From the therapist's side, the sense of safety comes from having established a relationship with the patient in which the therapist does not *have to* reveal herself. The therapist, in effect, reserves the right at all times to withhold information about herself, and indeed, as I shall describe shortly, she should be able to state this fact quite explicitly and even to explain why. For in fact this protection for the therapist *is in the patient's interest.* It is what enables the therapist to feel free to explore matters that in ordinary social intercourse she might well drop (in good measure precisely because of what such a discussion—under more conventional assumptions of symmetry or mutuality—might eventually reveal about *her*).

But it is one thing to be *free* to not reveal oneself and it is quite another to be *compelled* not to. Rules that make such self-revelations clinical taboos needlessly restrain and hamper the therapy.[5] Psychotherapy is an event taking place between two people, not a circumstance in which one person experiences and the other merely observes.

To be sure, some—even considerable—limit on how much the therapist reveals of her reactions is appropriate. But to move from the need for reflection and discretion to an almost blanket rejection of self-disclosure altogether, to a general negative predisposition that is independent of the particulars of the clinical situation one encounters, is unnecessary and unwise. It is perfectly possible to reveal certain aspects of oneself where that is deemed clinically appropriate without opening every back room of one's psyche for the patient's inspection. Some therapists feel they had better not reveal anything about themselves or answer any questions because once they do, they are then obliged to answer all. Such a contingent obligation may hold for those who take the Fifth Amendment in a legal proceeding; a witness may decline to answer *all* questions, about a topic, but cannot choose to answer some and not others. Psychotherapy, however, is not—and shouldn't be—a legalistic enterprise. There is good reason why the therapist might choose to answer some questions and not others, and she cannot be held in "contempt of therapy" for so doing.

It is perfectly consistent with good therapeutic practice—and indeed, since it entails sharing more fully with the patient the *rationale* for what one is doing, it is as well an indication of the highest ethical standards of professional conduct—to explain quite explicitly why one will answer some questions and not others. One might say, for example, something such as the following: *The work we do in here involves examining very uncomfortable kinds of feelings, taking a look at hurts and pains and rages and all sorts of things that it's easier and immediately more comfortable to put aside. And as a human being, I too have my anxieties and conflicts. There are feelings that it's easy for me too to want to put aside. If I have a stake in our not talking about certain things because if we do it's going to require me to talk about them in myself as well, that's not going to leave me free to focus with you on*

---

[5]They are also usually based on a false understanding of the possibilities for following through on self-disclosures by the therapist. As Gill has particularly emphasized, if disclosures occur, their meaning for the patient can and should be explored.

difficult issues when we need to. So in a certain sense, part of what the structure of this relationship is, is that it protects me, because when I'm protected I can be more courageous about bringing things up with you.

I believe the therapist should use this self-protective feature of the therapeutic relationship liberally. Not only should one not, in most instances,[6] answer questions or offer observations that reveal aspects of oneself about which one feels uncomfortable; in addition, I believe it is useful for the therapist to create for herself a comfortable "safety zone." By this I mean that one's revelations should not skate right up to the edge of what one dares to reveal but rather should leave one a margin, so that even relatively mild indications of increasing discomfort should be enough for the therapist to shift away from the mode of self-disclosure.[7] It is well for the therapist to keep in mind that although she is indeed a *participant* observer, and in a real and powerful relationship to boot, she is nonetheless a participant observer in a relationship that is asymmetrical. If one begins to move too close to symmetry in the relationship, it ceases to be psychotherapy.

The explanation I suggested offering to the patient is, of course, an instance of self-disclosure in its own right in a number of ways. At the simplest level, it is a disclosure simply by virtue of the fact that the therapist is, after all, spelling out her thinking and her rationale in front of the patient. She is, moreover, stating quite explicitly that she too has anxieties and that if she were not protected she would hesitate to go into some areas. In addition, however much she may exercise the general principle noted above of stopping well before we have gotten to the heart of her most difficult conflicts, the patient might very well gain some general notion about their outlines from where the therapist

---

[6]The modifier "in most instances" here is not just a casual afterthought. One key meta-message, if you will, of this book is that if one does therapy solely according to "rules," rather than with one's heart and one's head, the results will be meager. There will be times when the therapist senses that, indeed, openly revealing something one is ashamed about will be a powerfully therapeutic experience for the patient. In such instances, if one does not feel it will compromise one's ability to be available to the patient in the ways he needs as the therapy proceeds further, it may be appropriate to introduce the disclosure. I suspect such instances will be infrequent, and the general rationale offered above more commonly applicable, but I do not wish that rationale to be taken as a straight jacket constraining one's clinical creativity and sensitivity to the individual needs of any particular patient.

[7]These experiences of discomfort have a positive function as well, to which one should also be alert. They can be potential clues to the therapist about important issues and conflicts for the patient and about the feelings the patient is likely to elicit in those with whom he interacts. (Obviously, the ways in which the discomfort is related to specific vulnerabilities of the therapist that are not likely to be as relevant for an "average expectable other" must be taken into account.)

draws the line. Since, however, at the level of such general outlines, we are, all in all, much more simply human than otherwise as Sullivan (1953) put it—and since, moreover, as noted earlier, little more is likely to be revealed via this route than through the patient's perceptions of the issues one selects to interpret or ignore and the idiosyncrasies of how one does so—there is little in this degree of self-exposure that ought to be threatening to most therapists.

In describing to students or supervisees this approach to the boundaries of self-disclosure, and to *selectivity* in self-disclosure, I have occasionally had raised the question of the fairness of this approach: is it arbitrary or high-handed for the therapist to decide what she will answer and what she will not? (Interestingly, it has been my experience that this concern is almost never raised by patients, including by patients who are by no means shy about giving me a hard time or uncreative in that enterprise. I think this rationale for my answering some questions and not others makes sense to them because they recognize that in fact it enables me to answer *more* of their questions than I would if I maintained a more "consistent" stance.)

In thinking about this issue of fairness or arbitrariness, several considerations seem to me apposite. To begin with, it seems to me that answering *some* questions is less high-handed than not answering any at all (especially if, as recommended here, one is willing to explain to the patient one's rationale for doing so). Moreover, the decision about whether to answer questions and when to do so is not really arbitrary; it has a clearly thought out rationale and is, moreover, in the service of protecting not only the therapist but the therapy as well. Finally, and perhaps most important, the patient too has the right to decide what he will and will not reveal. Although the therapist certainly tries to encourage the patient to push back the borders of discretion and repression, and though she is ready as well to question and call attention to the patient's hesitations, she nonetheless must recognize and honor the patient's own right not to discuss something if he so chooses. And indeed, just as the process of therapy is enhanced by the therapist's feeling free to draw a line as to what she will reveal, so too at times is it advanced by the patient's freedom to do the same. Although the therapist hopes that the patient will eventually feel freer to discuss matters he once found too threatening, the sense of safety that can enable that to happen has as one of its components the therapist's commitment not to try to coerce the patient into discussing anything. Thus, although in the ordinary course of therapy the patient will disclose a great deal more than the therapist, in principle both parties have the right to "arbitrarily" keep something to themselves.

INDIVIDUALIZING THE THERAPY

The approach to partial self-disclosure by the therapist described here enables the therapist to approach the question with flexibility and sensitivity to the differing needs of different patients. If, for example, you sense that a patient needs at some point in the work to maintain an idealized view of you, or needs to feel he is in strong hands and would be uncomfortable to see you as a three-dimensional (and hence inevitably flawed) human being, you can be very sparing in your revelations. For such patients—or better, at such points in the work, for patients' needs change if the process is working as it should—considerable discretion is required to develop the sense of safety that is the foundation of effective therapeutic work.

For many other patients, however, the therapist's revelations have a quite salutary effect on the therapeutic process and on the patient's sense of safety. So too does presenting the rationale for why disclosure will not be complete. That rationale makes it clear that *all* people are motivated to avoid topics that make them anxious, and that the resistances that will inevitably be encountered in the course of the therapeutic work are not signs of the patient's recalcitrance or weakness but are, rather, manifestations of the human condition. This can be a key message in helping the patient maintain his self-esteem in the face of the challenges to it that the explorations of therapy can potentially represent. Consequently it can also be an important aid in maintaining the therapeutic process itself.

Once again, the pivotal point is that the particular requirements of a given patient at a given moment in the work must guide the therapist's choices. Many of the global rules that have been passed down from generation to generation of therapists are insufficiently differentiated to be of much help in this respect, and they can, in fact, actually get in the way of sensitive attention to the individual patient.

THE PATIENT'S QUESTIONS

I wish to turn now to a matter, introduced at the beginning of this chapter, that has been implicit in much of the foregoing discussion of self-disclosure—what to do when the patient asks a direct question about the therapist. It is useful to think of the questions the patient asks as presenting a kind of, "crisis" in the Chinese sense. The Chinese character for crisis, I am told, contains the characters that signify both opportunity and disaster. Patients questions are a bit like that. Their element of opportunity is derived from the explicit warrant they provide the therapist for introducing something about herself. If the patient has asked, then one's comment about oneself is not gratuitous or a diversion from the interests of the patient. In this sense, the patient's question makes it easier.

On the other hand, questions also put more pressure on the therapist. They can "concentrate the mind" in the rather unpleasant way that hanging is supposed to do. Questions can at times introduce a coercive element into the picture, diminishing the therapist's sense of autonomy, making her feel *forced* to answer instead of feeling she has *chosen* to do so. When this element is present, it is an important issue to address in its own right. One of the first things I would do is to reflect on what I already know about the patient and his life, with an eye toward the question of whether other people too feel coerced by him and, further, whether their feeling of coercion contributes to the dynamic behind the problems that are most troubling to him. Where this is the case, such an experience of coercion can be in fact a valuable entree into the very issues that most need clarification and attention.

How one responds to a patient's questions depends considerably on one's estimate of what function the question serves. With an externalizing patient or a patient whose style is to deflect away from himself and his own experience onto someone else, one would be very concerned about his shifting the focus to the therapist. But there are other patients—for example, shy people who are afraid to be intrusive or to make requests or convey feelings—for whom asking the therapist personal questions is an important sign of progress. When such patients ask questions of the therapist such as "Are you married?" or "Where are you going on vacation?" or even (especially) "Were you paying attention to what I just said?" it can be a groping toward intimacy that it is important for the therapist to nurture.

Some therapists are hesitant to answer patients' questions because they are concerned that to do so will cut off further inquiry. In part, this concern replicates a concern discussed earlier—that if the patient knows what is "really" true about the therapist (whether it be what the therapist is presently feeling about him, or something about the therapist's life outside the office) this will lead the patient to suppress or fail to elaborate fantasies that might be "unrealistic" or "untrue." I have already discussed this concern in general, but I wish to turn specifically to its relevance to answering questions, for here another wrinkle is often introduced. The question, we are reminded, does not necessarily mean what we think it means. Or put differently, the therapist may be unclear just what it is the patient really wants to know when he asks if the therapist is married, what her religion is, whether she watches television much, and so forth.

This caveat is well taken, up to a point. The patient who asks if the therapist is married, for example, may really be most interested in finding out if the therapist appreciates how miserable the marital state really is; or whether, in contrast to the patient, she has managed to establish a good relationship and can therefore guide the patient toward the same; or whether the therapist is homosexual; whether the therapist is conventional; and even, simply whether the therapist is willing to answer the question or rigidly sticks to rules. Moreover, the patient himself may be only dimly aware, or not aware at all, of what he is actually trying to find out.

One important guideline, which can help the therapist to approach as a human being rather than as an automaton the matter of how to deal with patients' questions is simply to keep clearly in mind that it is important to understand why the question was asked and what it means *regardless of whether you answer or not.* That is, one should not equate answering the question with abandoning one's interest in understanding its meaning and, conversely and equally importantly, one should not assume that the only way to discover its meaning is to refuse to answer it.

This is not to say that one must explicitly inquire about the meaning of every single question. To do so can feel rather tiresome to both patient and therapist and can feel to the patient as if he is being badgered. Moreover, the effect of such a repetitive and stereotyped approach is to give the whole endeavor a rote feeling that renders it lifeless. Without some variation, novelty, or spontaneity, one's questions and comments all fade into a gray haze such that none of them have much meaning or impact. By and large, it is well for the therapist to trust her feelings in this regard as she does in other aspects of the therapeutic process. Some questions that the patient asks are likely to feel rather straightforward and to be answered as such, whereas others will make the therapist uncomfortable. Respect for those feelings of comfort or discomfort—we must always bear in mind, of course, that such feelings may reflect as well ways in which the question touches on conflictual issues for the therapist—can enable the therapist to inquire more fully when there is some indication that something else is "up." Indeed, one further benefit of the therapist's being willing, at least in principle or on some occasions, to answer the patient's questions is that it provides further data for understanding the patient in depth: if one has to *consider* whether to answer the question (as opposed to having an automatic stance that the question is simply to be regarded as one more bit of therapeutic "material" to be interpreted or inquired into), one is likely to be more in touch with which questions make one feel uneasy, and that can alert the therapist to important variations in meaning that might otherwise have been missed.

When the therapist does feel some uneasiness about the question, or simply a heightened curiosity or sense that this may be something worth exploring, there are several ways to approach the inquiry. Crucial to appreciate is that the fact that one sometimes answers the patient's questions in no way interferes with the inquiry. Sometimes, indeed, I find that I can inquire quite fully even after having answered the question. Having given an answer, I then simply say something along the line of: *How do you feel about that?* or *Does that tell you what you really wanted to know?* or *What difference do you think it might have made if I were not married/if I had an M.D. instead of a Ph.D./if I were Catholic instead of Jewish?*

Much of the time I find little if any indication that my having answered the question has inhibited the patient's fantasies or locked him into a fixation on what "really" is the case. Indeed, it seems to me that when I compare the openness of my patients now to how they responded when, during my training, I felt more of a necessity to put off the patient's questions and turn them into "material" to inquire into, they seem much more ready now to follow the flight of their fantasies. That is, the idea that the patient won't say what your being married or not married, religious or not religious, and so forth means to him because now he *knows* that one or the other is the case and either (1) will fear to insult you or (2) no longer finds the discarded alternative relevant, does not seem to me to weigh as heavily in actual practice as it did in the theories of my supervisors.

To the contrary, the implicit power struggle that can go on when therapists refuse to answer patients' questions, and the adversarial tone this gives to the relationship, can often do more to inhibit the patient's fantasies, and certainly his willingness to share them with you, than whatever bit of information you supply. "I'm glad you're married because if you weren't I'd worry you were homosexual or unable to sustain a relationship" or "I'm sorry to hear you're married because I had hoped to have a therapist who could understand my loneliness" are not responses that answering the patient's question necessarily inhibits if trust has been built along the way; whereas repetitive preemptive inquiry, question after question, into what the patient *thinks* might be the case, or why he is asking, might impede that very trust. Persistent refusal to answer questions can generate what one might think of as "surplus resistance," resulting from the patient's feeling warded off and experiencing (consciously or unconsciously, but perhaps not inaccurately) that the therapist is playing a kind of cat and mouse game about answering his questions.

To be sure, there are times when one wants to get a better sense of why the patient is asking or what he wants to know *before* answering— and indeed, as already suggested and as elaborated further below, when one decides for one reason or another not to answer the question at all. In such instances, it is helpful for the process for the therapist to have established a "track record" of not reflexively putting the patient off. Because my patients know that I do not automatically refuse to answer their questions, if I say to a patient, *I'll be happy to tell you, but I don't feel clear about what it is you're really interested in knowing,* my experience is that the patient is usually quite ready to accept that at face value and take it as an invitation to explore. If, in contrast, one hides behind some notion that "the therapist is not supposed to answer questions," *then* a power struggle is likely to ensue that does indeed get in the way of under-standing what the question is about (and that is likely, moreover, to introduce the *artifact* that everything now seems to be "about" manip-ulation, power, control, and similar themes).

The example just noted is but one of many ways of inquiring about the meaning of a question. These inquiries at times will be linked with a preface that indicates that you do intend to answer the question, as with the first example above. At other times, it is clear to both patient and therapist that that is the intent, and explicit statement of it will feel redundant and stereotyped. At still other times, the inquiry so alters the nature of the question as understood by the two parties that a different question altogether is finally answered, or the original question feels beside the point to both, and the dialogue continues on the basis of the new direction it has taken. And sometimes, of course, regardless of the nature of what is clarified in the inquiry, the question turns out to be one of those that the therapist would rather not answer. Here again, the considerations in this regard described earlier hold. Often the patient will accept the therapist's setting of boundaries. At other times, that issue is once again up for grabs, and the issue is addressed both in the explanatory terms discussed earlier and in the more general terms of examining the patient's experience of the therapist and the relationship (e.g., *You're having a hunch here about one of my vulnerabilities. What thoughts come to mind?* or *It's feeling to you like I'm pulling rank here. Can you tell me more about that?* or *I have a sense that even though you're pushing for me to answer your question, you're also feeling relieved that I won't. What are you afraid I might reveal?*).

The actual focus of the inquiry into the patient's question can take many forms, which are mostly familiar to the experienced therapist. For example:

I'd be happy to answer your question, and I will in a short while. But first I'd like to understand better just what it is you really would like to know. Any hunch what it would mean to you if I said yes to that question?

It sounds like this question is one that you've been thinking about for a while. Can you tell me some of what you've been thinking?

I somehow get the feeling you're hoping I won't answer that question. Is there anything to that?

That seems like a perfectly reasonable question and I'll answer it in a moment. But I wonder if you have any hunches as to why it occurred to you to ask that question just now.

Clearly where I went to school is something you have a right to know, and your interest in it is perfectly natural. But I wonder if you have any ideas about why it occurred to you to ask me that today? Do you think there might be something else as well that you're wanting to know about me that has to do with what we're discussing today?

If, say, in response to the last example, the patient is not yet engaged by the question (saying, for example, something like "I don't know. I just wanted to know where you went to school."), and you still have a hunch that there's something more involved that may be worth exploring, you can say something like, *You know, often in this work we find that people ask a question for more reasons than one. Certainly one reason you're asking is you want to know where I went to school; but what would it mean to you if I went to one place rather than another? What's your guess, what else will it tell you about me?*

Now questions such as where the therapist went to school, how much experience or training she has, what her general orientation to therapy is, how much experience she has with problems like the patient's, and so forth, are questions that I believe the therapist is ethically bound to answer. *Whatever* one's orientation to questions in general, such matters, having to do with one's credentials and qualifications, are information the patient has a right to know. They are useful for illustrating the issues under consideration here precisely because of that. Here is an excellent arena to clarify further that interest in what the patient is "really"[8] wanting to know, or in what the *meaning* is of the patient's asking the question, is not in any way inconsistent with a commitment to answering the question. It is often indeed unclear what it means to the patient that one went to one school or another, that one is more or less experienced, etc., and it is often especially unclear what it might

---

[8] The reader should bear in mind here the discussion in Chapter 8 about the difference between comments that purport to be about what the patient "really" means versus those that refer to what the patient may "also" mean.

mean that the therapist is "Freudian," "behavioral," "Sullivanian," "integrative," "cognitive," or what have you. Indeed, the answer to this last question is often not clear even to the therapist. Many therapists can quite honestly claim that they do not operate according to some label, indeed even that they "don't know" what their orientation is. Nonetheless, it is much less productive to claim one does not operate according to any standard label (a reply that can have a vaguely arrogant or disdainful quality and that combines the worst features of both answering and not answering the patient's question) than to say something such as: *I'm not quite sure how to answer that question. Are you interested in whether I will be silent or will respond to what you say? Is there a certain approach you feel more in tune with? Could you tell me a little more about what aspects of the way I work you're most interested in? That way I can give you a fuller answer.* This latter approach—assuming one is appropriately responsive once the patient describes further what he is interested in knowing about—combines the twin principles of not being needlessly evasive and wishing to understand as fully as possible what it is the patient wants to know.

SHARING ONE'S DILEMMAS WITH THE PATIENT

Doing psychotherapy, by its very nature, entangles the therapist in the conflicts of another human being. Short of maintaining a degree of distance I have argued throughout this book is unproductive, there is no way the therapist can entirely escape from the trials this introduces. The consequences of this enmeshment in the patient's conflicts are not entirely negative, however. If the therapist can skillfully maintain the proper balance of engagement and reflection, such immersion in the patient's interpersonal world can be a primary medium for understanding the patient's experience and the sources of his difficulties. And not infrequently, discussing with the patient the dilemmas one experiences in relation to some aspect of the work can not only free the therapist from some of the sense of being ensnarled in twine, but it can promote insight for the patient as well.

An instance of this came up in the case of José, discussed in a different context in Chapter 8. After failing to get into any of the colleges he applied to, José was not only quite depressed, but he was also almost frantic to get advice from his therapist. And indeed, the therapist in this instance did have some pretty clear ideas about what would be useful for José to do in the interim period between now and reapplying to colleges again. Nonetheless, she was hesitant simply to respond to José's request for advice, because she felt that much of the difficulty that

José had gotten into originally stemmed from the excessive efforts his parents made to plan out his life for him. José was hypersensitive to the possibility that others too would try to manage him as his parents did, and his rejection of the much more limited efforts by his teachers to "help out" this worthy minority student was in large measure responsible for the image they had of him that led to his rejection by the colleges he wanted to attend.

José's therapist felt that if she too fell into the role of advice giver— at least in the way her teachers did—her efforts would similarly prove counterproductive. Yet at the same time, she saw that José was clearly asking for such advice, and that he was in a good deal of distress and would likely feel abandoned without it (even if, at the same time, he was likely to feel intruded upon if it came). Adding to the therapist's dilemma was the fact that she felt she actually did have useful things to say.[9]

After discussing the conflicting concerns and indications in a supervision session, the therapist decided to deal with her dilemma by sharing it with José. What she said to him was:

"You know, José, I'm having a problem at this moment that I'd like to share with you and get your opinion about. I know that much of the difficulty you've been having, that we've been discussing, is that just about everything you've done you've done for someone else, you've done because *someone else* thought it was a good idea. And clearly you're very sick of that. So when I think about your question about what you should do now, I feel in some conflict about it: I do have some ideas about what I think might work better for you at this point, what would be some constructive ways to put things back together and get back on track; and I'm even willing to share them with you. But I have to share with you also my real fear that if I do it's going to feel to you like one more demand, like one more thing you're doing to please someone else, and we've seen what happens when you feel that way."

This comment gave the therapist a greater feeling of freedom to proceed in the work, and it highlighted for José the dilemma *he* had created for himself. Eventually it contributed to his being able to discriminate better between the demanding and engulfing demands of his parents and the advice of others that was less coercive and more genuinely helpful. Among other markers of this was his grappling with the

---

[9]Recall that the overall approach described in this book (and followed by the student therapist in this case) is one that does not automatically regard the giving of advice as countertherapeutic or as rendering the therapy superficial or "merely supportive." From a cyclical psychodynamic perspective, advice can enhance or impede the resolution of deeper conflicts, depending on a host of specific clinical considerations in any particular case. The example cited here illustrates one of those considerations.

bind that the therapist had highlighted and his eventually being able to be genuinely interested in what the therapist had to say.

A different kind of self-disclosure by the therapist proved helpful in the case of Ben—in this instance highlighting the *patient's* dilemma, but in a way that relied centrally on the therapist's sharing his own feelings. Ben was someone who had experienced a great deal of hurt and disappointment in his life, and who had learned to deal with it by not letting himself care too much and by putting down any person or any relationship that threatened to mean too much to him. He communicated in a variety of ways an attitude of disparagement and indifference toward the therapy and the therapist. He would frequently come late, miss sessions, or have to leave early for one engagement or another, and he dealt with all of this with a kind of aggressive casualness that left the therapist feeling diminished and unimportant.

We discussed in supervision what was happening, and it became much clearer to the therapist just how angry he had been about how Ben had been treating him. Prior to this discussion he had taken up with Ben on a number of occasions the issue of Ben's missing or cutting short the sessions, but he had done so in a way he sensed was stilted, vaguely accusatory, and overly controlled. In the supervisory session, we worked on how he could be more direct with Ben about what he was experiencing and do so in a way that would further the aims of the therapy rather than be just one more instance of the kinds of interactions with others that had maintained Ben's wariness and haughty unapproachability. He first said to Ben, "I've been thinking about our sessions, and I realize that I haven't been sharing with you how much it bothers me that you come late. It must seem to you that I don't care that much." When Ben was able to acknowledge this at least a bit, the therapist elaborated further on the vicious circle Ben was caught in:

"I can sense the bind you're in, and I feel for you even though I also feel angry. I can see that when you disparage people it's to protect yourself from being hurt. But when you do that, people are likely to feel resentful toward you—I'm realizing that I've been feeling that way myself—and then I can understand that that feels to you like *proof* that people can't be trusted, that you better *not* open up and care and get involved. But the problem is that the proof that you're getting is highly selective, it gives you a picture that keeps you stuck in a very ungratifying and frustrating way of life, and it doesn't let you see other possiblities."

The therapist's acknowledgment of his own reactions to Ben's missed and shortened sessions was crucial in a number of respects. At the most surface level, it broke through Ben's stance of indifference and *interested* him in what the therapist was saying. The therapist's revelation of anger was dramatic enough to get his attention.

It also helped to get the message heard in another way: by being honest and owning up to a feeling that was in a certain sense not quite acceptable, the therapist both demonstrated that it was possible to be less than perfect without disastrous results and took the onus off Ben. Whatever was going on, though Ben had some responsibility for it, was not just about Ben; the therapist too had a part in it. Thus, the therapist's comment, although about a difficult feature of Ben's way of relating to others, could be experienced as not simply an accusation. Finally, by taking the risk of departing from the safe ground of what a therapist "should" say (or not say), and by acknowledging Ben's impact on him, Ben's therapist was evidencing caring for him, something that tended to happen rarely in Ben's life.

Ben's offhand manner was well designed (if unintentionally so) to elicit unreal reactions from others. Ben was used to experiencing people as vaguely not liking him or not warming to him. (I say vaguely, because his style diminished the likelihood of the other person's being up front about what was happening; Ben himself was so casual that the *other* felt humiliated at acknowledging caring enough to feel angry.) Ben was accustomed as well, for reasons similar to those just adduced, to experiencing people both as unreal and as indifferent. The therapist's frank acknowledgment of being angry at Ben provided a much needed dose both of reality and of caring, which I believe was a necessary element in Ben's being able to begin to address the predominant pattern in his life.

VALIDATION OF THE PATIENT'S EXPERIENCE

The example of Ben can be understood in slightly different terms as well that highlight another important dimension relevant to questions of disclosure of the therapist's feelings. The "standard" stance of nondisclosure by the therapist can leave the patient feeling that his experience is not being validated. For some patients, this is a replication of one of the most painful and undermining patterns of their childhood. Many aspects of parental behavior and demeanor can contribute to the experience of not being validated. And much that goes on in therapy under the label of letting the transference emerge or unfold, or under related rubrics of neutrality, not imposing one's own concerns or reactions on the patient, or attending exclusively to the patient's experience, can in fact have the effect of adding to the sense of being invalidated. When the therapist refuses to answer questions, or reponds to them with a version of *Why did you ask?* or ignores them altogether, or when she fails to acknowledge in any way that what the patient thinks he has perceived in her has any basis, she again adds to the invalidation. Indeed, for some patients, the entire structure of the therapeutic relationship can be not so much a therapeutic experience as a "crazy-making," invalidating one, confirming that one's perceptions are "off," that one cannot trust one's own eyes and ears, that one is in some way "crazy," or that one is seeing things or is interested in things one is not supposed to (cf. Laing, 1960, 1969).

A brief and simple clinical vignette by Basescu (1990) illustrates well how the therapist, by a considered disclosure, can contribute to the overcoming of such experiences of invalidation rather than their perpetuation. A patient of his said, "I was trying to read the meaning of changes in your tone of voice last time when we were talking about makeup appointments. It felt like you thought I was a pest." Basescu responded, "You read correctly that something was going on with me, but it had to do with my realizing I was uncertain as to when I wanted to make the appointment." The patient's response in this instance was significant: "I'm glad you told me. It's so easy to feel crazy—like adults aren't supposed to react to changes in the tone of voice" (Basescu, 1990, p. 48).

Patients who are prone to "feel crazy" in this way, or who are overly ready to assume that their perceptions are "off" if the other doesn't seem to acknowledge them, or if they sense they have seen or picked up something that they "shouldn't" have noticed, experience a sense of falseness and a lack of that inner confidence and firm sense of self-directedness that are crucial to satisfying living. For many such people, experiences that replicate this pattern are numerous in the course of living their lives, because they tend to convey their perceptions in a very tentative way that makes it easy—especially if they have seen something that is in any way uncomfortable for either party—for the other to ignore or deny. When the therapy becomes one more experience in which this occurs, if only by a scarcely recognized conspiracy of silence, the therapy can actually be a contributor to the continuation of the patient's difficulties rather than to change.

THERAPISTS HAVE CONFLICTS TOO

The final example I would like to discuss in this chapter was actually the original impetus for the chapter and part of the impetus for the volume as a whole. One of the key experiences that led me to see the topic of this book as being a central one in the practice of psychotherapy was the seminar described in Chapter 5, in which the therapist said to a patient who was sitting in silent distress: *I think you're silent because you're trying to hide a lot of anger.* The reader may recall that the class at first generated a number of alternatives that were equally problematic, and then devised a number of more facilitative ways of helping the patient to understand her conflicts over expressing anger and their relation to her silence. There was one possible intervention we considered in some detail then that I did not include in Chapter 5 because I felt it would best be examined in the context of the overall discussion in the present chapter. The comment to be discussed here, like those offered in Chapter 5, conveys basically the same focal message as the therapist's original comment, but it has a number of features which enable it to accomplish certain things that the other alternative comments do not. The comment, which includes a self-disclosure by the therapist, was the following: *I find that sometimes when I have nothing to say, after a while I realize it's because I'm angry.*

Several things are accomplished by such a comment. To begin with, a comment phrased this way does not set the therapist apart from the patient, does not implicitly communicate that such experiences are part of being a "patient" and that the therapist has, in effect, only encountered them in textbooks or from watching impaired others. Moreover, in this last version, the therapist is acknowledging not only that she gets angry but also *that she is sometimes unable to acknowledge it at the time.* Thus the patient's defenses do not set her apart any more than her anger does, and she is more able to examine both without a great loss of self-esteem.

At the same time, such a comment by the therapist conveys to the patient that it is possible to cope with and overcome such conflicts. The therapist presents to the patient a coping model (Bandura, 1969; Meichenbaum, 1977). She has been in the situation and has emerged from it intact and able to discuss it. Moreover, the therapist's describing her reaction as one in which the anger was at first not experienced, but was later recognized as such, enables her to engage the patient's interest even if the patient is not at the moment feeling that she is angry. Even if the patient's subjective experience remains the (presumably) defensive one of simply having nothing to say, she is encouraged not to consider the matter closed and perhaps to examine with interest and curiosity the marginal thoughts and associations that may well lead her to a clearer sense of both sides of her conflict. In disclosing an aspect of the therapist's humanity as part of an effort to help the patient reappropriate the full experience of her own, this comment illustrates well the issues with which this chapter has been concerned.

CHAPTER 12

Achieving Resolution of the Patient's Difficulties
Resistance, Working Through, and Following Through

The therapeutic strategies and styles of communication described in the preceding chapters illustrate how the therapist can convey her ideas to the patient in a way that minimizes counterproductive resistance. Approaching the therapy in this fashion can, I believe, considerably enhance one's effectiveness and increase the likelihood that the patient will have a positive and productive experience. It is essential to be clear, however, that the matters discussed thus far are by no means all that effective psychotherapy entails. If the therapy is to be successful, a variety of efforts must be made to enable the patient to rework his internal representations and change his manifest patterns of interaction with others.

In psychotherapy, as in life, it is usually follow through that makes the difference. The blinding insight that changes a person's life is far more common in the movies than in the consulting room. In daily practice, much of the therapist's effort is directed not so much toward opening up entirely new directions as toward enabling the patient to find ways to travel along the paths he has begun to glimpse.

Much of this effort is unspectacular and workmanlike. Steadiness, persistence, and a readiness to go over familiar ground again and again from slightly different angles are qualities as important to the therapist's success as the capacity to plumb the depths of human experience with empathy and insight.

This is not to say that following through effectively does not require skill. Indeed, it may well be that what most differentiates the effective therapist from her less successful counterparts is precisely the ability to follow through effectively. It is perhaps most of all in the effort to assure that the patient's participation results not just in verbalized understanding but in genuine change that the therapist is likely to encounter her most severe challenges and her greatest potential frustrations.

This aspect of the work, often referred to as the process of "working through," tends to be time consuming and difficult. It is likely that the most common cause of therapeutic failure is not a failure to achieve some degree of insight but rather the failure to carry through with that insight into new ways of experiencing oneself and new ways of relating to others. In this chapter, I address some of the considerations that enable the therapist to be effective in the stage of working through, and will try to show how variations of the principles and strategies described in this book can be useful in this aspect of the work as well. Indeed, perhaps nowhere are the strategies for reducing resistance described in the preceding chapters more essential than in helping the patient translate his increased understanding into genuine therapeutic change.

TWO FACES OF FOLLOW THROUGH

The process of working through can be conceptualized as having two main components: the patient must change the manifest patterns of his interactions with other people, and he must rework the internal representations of self and other that underlie those interactions. Both processes of change are built on the patient's greater understanding or insight, but both go well beyond insight alone. As will be apparent from the discussion that follows (and should be clear from the guiding overall perspective of this volume), these two dimensions of change are not really separate or independent. Each contributes to the other and is almost impossible to achieve *without* the other. But for purposes of presentation, it can be helpful to make the distinction.

REWORKING INTERNAL REPRESENTATIONS

I will turn first to the reworking of internal representations. Notions of representation are prominent across the spectrum of theories and orientations, ranging from Sandler and Rosenblatt's (1962) discussions of the representational world, Kernberg's (1976) emphasis on internalized self- and object-representations, and Bowlby's concept of generalized working models (1967), to Sullivan's (1953) accounts of personifications, to the various conceptions of cognitive behavioral therapists regarding personal constructs, schemas, and generalized expectations. Common to these various conceptions is a recognition that we experience the world, and respond to it not in terms of what is "actually" occurring but as we perceive it. The mediation of complex cognitive and perceptual processes virtually assures that changes in the contingencies of daily living and in the responses we encounter from others—as important as they are in the overall set of influences bearing on the therapeutic process—will not be reflected in any simple or direct way in changed behavior or experience on the patient's part. Changes in the images and processes whereby we represent the world are necessary for the changed circumstances truly to register.

Theoretical accounts of the "representational world" vary in the degree to which it is portrayed as an exclusively "inner" world or as in continuing and reciprocal transaction with the manifest occurrences of daily life. It will certainly be apparent to the reader by this point that I do not subscribe to those views that posit locked-in internal objects having little to do with what is going on in the patient's life. But I can well understand why the world looks that way to some theorists. There is certainly a stubborn persistence to our behavior and our experience that can give at least the appearance of imperviousness to the input from our day to day encounters and transactions. Whether one theorizes in terms of internal images, voices, attachments, introjects, objects, or what have you, it is easy to observe people persisting in beating their heads against a wall whose outlines have seemingly been drawn somewhere between their right and left ears. Helping people to examine and disentangle themselves from loyalties and attachments they were not even aware they had, and to revise and modify the cognitive/affective building blocks through which they construct their world and their lives, is not an easy matter. Much of what goes on in psychotherapy can be understood as a process of helping the patient construct a different set of categories and psychological structures for apprehending and experiencing the world, a set that, as Rogers (1961) put it from within his particular theoretical framework, is more consonant with lived experience.

Identification and Disidentification

Central to the effort at modifying the patient's representational world is helping him to rework the identifications that form the core of his sense of self and of his place in the world. These identifications mostly operate outside the range of critical reflection, shaping and constraining our sense of life's possibilities, imperatives, and desiderata. Beneath the level of awareness, and soaked in the psychic import of the early parent–child matrix, these identifications are highly value-laden. They impart a sense of compelling necessity to our experience and lay out boundaries that we are forbidden to transgress. These boundaries are not merely with regard to behavior; they dicate what we may hope for and what we may believe. To see around them, much less to live on a different basis or with different assumptions and different internal imperatives, is extremely difficult. The distinction between description and value disappears at this level; it is the level of what *should* be, what *must* be.

None of us can live without such identifications, but in some circumstances they may be tenuous or lacking in substance. When they are, a sense of living without meaning or with a sense of isolation and inner emptiness results. In such instances, the relationship with the therapist becomes especially important. The therapist must be comfortable in permitting herself to be an object for identification and skillful in the balancing act in which such identifications are fostered while at the same time the patient's capacity to rework those identifications and achieve a unique and independent selfhood is fostered as well. This task is especially difficult with such patients because with them the relationship tends to be not only especially crucial but especially problematic as well. It is likely to be hardest to offer oneself as a good object to the very people who need it most. Difficulties in committing themselves or investing themselves emotionally, volatility, boredom, extreme demandingness or extreme unwillingness to expect anything at all—these and other traits either separately or in combination make the establishment of a relationship very difficult.

Although some commentators have suggested that the pattern just described is more prevalent today than in prior eras, it nonetheless clearly remains the exception. Most of the time, the patient will give evidence of a host of conflicting identifications and attachments, some of them adaptive, some clearly pathogenic, and many both at once. The task of aiding the patient in reworking these inner building blocks is an important part of the therapeutic process and a central aspect of what is meant by working through. The annotated clinical excerpt described below illustrates some of the ways in which this process is facilitated. The excerpt depicts a piece of "ordinary" clinical work in the later stages of the therapy, a mostly unspectacular process of repetitively addressing the assumptions by which the patient lives and their connection with the parental figures with whom he identifies. It is noteworthy in the present context, however, for a number of reasons. First of all, it illustrates the use in the working through process of a number of the principles and strategies that were discussed in earlier chapters. The roles of reframing, attributional comments, and building on the patient's strengths, for example, will be readily evident. It illustrates as well how the therapist can consciously direct his efforts to modifying the patient's identifications. It will be clear to the reader that the therapist's aim is to help the patient *disidentify* with certain aspects of his mother, to free himself to pursue a way of living less burdened by the shadow of the past. At the same time, the therapist attempts to foster and amplify other identifications, aiding the patient in selectively reworking the grounding of his self, so that he may at least to some degree take from his parents what is valuable for his growth and leave what is not.

Conceptualizations about introjects and internalized objects figure prominently in much current theorizing influenced by the range of viewpoints commonly described as object relations theories. Little in these theories, however, gives much in the way of guidelines for what the therapist can actually do about these introjects. Moving beyond the level of speculative theories about their developmental origins, what can the therapist actually *say* that will contribute to the assimilation or the reworking of these representations? It will be clear in the excerpt that a major thrust of the effort was to enable the patient to separate himself from the internalized attitudes of his mother, to put them outside himself. In part this is a matter of positioning himself so that he can *examine* them. But it is not so intellectual a process as the term examine seems to imply. As will be clear, some of the comments made in the session were designed specifically to *alienate* the patient from these attitudes, to actively place them outside the self and remove the quality of ego-syntonicity from them. In effect, the patient was being helped to redraw the boundaries of self and other, to shift his representation of certain emotional attitudes from the realm of self to the realm of not-self.

As will be apparent as well, the process of modifying representations in this way—and of disidentification—entails as part of it helping the patient to understand *the other* better. Discussions of insight's role often are too narrowly focused. Insight about others is often almost as important as insight about oneself, and, as this excerpt will illustrate, here as in so many other aspects of psychotherapy and psychological theory, the dichotomies with which we have become familiar can distort the unitary reality they attempt to address. Understanding of others and understanding of oneself are actually *not* two separate realms. As this case excerpt well illustrates, one understands *oneself* better through understanding the key others in one's life, and vice versa.

The patient, Mark, was a successful executive in his late 30s. His job as a high-functioning executive in the medical insurance division of a major insurance company provided him with a six-figure salary, but he nonetheless felt much of the time that he had not really "made it." He often felt that his job was boring and brooded over the fact that some of his classmates at Stanford Business School had achieved the sort of success that put them on the front pages of the business section, whereas he just plodded along, being competent but not taking risks. Much of the work of the therapy had focused on Mark's low-grade depression and his persistent tendency to be very self-critical. Though he was in fact a rather active and energetic man, he frequently saw himself as lazy and almost inert and perceived ominous signs of slothfulness whenever he relaxed.

Mark had grown up in a Midwestern suburb, in a neighborhood in which his father was economically one of the less successful men. His mother's income as a bookkeeper had always been necessary for the family to maintain its standard of living. Mother had been rather disparaging of his father, who did not seem to have the "get up and go" that she did (and that Mark was supposed to have). Mother herself, as will be clear from the excerpt, was a woman who had struggled with depression all her life. In recent work in the therapy, Mark had begun to appreciate that her compulsively active life style was a way of warding off the depression, an effort that was not always successful but that usually had, as its final maneuver, either a projecting of the depression onto his father ("Your father just has no vim and vigor; he's not like me"), or, when her final efforts at warding it off failed and she experienced the depression directly, an outright blaming it *on* the father ("If I hadn't married someone like your father, I'd be a happy woman").

These sequences and mechanisms had not been evident to Mark when he began the therapy. He had simply seen his mother as energetic and his father as depressed. He could experience considerable annoyance at his mother, sensing that she was generally "after" his father a lot and that she was frequently an irritant to himself as well. But he had little real understanding of just what the irritation was about or of what really went on between his mother and father. His view of his father was also one-dimensional. Father was perceived as a depressed, passive man and as the image of whom Mark needed to work not to be. In more recent sessions, he had begun to recognize some of the complexities and hidden elements in these family patterns, and the session reported here was an effort to follow up on that new understanding.

A central theme of the session was the carrying forward and working through of a modified understanding of what mother and father were like and of what was involved in the ways he saw and reacted to them. A particular focus was Mark's seeing his father as more depressed than he actually was—thereby increasing both his fear of *being like* his father (which his mother implicitly accused him of if he relaxed or didn't go out and do) and his fear of *destroying* his father (because the father was seen as more fragile than he really was). Mark also came to recognize in the session how he exaggerated his own depression and inadequacy, both *in contrast to* his mother's exaggerated energy and as a passive–aggressive tactic in fighting back *against* his mother's pushing. As part of this, he recognized that not infrequently he had actually had to not feel well in order to have a right to relax.

Mark began the session, as he often did, with a brief summary of where we had been last time. This could sometimes be a stilted, "business-like" way of beginning, but it did not reflect a deep-seated resistance of any sort and was often a useful way of promoting continuity between sessions.

PATIENT: Well, we were talking last time about my family history and you were posing the possibility that, uh, I guess we should try to separate this out. One is that I was right that my mother thought my father a failure but that maybe I was wrong in thinking that he really *was* a failure. And you were posing the possible alternative scenario that he was a good guy who just didn't have high ambitions and his goal was to lead a balanced life without putting in more effort than was necessary. And you said perhaps this was a whole new way of thinking of my father, and that's kind of where we were. I talked to a couple of people about it and they said, well do you feel better now?

As the reader will probably gather, "good guy" was not quite how I had put it. But it will be clear as the session proceeds that I was indeed trying to suggest an alternative way to understand his father; and one in which the father's lack of ambitions—or, put differently, his ability to be content and to relax—could be seen as a valuable trait that Mark had taken on with good reason. Mark struggled terribly with whether it was OK for him to relax, to spend an evening at home watching television, for example. The inner voice of his mother's struggle with depression made any such occasion of relaxation a source of considerable conflict, and I was trying to help him clear some space for the legitimacy of the moments when he laid his ambition aside.

THERAPIST: What did they mean?

P: Well, you know, now that you've made this big breakthrough.

T: Were they saying it ironically?

I mistakenly heard this as an ironic comment because of my own conviction—apropos this chapter—that rarely is significant change produced by just one comment or one "breakthrough." Mark's comment that follows is correct: you have to integrate it into your life.

P: No, no. They were asking was I all better now? And the answer was no, I have to somehow integrate this more into my life.

T: There was another important piece to the pattern we discussed, a part of the same package: if this line of thinking has any validity, part of why you might have distorted to some degree—and by distorted I don't mean you made it up out of whole cloth and there's no validity; you chose one of several possible ways of viewing it—part of why that happened is that you were participating in something with *your mother*; not just about her judgment about your father, but also about her struggle with her own depression. So putting it together with some of the things you've been saying for the last couple of weeks, part of the same pattern would be that when she says to you "how can you be in the house on such a beautiful day," it's not just are you a stay-at-home good for nothing like your father but also how can you do that when it would make *me* (your mother) so depressed.

My comment here was designed to point out that Mark's misperceiving his father was not simply an error on his part but part of a process with his mother. The comment is a bit long-winded, but as will be apparent as the excerpt proceeds, it did bear fruit. I think I said all this because, in responding to his summary of what the last session was about, I wanted to broaden his recollection of what we had been addressing, not to let an important part of what we had been discussing disappear. But I was trying to do too much with one comment. By packing so much into the comment, it became much too cognitive, too much of a "formulation" that couldn't really be grasped emotionally at one sitting. At best it would leave the patient with an *explanation*, which is not enough for change to occur. But the relevance and importance of what I was trying to get at (albeit poorly at this point) will be apparent shortly.

P: Yes, and it makes *me* depressed too. It gets passed on in that fashion.

T: But it makes *you* depressed, it

In this extended comment, I'm

seems to me, by proxy so to speak. What I mean by that is that depression seems very centrally woven into your mother's personality. She's not responding to *someone else's* voice when she feels depressed about it, whereas when *you* get depressed when you're sitting at home, that depression is not your inner nature; it's another voice telling you something about another part of you.

P: Well, I guess what the voice is saying is it's just not worthwhile to sit around and relax. You know, it's this thing about valuable and not valuable and so forth. It's not valuable . . . it's not accomplishing anything. You must always be accomplishing something. And maybe this goes to this question of spending time with valuable people, and I guess that leads somewhat to this fantasy I have, this gets to the shoulds, that if I only did *x* instead of *y,* or if only I went to this party instead of staying home, I might have met someone who would change my life, who would make everything more wonderful. Or if I had gone to this movie instead of staying home watching the ballgame, it would have changed my life in some way. All of which is highly unrealistic.

T: What it sounds like is nagging.

working at breaking the identification with the mother's depression: when *she's* depressed, she's responding to her own inner voice; when *he's* depressed, he's responding to a voice that's someone else's. Although the distinction is perhaps being drawn somewhat more sharply than is strictly warranted—the depression, after all, is by now also "his"—the aim is to contribute to making ego alien the inner voice that drives depressive thoughts. Put differently, the introject is being pushed out of the realm of the self.

This comment is a further effort to facilitate the process of disidentification. The reframing of the message of his inner voice (in this case negatively rather than positively) contributes to alienating him from it. It is important to be clear (and will be apparent as we proceed) that the aim is not to alienate him from his parents as real people, but rather to free him from the inner voices that impose an automatic constraint that interferes with his capacity for happiness and maintains painful inner conflict.

P: Me nagging myself, yeah. Yeah, that's true. You know, at work when I have a task to do, even if it's something I know I can do well, a lot of times I still *drive* myself to do it. I don't let up. More and more I'm finding I can enjoy it, but still I push myself very hard. But I realize when I talk with younger people at the office—and maybe I was once that way, you know—that they can't relax on the side; they only know one way and that's to keep moving forward, and when hours end they can't just let it go. And it probably is true that I'm better than most in terms of goin' home, havin' a beer, turnin' on the television, and giving absolutely no thought about what's going on at work. You know, when I think of my mother and her work, and if there was any sort of problem at all, she wouldn't sleep over it, worrying if she was doing things properly. And that's the kind of thing I can easily get into. If something bad happens to me during the day that has to be attended to the next morning—not jobwise so much, though for a long time it was school and all of those things that kept me up; some difficult thing that has to be dealt with, Stephanie [his girl friend] or

My previous comment "took" only partially. On rereading this, I wish I had said at this point something such as *It's more someone else's voice nagging you than your own. That nagging attitude is not really yours. It's your mother's, and you took it on.*

The earlier attributional work seems to be bearing fruit here. Mark is able to value positively and reframe this aspect of himself. (In a previous session I had said to him, as a further example of the effort directed toward this reframing, "I think your father had something very valuable to offer you, which you did take in and is an important part of you. You seem to have taken in some of the healthier parts of your father— being able to relax, not drive yourself all the time; and you've done it in a very useful way because you've combined it with a good deal of drive and ambition." This comment had had a number of dimensions and intentions. First of all, some of the father's traits had been reframed as positive and, implicitly, an inner voice that *values* Mark's more relaxed, self-accepting side is being substituted for the critical voice. There is an attributional dimension as well (see Chapter 9) in the comment's implicit suggestion that when Mark relaxes it does not mean he has lost his drive or ambition.

something like that—I will not be able to sleep. I'll get myself all tense, and I can't sleep. And it's just my mother, you know my mother just carries this everywhere, and it's true she . . . [*pause*] But it's funny, when you talk about depressed being central to her personality, I see what you mean, and I can even feel that. But I'm also a little confused because when I see Stephanie or Stephanie's mother, where depression *is* really central to their personalities, I just don't think of my mother in the same way, because she's always got a smile on her face and is always going somewhere. You know, I think of depression as making you like Stephanie, unable to do things.

At this point he is carrying forward on the work of the session, separating his representation of himself from that of his mother. But the distance achieved is as yet unstable, and he pauses and then questions the perspective he has just gained.

Stephanie's depressive makeup was very obvious. Apropos the dynamic that gets elaborated further as the session proceeds, this was in a sense part of her attraction for him; he could quell some of his fears of being like his father by noticing the contrast between him and Stephanie. At other times, Stephanie's depression would instead add to his guilt. He would feel it was his fault that Stephanie was depressed.

T: Right, your mother is not someone who *succumbs* to depression; but she's someone who's constantly *struggling* with it.

This comment returns to the central task of the session, helping Mark work toward a representational differentiation between self and mother. Notice that the comment is not about the patient but about his mother. Some of the most important interpretations in the course of a therapy are interpretations regarding significant others rather than about the patient himself (see Wachtel & Wachtel, 1986). In this instance, the comment was directed toward helping Mark to make more sense of his experience by clarifying something that been confusing and confused all his life. It was designed as well to carry forward the reframing and disidentification.

P: Maybe that's true, maybe that's true. I mean, she actually has said that sometimes. I guess I always thought of my *father* as unhappy because he looked unhappy and he sat around the house watching television.

T: It may also be that he looked unhappy *in contrast* to your mother, who was being compulsively and exaggeratedly *non*depressed.

Here again I am offering a reframing that provides a different way of interpreting his experience. Part of the context for this comment was that much of the work in the sessions of the past few weeks had been directed toward exploring a revised view of Mark's father. Although there was clearly some truth in the perception of him as depressed and passive, there was another side to him that Mark had begun to recognize. It turned out, for example, that father had been an accomplished amateur fencer and that he continued to go to the gym quite regularly. He also had completed a college degree because he was genuinely interested in learning, even though the degree had no relevance to the work he did or to his possibilities for earning a higher income.

P: That may be true. I mean one of the things that struck me about my mother some years ago, when her father was dying, we used to go to the hospital, and my mother's behavior can be quite strange. In that case, and I notice this is quite typical of my mother, she would spend a lot of time with all the other people in the hospital; she found it a lot easier to spend time comforting all the other patients, who were strangers, than to deal with her mother and father, which would be hard for anyone to deal with. But someone else might sit around crying or even avoid going to the hospital, say I can't do it, it's too painful to see my father that way. But my mother says, she goes and she just goes around helping everyone else out, people who have no relation to her. And so she has all these zillions of friends, and she loves meeting new people. I can't believe they keep up with all the people they know. It's not a case that when you go out there they're always doing something with other people. These are friendships that last for some period of time. They're not close friendships, but she likes that, as opposed to, I think, dealing with very close personal things. So you're right, she calls me up and she's still chipper, "how're you doing, everything going great?" She always wants to hear everything's going well. And the more she wants to hear it, the more somehow it's always been that I say things suck, everything's terrible. And there seem to be two things coming together in that. One is to displease my mother—there's a lot of anger at being pushed—and the other was not to exceed my father. Both kind of led to the same thing. You know, if I were miserable I'd upset my mother and make my father feel better, because after all I hadn't really outdone him. And I was thinking on the way over here about the idea that my father, of his being an admirable guy, and leading a reasonable life that he had some control over.

Mark seems here to be showing signs of having begun the work of internalizing an alternative voice taken from the therapy. To begin with, he lets me know he has been thinking between sessions about the

And I thought how come I didn't do that—although you would say maybe I *have* to some degree led a balanced life. But the answer is that when you're 3 or 4 years old it's a lot harder to fight back than when you're *24* years old. What happened was that I fought back but in the wrong way. Instead of becoming a rounded guy— although I think the world probably does see me as a rounded guy; maybe I *have* become a rounded guy—I became a succeed–failure guy. I couldn't help but succeed I was so driven. On the other hand, instead of saying now I'm gonna sit back and relax and enjoy my success, I'd say now I'm gonna fuck up to show my mother she really didn't win, which is I guess a natural thing for a kid to do. You know, "eat your food," and you say "No I'm gonna hold my breath." It's not "I've had enough mother, that's enough food, let's go on to dessert," or something like that. Kids don't talk that way. They take the food and they throw it on the floor. And that's probably long been my reaction to my mother's pushiness; she pushes and so I push back. Whereas my father was in a position to do something else, although not without unhappiness.

T: It's interesting, along the same lines but from a slightly different angle, that when you interact with your mother you find yourself coming off as more down than you ordinarily think you are. That may be another part of why your father looked depressed to you.

issues we have been discussing. The internalization is still clearly incomplete: he can bring to mind the idea that perhaps he has led a balanced life, but he still identifies it as something *I* would say. He continues the struggle productively as he proceeds. First he defends himself (immediately below), pointing out how hard it is for a little child to fight back. Then he alternates between saying he has become a "succeed–failure" guy *instead* of becoming a "rounded" guy, thinking that the world probably does see him as a rounded guy, and thinking maybe he really is a rounded guy. All of this reflects both the taking in of countermessages from the therapy and the transience and partial nature of that taking in, the fragile, delicate nature of the balance at this point. All in all, he seems to be moving toward a kinder, less judgmental and more forgiving attitude toward himself that reflects progress in the therapy. This back and forth shifting is characteristic of the process of working through. It is rarely an uninterrupted series of triumphs, but rather a reworking of conflicting images and attitudes that only gradually becomes more stable and solid.

P: Why's that?

T: He may have done what you did.

P: Oh, you mean he got down because of her constantly going on?

T: Because of it, in response to it, and almost as a way of saying fuck you to this compulsive "being up" that didn't have any relation to reality.

P: Yeah, what you're saying is you can, I mean one of the things that my mother was against was sleeping late. You know, my father got up at 4:30 in the morning to go to work for years and years and years. So on weekends he liked to sleep late. And my mother would go nuts. She'd wake you up and say you gotta get up, the day's a wasting, you're gonna miss the day. And so probably my father would start out by saying I wanna watch the ballgame this afternoon, and my mother would say "Ed how could you do that, it's a beautiful day out there, we gotta go, we gotta go out, we gotta go this, we gotta go that." And you're right. It makes you feel like saying, "no I wanna watch the game."

By caricaturing and exaggerating here, he is showing evidence of having gained some insight, or some different perspective or attitude; or put differently, of having alienated himself some from these attitudes.

T: The sense I get from what you're describing is that to protect your own integrity—whether it's you or your father—against the intrusion of a kind of false enthusiasm you have to kind of hold on to the part of you that's not swept up in that same swirl and that the feeling comes off, maybe even to yourself, as depression, even when that's not quite what it is.

We have another reframing here. It wasn't depression; it was rebellion.

P: Yeah, it does to me, it definitely does to me. I mean I almost have to say—it's a big relief almost; I'm embarrassed to say it—but in the last 6 weeks I had two weekends—ironic it was weekends; no, not ironic—where I got, well one weekend I got very sick and then two weekends ago, I just lost my voice. But one weekend I clearly was very sick, and I had to go to the doctor, and the doctor said I couldn't fly. And it wasn't just for a weekend, it lasted, well all week, although I went to work during the week, as I do. But my mother called and said "how're you doing" and I said "I've got a bad cold," and you could hear it, I sounded awful, and there's this kind of relief I don't have to go out, I don't have to push. And even then I had, you may remember, I had this ridiculous discussion with her where she said, "well what does it look like for the week," and I said, "well Sunday is the company picnic but I think I'm gonna stay in for the day and try to get over this cold"—you've heard people say that. And she says "No you should go to the outing, much better to be out in the sun, much better for you." What does she know? She went to medical school? I mean, certainly some people think rest is useful for a cold! So even then there's not even an exit. And even today, if Stephanie says it's a beautiful day, and I feel I want to watch television, I'm afraid she'll say "Gee it's much too nice to do that," and so I'll say "Well, I'm not really feeling so well." Now that could be a cold, that's easy to demonstrate, but it could also be I'm feeling a little depressed.

It is a measure of how hard it is for him to extricate himself from his mother's view of the world that he feels a need to seek my reassurance that people indeed sometimes stay in when they're trying to get over a cold.

So in other words you couldn't
sit around and watch television
and say boy isn't this great, I'm
really feeling great, because if
you're really feeling great you
should be outside. You have to
be feeling shitty. My memory is
of my father being depressed
when we were in the car driving
somewhere. Every Saturday we
went to see my mother's parents
and sometimes we'd go see my
father's parents, either on Sunday or on Saturday after visiting
my mother's parents. And probably part of why my father was
depressed was that that wasn't
what he wanted to do on a Saturday or Sunday. You know, he
worked his tail off during the
week. The funny thing is he
didn't even like seeing *his* parents. Part of the reason he saw
his parents is because my mother
would say we *should* see your parents too. He felt his parents
hadn't been so good to him, and
they were all the way at the other
end of Chicago, and it was a hassle getting to them, and he really
would have preferred to see
them a lot less. And my mother
would say Ed, we really have to
go see your parents too. Not that
my mother gave a shit about my
father's parents; neither of them
did. But they had to go see
them. So you had to do this and
you had to do that, and there
could never be a Saturday where
he could say Mark what a nice
Saturday, let's go fishing. We had
to go to my grandparents. And I
thought as a kid that's what my
parents wanted to do; after all we
were doing it. So I couldn't understand why my father looked

so miserable. It probably wasn't
what he wanted to do. And in
fact it probably wasn't even what
my mother wanted to do. My
mother doesn't know what she
wants to do; she only knows
what's on the calendar.

T: And what she has to avoid.

Here I'm refocusing us again on her
compulsive avoidance of depression,
which has been the central thrust of
the session's work. Mark's last comment offered further evidence of his
distancing himself from his mother's
attitudes. At this point the work of
disentangling himself from mother
is primary. But it is important to be
clear that the aim of the therapy is
not parent-bashing. At a later stage
of the work, he will be able to temper his disaffection with compassion
and be able to relate to her without
going along with her, especially by
internalizing his reactions to her.

P: Right, and what she has to avoid.
So for her, you know, she also
worked hard during the week,
but for her the worst possible
thing was to do nothing on the
weekend.

T: And she had a very hard time
being clear about the difference
between her and other people.
She attributed her needs and her
desires to your father, and she
does the same with you.

P: How so? Oh, you mean she pro-
jects them onto other people,
yeah, yeah. Oh definitely. Yeah,
in my case it may even be relatively true. I mean, she was able
to influence me obviously much
more than my father. I thought
by far my mother was the greater
influence on my life, and so
there is some truth. I do feel depressed when I don't do things,

and so I overschedule myself. We've talked about that. Even now, even since we've talked about it.

T: What I'm also hearing is two things in addition. One is that when you can get that external voice—and it is significantly an external voice even if it's in your own head—off your back, you *enjoy* relaxing.

P: (*interjecting*) Yeah, I do, I really do.

T: The other thing is that along with that I don't hear any danger that if you indulge that you'll never go out again.

P: (*interjecting*) No.

T: The desire to relax, to stay at home, to watch TV, to watch a ballgame, whatever, is very real and a very important part of you. And the desire to go out is real and an important part of you.

P: (*interjecting*) True.

T: And they would naturally achieve a kind of balance. The problem is that you kind of get scared either way, and the balance doesn't quite work well then.

P: Well, and it becomes very awful making choices. That's where I really have problems. When I had these two big weekends come up, Memorial Day and July 4th weekend, I wanted to relax and catch up. I had been working very hard and running around also. I really *had* been doing a lot. But I felt very uncomfortable at that idea. But it felt great last weekend when, at a certain point, after being with friends, I went home, bought a roasted chicken, had a glass of wine, watched a ballgame and had a great time. I really enjoyed doing that.

T: Now your *mother* would *not* enjoy that.

I am further fostering differentiation here.

P: No, she would hate that.

T: And she hasn't got it clear what that difference is about. It would be very different if she were to say to you "Gee I wouldn't be able to enjoy that." That's true. She wouldn't be able, and it's a shame she can't. But she assumes that *you* shouldn't also. And she lets you know she loves you *because* (as she sees it) you *don't* enjoy that either. And that makes it very hard for you to keep clearly in mind that you *do* enjoy it sometimes.

P: Right. And there's a large part of me that finds it difficult to do, because she would say that is not valid. What you are doing is not valid. What your father does is not valid. There's something wrong with your father. Real people, valid people, valuable people, *do* things. . . . [*pause*] But you know, it's also true that she's not just depressed, or fighting depression. She does useful things with what she does. It brings happiness to a lot of people.

The balance has shifted a bit too far here for Mark's comfort. He's feeling a bit too alienated from his mother and feels a need to preserve some of the connection.

T: I know. There are many admirable things about your mother, and they've been a source of strength for you too. What I think you're working toward, what you're becoming clearer about, but it still gets confusing sometimes, is that you got different and

equally valuable things from
mother *and* father. The problem
comes up because your mother
doesn't seem to recognize that
what you got from your father was
also valuable. That's why you feel
the conflict. The one thing you
got from your mother that *wasn't*
so valuable is the compulsive nature of it. That's what you're
working to get rid of; that and the
fear that if you're not constantly
pushing yourself you will run
down totally, a fear that's really
your mother's fear, not yours. It's
almost like you've taken on this
notion, which doesn't really make
sense to you when you look at it,
that if you watch television one
night, that's all you'll do for the
rest of your life.

This last, rather lengthy comment incorporates a number of the
elements that have been important in the entire extended segment with
Mark presented here. Describing the fear as *a fear that's really your
mother's fear, not yours* is at the heart of what the therapeutic work with
Mark in this segment has been about. The comment includes as well
several attributional elements of the sort discussed in Chapter 9 (e.g.,
which doesn't really make sense to you or *that's what you're working to get rid of*).
Perhaps an indication of the value to Mark of this effort to aid him in
gaining freedom from the shadow of his mother's imperatives is that at
the end of the session he made a special effort to rearrange his time so
he could come in for a session he thought he would miss because of his
vacation.

FACILITATING CHANGED BEHAVIOR IN DAILY LIFE

As crucial as it is to enable the patient to rework the affect-laden representations that shape and mediate his life experiences, enduring and
meaningful change cannot be achieved from this direction alone. Unless
change in the patient's manifest behavior proceeds apace, unless the
vicious circles that have been at the heart of the patient's difficulties are
modified, any changes in internal representations will be unstable and

transitory. Internal change and change in overt patterns are not really alternatives. They are two facets of one process, and neither alone will yield reliable and satisfying results.

Put differently, and considered more broadly, the primary focus of the book thus far has been on what transpires within the sessions, particularly on what enables the patient to hear what the therapist is saying with a minimum of resistance and a minimum of damage to his self-esteem. Much of the process of change in psychotherapy, however, takes place *outside* of the therapy sessions. For meaningful therapeutic change to occur, the patient must *apply* his insights in his daily inter-actions with others. A central premise of the cyclical psychodynamic point of view is that psychological difficulties are maintained most of all by the cyclical patterns of interaction in which the person repeatedly engages. As critical as intrapsychic processes are to the maintenance of the patient's difficulties, the unconscious motives, conflicts, defenses, and fantasies must themselves be understood as part of a larger circular pattern in which they are at once cause and effect. To attempt to work on the patient's internal representations without also addressing the patterns of living that both reflect and sustain them is to engage in a task worthy of Sisyphus.

To be sure, not infrequently the patient seems to make changes in daily life relatively spontaneously, with little apparent need for the therapist to monitor or promote them. When this happens, however, closer inspection is likely to reveal that the therapist's comments have in fact pointed the patient quite clearly toward engaging in certain actions or attempting certain experiments in daily living. Indeed, although the therapist may not have been explicitly aware of doing so, it is not unlikely that she has employed, in an informal and unexamined fash-ion, some of the principles that have been central to the discussions in this book.

In many cases, however, more explicit attention to overt change in behavior and relationships is necessary, and failure to attend to this dimension systematically may seriously impede the patient's progress. The manner of addressing this aspect of the work can vary—depending on the therapist's personal style and theoretical orientation—from ques-tions and comments that have a subtle structuring or suggestive element (see Chapter 9), to more explicit suggestions or directions, to methods such as role playing, modeling, rehearsal, graded *in vivo* tasks, and the like. (For a more detailed examination of these methods and how they may be adapted to fit into a therapy that is psychodynamic in its basic orientation see Wachtel, 1977; Frank, 1990, 1992.)

In attempting more explicitly and systematically to help the patient change his daily patterns of interaction, most of the considerations introduced in this book play a significant role. It is as important, for example, for the therapist to attend to and build on the patient's strengths in this stage of the work as it is in earlier stages. The working-through process is greatly enhanced when the therapist is alert to underlining and calling attention to those occasions when the patient is doing things differently. Comments such as *It sounds like you were able to be a little more open with Jim about some of the things he does that hurt you, even though talking about it made you anxious,* or *You may not have noticed the change, but I can see that in the past few months you've been much more determined not to get back at Susan by acting depressed but have tried to say what's on your mind instead,* or *You know, you used to get silent if you thought something I said was not on the mark, but now you're beginning to let me know in a very straightforward way; I'm really struck by the difference* can enable the patient to recognize change that might otherwise go unnoticed and, in the process, can help maintain and encourage it.[1]

Often a part of the same process entails *reframing* the patient's behavior in a way that highlights the change. Sometimes this is primarily a matter of emphasis, of a figure–ground shift—e.g., *I know you think of what happened as just another example of Ted's not taking your feelings into account, and I agree that it's very important for you to find a way to get him to hear you. But part of the process of getting there is to notice that, even if Ted ignored it this time, you did say what was on your mind. You used to not do that.*

On other occasions, the comment that encourages and amplifies change may entail not just a shift in figure and ground but a more thorough reinterpretation of the meaning of the occurrence—for example, *I suppose one could see it as a cop-out, but it seems to me not only fairer but also more accurate to say that you made a conscious decision to spare him something you thought he really couldn't handle.*

EXPLICIT ATTEMPTS TO ENCOURAGE NEW BEHAVIOR

In the examples just cited, one might describe the therapist's behavior as a kind of *following* or *tracking* of the patient's behavior: the patient takes the step on his own, and the therapist's role is to pay attention to the steps taken and to assure that the patient does also. Sometimes,

---

[1]The reader may recall at this point the interesting work of Tenzer (1984) discussed in Chapter 7. Tenzer stressed the critical importance of the patient's *noticing* changes that are taking place if they are not to evaporate, and illuminated how fundamental features of human cognition—especially the tendency to discount what does not fit in with prior expectations—can mitigate against that noticing. Without explicit effort on the therapist's part to promote the patient's awareness of change, the patient is likely to assimilate what has transpired into his old structures and schemas, and the change will be short-lived.

however, the therapist must make a more active effort if the patient is to follow through on the new understandings achieved. This necessity was recognized as early as 1919, in one of Freud's last papers explicitly directed to technique. Exhibiting a clear appreciation of the need for psychoanalytic technique to evolve beyond its classical contours, Freud noted that standard psychoanalytic technique "grew up in the treatment of hysteria and is still directed principally to the cure of this affection. But the phobias have already made it necessary for us to go beyond our former limits. One can hardly ever master a phobia if one waits till the patient lets the analysis influence him to give it up" (Freud, 1919/1959, pp. 399–400). Rather, Freud stated, the patient must be encouraged to expose himself to the object of his fear. Only when a considerable moderation of the phobia is achieved in this way, Freud maintained, will the associations and memories necessary for the full solution to the phobia come forth.

In discussing severe obsessional patients, Freud went even further in advocating the use of active intervention techniques. With such patients, he argued,

> a passive waiting attitude seems even less well adapted; . . . in their analysis there is always the danger of a great deal coming to light without its effecting any change in them. I think there is little doubt that here the correct technique can only be to wait until the treatment itself has become a compulsion, and then with this counter-compulsion *forcibly to suppress the compulsion of the disease.* (Freud, 1919/1959, p. 400; italics added)

Much as his first recommendation anticipated modern exposure-based treatments of phobias, this second points toward contemporary response-prevention techniques for dealing with compulsive behavior. Though Freud certainly had in mind that full and effective resolution of these patients' difficulties required psychoanalytic exploration as well, he did not share the antipathy to active intervention methods shown by some contemporary analysts.

In recent decades, a variety of methods have been developed to enable exposure to be more efficient and precise. A considerable literature has accumulated documenting the therapeutic effectiveness of exposure to the object of one's fears, and a wide array of methods have evolved, both from behavioral and from psychoanalytic sources, for effectively enabling the patient to confront the source of his fears and avoidances (see, for example, Marks, 1989; Wachtel, 1977, 1991b).

As effective and important as promoting exposure is, however, it is not the only means of actively aiding the process of working through. As discussed in Chapter 2, deficits in crucial interpersonal skills tend to accrue in the course of development as a consequence of early anxieties and avoidances, and they persist as part of a web of reciprocal influences that maintain the patient's difficulties through the years. If the patient is to successfully extricate himself from this web, he must not only understand it, he must take steps to modify his ways of interacting with others and to overcome the gaps in his development. This reworking of interpersonal relationships and overcoming of interpersonal anxieties is made difficult, however, by the fact that more is involved than simply exposure to a situation that remains constant. Unlike elevators, heights, or open spaces, other people *react* to our anxieties and to the particular behaviors we manifest in relation to them. As a consequence, it is perfectly possible—even common—for people to be exposed to the interpersonal situations they fear and have their fear confirmed rather than diminished. If we fear that expressing anger, or love, or need, or ambition to another person will result in rejection or humiliation, there is no guarantee that that will not be the case. The particulars of *how we go about* expressing those feelings, and the mood and proclivities of the other person, can make a crucial difference in whether the experience is one in which our apprehensions are confirmed or disconfirmed.

Instances in which the patient dares to be more open and is psychologically battered as a result scarcely can be regarded as therapeutic. Thus, an important part of the therapist's responsibility is to help the patient to structure the challenges he takes on so that they are consonant with what he can handle and are likely to be the foundation for further progress rather than a discouraging step backward (see Chapter 4). In this effort, such methods as modeling, role playing, rehearsal, and helping the patient plan out a series of graduated tasks and challenges in daily life can be very helpful.[2]

Such procedures—or at least their explicit and systematic use—are not common in therapies that are guided by a psychodynamic or other exploratory orientation. They can be introduced, however, in a fashion that is much more consonant with such approaches—both theoretically and stylistically—than is commonly appreciated; and when they are, the process of working through, of translating understanding into enduring change, is greatly facilitated. One key to forging effective links between these methods and the procedures and orienting ideas of exploratory psychotherapies lies in modifying their application so as to highlight generally unrecognized congruities between them and the interventions we call interpretations. Like more traditional interpreta-

---

[2]See Wachtel (1977) for a detailed examination of the objections that have been raised to the use of such methods in the context of a psychodynamically oriented therapy and a review of the clinical and theoretical considerations that point to the appropriateness of their use. See also Arkowitz and Messer (1984) and Frank (1990, 1992).

tions, these interventions address inclinations about which the patient is conflicted and which, although they are incipient, have not yet "occurred" to the patient.

Good interpretations do not address material that is still alien to the patient's consciousness but rather material that is almost—but not quite—accessible. In similar fashion, the actions that the therapist encourages and facilitates in appropriately structuring a program of assertiveness training or some other effort at helping the patient express his feelings more directly must be consonant with the patient's values and with his basic sense of what he is up to. What the therapist's suggestions or the program of modeling, role playing, and graded challenges add is a way of giving voice and shape to the patient's emerging inclination. The ideas or suggestions the therapist presents are likely to be somewhat beyond where the patient has already ventured—if they are not, they are unlikely to be a real contribution to the person's effort to change—but they cannot feel alien. Like a good interpretation, they make more explicit what is implicit and point the patient in the direction he is already inclined to go.

The comment that points the patient toward more assertive or effective behavior often is most usefully put in a form that is midway between that of an interpretation and that of a suggestion or assignment. One might say, for example: *It sounds as if you'd like to tell your husband that you enjoy spending time with him and wish he'd come home from work a little earlier, but you're afraid it will come out sounding as though you're just being critical and wanting something from him.*

This comment by the therapist does several things at once. If it is an accurate statement of how the patient feels, it conveys to the patient the therapist's understanding. Like any interpretation, it puts into words what is incipient and leaves the patient feeling both better understood and more able to understand herself. It does so, however, in a form that also offers the patient a model of how she herself might express her feeling *to her husband*. In this it implicitly carries the interpretive thrust into interpersonal action, providing the patient with tools that can modify her cycles of interaction with the other.

In addition, the comment also acknowledges the anxiety and conflict that has prevented the patient from expressing herself to her husband in such a fashion (or even from quite articulating *to herself* how she feels or what she wishes she could say). Because it casts her request as deriving from her *liking* spending time with her husband, the comment provides the patient with a model of how to speak to him in a way more likely to elicit a positive response. At the same time, by discussing how she is *afraid* her comment might sound to him, it acknowledges and illuminates her conflict (and, by clarifying how she does *not* want to come across, it enables her to be more alert in choosing and framing what to say).[3]

Statements by the therapist of the sort just described address inclinations in the patient that have not yet been fully experienced or articulated and aim both to make them clearer and more conscious and to help structure them in a way that will be interpersonally effective. Unlike interpretations carried out from a more classical psychoanalytic framework, this sort of comment does not aim at insight alone but attempts as well to help the patient give shape to his thoughts in a way more likely to achieve his aims or have an experience of satisfaction or effectiveness. These two purposes are complementary and mutually supportive rather than antithetical. The more confident the patient is that he can express his thoughts in a fashion that will have reasonably salutary consequences, the more able he is to relinquish the anxiety-motivated defenses that keep him from being in touch with his feelings and desires.

Given the complexity of interpersonal transactions, and the ways in which affective reactions and imputed meanings are inevitably filtered through layers of past experiences, it is likely that the patient's initial efforts to give voice to his recently expanded sense of his feelings and wishes will encounter at least some difficulties. By utilizing role playing and other such procedures to complement the more interpretive aspect of the work, the therapist is able to help the patient anticipate and come to grips with potential problems in a safe context before he tries out new behaviors in the more demanding and less forgiving situation of real life. After the patient's initial efforts at role playing how he might express himself more directly or effectively in some interpersonal situation he will encounter, the therapist can then raise (or the patient may himself spontaneously raise) a question such as: *What if your wife were to say such and such in response?* Patient and therapist can then go through various scenarios in the relative safety of the role-play situation, where ineffective or ill-considered responses by the patient can be reexamined and become part of a valuable learning experience rather than having immediate real-life consequences. They can then "take it from the top" and try the same scenario again after discussing together other responses the patient might make to the situation. As the patient builds both confidence and skills, the sources of his anxiety diminish, enabling him both to increase his awareness of his own feelings and inclinations and

---

[3]Sometimes, of course, the patient's putting things diplomatically or emphasizing the positive is not appropriate. There are clearly times when a direct expression of anger or a tough stand is called for. Most often, however, efforts to teach patients assertiveness and expressiveness skills begin with statements that give the other person the benefit of the doubt or stress the *common* advantage of the behavior desired, holding in reserve the possibility of later asserting one's wishes more aggressively.

to develop still further his capacity to give them effective shape in his daily life.

HELPING THE PATIENT UNDERSTAND HIS IMPACT ON OTHERS AND THEIR LIKELY RESPONSE

It is of course a central tenet of almost all approaches to psychotherapy that the patient must be helped to understand himself better. Sometimes overlooked, however, is the importance of his also gaining better understanding of *others*. Particularly from the vantage point of cyclical psychodynamics, which views psychological structures and processes contextually, it is essential to understand how the patient's experiences, conflicts, and anxieties are responsive to the actions and messages of those around him. The patient must achieve insight not only into what experiences, thoughts, or feelings he is warding off but also into his impact on others and their impact on him. The cyclical interpersonal patterns that are at the heart of most psychological difficulties, and the crucial role of "accomplices" in these patterns (see Chapter 2), make it essential that efforts to promote psychological change be rooted not only in an understanding of the patient's own psychological makeup but also in insight into the aims, vulnerabilities, and idiosyncratic ways of construing events that are characteristic of the key people with whom he interacts. The patient must learn to understand how others experience him and what the likely impact will be of various ways of relating to the principal figures in his life. Without such understanding, his efforts to carry forward into his life the nascent insights he has gained from the therapy sessions are likely to bear an unfortunate resemblance to the perambulations of a blind man in a mine field. If he comes out unscathed, thanks must go not to any skill in navigation but to sheer dumb luck.

It is my guess that if the practicing therapist looked closely at the comments she made in the course of a day's work, she would find that in fact a good number of them are addressed to the psychology of the other rather than exclusively to the experiences of the patient. Therapists implicitly recognize the importance of such a perspective both for themselves and their patients, and act accordingly, even if their theoretical orientation may not highlight such activity or may even make them feel vaguely uneasy about it. But in such instances this dimension of the work is likely to be somewhat casual and inadvertant, lacking in a clearly articulated rationale that can guide it in explicit and systematic fashion.

Almost inevitably, the therapist's comments about others will be more speculative than those about the patient, with whom the therapist has had much opportunity to interact directly. Nonetheless it is frequently possible to make a good enough guess about what is going on to be helpful to the patient in his efforts to break out of the repetitive cycles of maladaptive interactions in which he has found himself.

One might, for example, point out to the patient: *Given all that you've told me about your husband, he seems to get angry with you for the very things he himself is afraid of.* Or, in another situation one might convey: *Based on how ambivalent you've been and all you've told me about your girlfriend, it seems likely that she really is pulling away from you and that she's doing so in order to protect herself.* Or, in another context, one might comment: *Perhaps your wife is really expressing her own feelings of neglect by you when she complains that you don't spend enough time with the children.* Comments of this sort enable the patient to gain a clearer understanding of what is going on in his life. They fill in the gaps in much the way that interpretations of the patient's own unconscious motives and fantasies fill in the gaps, and they similarly contribute to the patient's gaining greater understanding and mastery in his life.

The ways in which understanding of the other's reaction to the patient contributes to helping the patient find a more adaptive resolution of her conflicts were interestingly illustrated in the case of Carla. Carla had been struggling for a while over her feelings regarding Jack, a man she had been going out with. Early in the relationship he had seemed to be the more enthusiastic pursuer, and she found him "very nice," "sweet," "considerate," and so forth, but not really an object of romance. Over time, though the terms in which she described her feelings remained the same, there was growing indication that the feelings themselves had begun to shift. At first the change was expressed through complaints. She began to feel, for example, that Jack was not spending enough time with her. And indeed, a certain amount of withdrawal on his part did seem evident. But there were also indications that his withdrawal was the result not of indifference but of self-protection, that he had not lost interest in her but rather felt very vulnerable.

As part of the effort to clarify for Carla what was going on between her and Jack, I pointed out to her that instead of saying to him, *I want to be with you more because you're wonderful*—which probably *would* result in his spending more time with her—she says, *How come you don't want to spend more time with me?*, a complaint that puts him off and makes him defensive.

Such a comment by the therapist not only helps her to see or understand what was happening, it also implicitly suggests an alternative path she can follow if she really wants to bring Jack closer. As a result, it raises as well, in a more alive and consequential fashion, the question of whether she really does want that. Here, as elsewhere, the therapist's attention to the patient's actual behavior and his active assistance in fashioning alternatives, far from obscuring or distracting from exploration of the patient's conflicts, enhances that very exploration.

In a similar vein, I made a comment near the end of the session that was also part interpretation (in that it illuminated a truth about her experience that she had been obscuring) and part suggestion or direction. I said, *I think if you were really being honest with Jack (and with yourself), what you'd say to him would be "I love you so much it scares me."* Such a way of putting it, of course, would feel very different to Jack from the kinds of things she had previously been saying.

Now, to be sure, Carla's maladroitness with Jack was not just a simple matter of "not knowing how." She was in *conflict*; in certain respects it would be accurate to say that she *wanted* to drive him away. But her conflict was mostly outside of awareness, and her unrecognized ambivalence reflected primarily her increasing feelings of vulnerability, which grew as her feelings for him did. If she could drive him away she would be saddened and hurt, but she would also be protected from the even greater hurt that would come if she lost him when her feelings had grown even stronger and when she had become even more dependent on him.[4]

Carla had had a long history of feeling panic when she started to get too involved and close to a man. Her feelings for Jack had grown to the point where she felt very susceptible to being hurt. As she put it, she was beginning to feel that her feelings had "outdistanced" his, and that she was now "in" the relationship in a way that was scary to her.

One of the ironies in the pattern just described is that, on the one hand, she had good reason to be cautious, because men *had* left her on a number of occasions; and, on the other, they had left her largely because of the very behavior she engaged in as a result of her fears they would leave.

An example of how this pattern worked came up in the next session. Carla reported having felt hurt that when she was telling Jack funny stories the night before, he didn't listen but went into the kitchen to take a snack. As we looked more closely at the episode, it became clear—to Carla as well as to me—that the real message of her stories was "men find me funny and find me attractive." She was telling such stories, with such a moral, because she felt insecure and wanted to make

---

[4]Sullivan (1953) has discussed the psychology of such preemptive strikes on one's own interests under the label of the "malevalent transformation."

Jack feel that he had a good thing and had better be careful to hold onto her. But the stories had the effect of making *Jack* feel insecure, and as a consequence he withdrew. This in turn further heightened *her* vulnerability and, without therapeutic intervention directed toward the pattern, might well have led to still other efforts designed to draw him in that actually drove him away. Helping Carla to appreciate the impact of her behavior on Jack, to understand how the world looked through his eyes, helped her to accomplish her goal of actually making a connection. Six months later they were married, and when I saw her for a followup interview 2 years after that, they were doing very well together.[5]

THE FEAR OF STEPPING OUT OF CHARACTER

One difficulty commonly encountered when the patient is being urged in one way or another to engage in new behaviors is that the patient experiences the new behavior as strange and as "not really me." In part the patient's hesitation and feeling of strangeness is the result of anxiety. What has been avoided is likely to have been feared, and so when it is approached anew, fear is stirred once again. But there is another dimension to this as well. In the course of development we all acquire an enormous stake in the image we hold of ourselves, and that stake— rooted in the well-founded perception that our sense of self is at the heart of whatever stability and security we are able to find in the world— leads us to defend ferociously whatever image or sense of ourselves we hold.

As Sullivan and Rogers in particular have emphasized, it is not just "bad" things about ourselves that we ward off if they are inconsistent with the self-image we hold. We can ward off "good" things as well. It can be as threatening to discover that we are smarter, or kinder, or more competent than we had imagined as it can be to learn their opposites. For, to appropriate a phrase from the poet Delmore Schwartz, "in dreams begin responsibilities." When we recognize ourselves as "better" than we thought, the basis for some of the ways we are living is called into question, and we begin to feel a push toward change. And change is threatening. It means sticking our neck out—for what if, in the midst of taking on new challenges commensurate with our newfound sense of

---

[5]Obviously Carla and Jack's success in getting together cannot be attributed solely to the interventions just described. But the vignette illustrates a process that I believe is frequently very helpful in turning around long-standing problematic patterns.

being smarter or more competent than we thought, we discover that we have gone out on a limb and that we were really right all along about our limitations?

Often, moreover, underneath this fear lies another, perhaps even more elemental. Stepping out of character can feel like breaking a serious taboo. The sense of identity is so fundamental, and yet potentially so fragile, that for many people there is a primitive sense of wrongness in altering it in any way. Often the patient will have a vague feeling that some new behavior or new mode of interacting with others or of carrying himself is perfectly acceptable for other people but not right for *me* to do it: "It just doesn't feel right; it just isn't *me*."

It is important for the therapist to be alert to these less welcome accompaniments of change and to help the patient understand that what he is experiencing is a common, and usually temporary feeling. The skillful use of paradox, attribution, and reframing can be very helpful in this regard.

An interesting illustrative example involved a couple that was being seen by a therapist I was supervising. One of the prominent features in the case was that although this man and woman seemed committed to staying together and to trying to work out a better relationship, they were unusually lacking in expressions of affection toward each other. They were also hypervigilant and averse to being "pushed" by the therapist. A previous session had highlighted the sense of alienation and deprivation they both felt because they hardly ever touched each other, and the therapist had thought of making the simple request that they make an effort to do so. He hoped that if they could begin to change their behavior toward each other in this way, it would contribute at least a small increment toward initiating a more positive dynamic between them. He worried about making such a request, however, because they were constantly on the alert for "phoniness" or "artificiality," and he felt they would experience touching each other "under orders" as gimmicky and insincere. (Interestingly, their overly keen concern with whether any expression of feeling was genuine or not was one of the reasons they were so distant from each other; they didn't trust either their own affectionate impulses or their spouse's.) I felt that the therapist's concern about how his recommendation was likely to be received was appropriate, and suggested that he instead say to them, *Can you each try to be more aware of when the other is touching?*

Such a comment, although addressing the same domain as the comment the therapist had originally thought to make, does not make the touching artificial or "unspontaneous." It does not leave the couple feeling that touching has been coerced or that they are going through the motions just because the therapist requested it. Indeed, there is no request at all for them to touch more than they have been. They are being asked only to *notice*.

In part, the request's purpose is to draw their attention to a dimension of their lives that they have been deficient in noticing. It is designed to foster both the sense of appreciating and of being appreciated. At the same time, however, it also makes more likely the *occurrence* of affectionate touching. Though it does not request it (and therefore minimizes the likelihood it will feel merely acquiescent and consequently unnatural or unreal), it does put the idea of touching into the back of their minds. By calling attention to touching and thoughts of touching, while removing the sense of compliance with an external demand, the comment heightens whatever inclination the couple might have to touch each other and makes an end run around the stultifying and interlocking obstacles to the expression of feeling. In addition, the request increases the likelihood of furthering and sustaining the touching because it renders the touching more likely to be reinforced.

INTERRUPTING VICIOUS CIRCLES

Almost all of the interventions described in this book can be seen as part of an effort to interrupt the vicious circles in which the patient is caught. But the full picture of the circle is not always clear. In many instances one works with whatever portion of the pattern is discernable at that point and applies whatever therapeutic principle seems to apply to that portion. In other instances, however, it is possible to grasp one or more complete circles and to address one's therapeutic efforts to the repetitive circular pattern as a whole. One such instance was in the case of Mark, discussed earlier in the chapter.

A key vicious circle in Mark's difficulties derived from his mother's life-long efforts to ward off depressive feelings, leading her to be compulsively active and on the go and to have little tolerance for any behavior that bore even the slightest stamp of what she would perceive (via her highly attuned state of the art radar) as slothful or lacking in vitality. As noted above, for example, his mother would be appalled if ever he were indoors on a sunny day, and even in his adult years, if he decided to stay home or cancel plans because he had a bad cold, she would respond in a fashion that was almost a counter-stereotype of the overly protective mother, making him feel like "a wimp" or a "cop-out" who was missing out on life.

Mark was in fact an active, successful, energetic individual, but he was plagued by doubts about whether he was really vital and active enough. He lived with a constant sense of what he "should" be doing, and his "shoulds" were oppressive enough to make this energetic man feel at times positively inert. He tried valiently to satisfy the voice of the "shoulds," but the results were (perhaps predictably) ironic: he was so focused on what he *should* be doing that he had little opportunity to sense or feel what he really *wanted*. As a consequence, he experienced little in the way of spontaneous desires and so had "evidence" for his purportedly slothful nature. It seemed to Mark that if he were not constantly driving himself through these phenomenologically external directives, he would do nothing at all.

Indeed, not surprisingly, the "shoulds" induced a kind of psychic counterinsurgency that took the form of *very strong* desires to "veg out" in front of the TV and be free of the need to *do* anything. This in turn strengthened the "shoulds" still further, as he felt the need to fight what he perceived as his passivity and lack of vitality by making himself do things. Of course, such a course was hardly successful; the new should would elicit a new resistance, a new longing to be left alone to do nothing, and then, reactively, still more "shoulds" and more of the same conflict.

Much of this was accompanied by a good deal of confusion, a sense of not being sure *what* he wanted to do. He would describe, for example, feeling he wanted to go hear music at a club but not being sure if he really wanted to or if it were just something he *should* do, something that the kind of person he felt he was supposed to be would do. He would start to feel it was a drag to get across town to the club, but then he would force himself to call, and would feel *relief* if they were sold out. It seemed to him that he didn't so much want to go out as to avoid being able to be accused of *not* going.

After a time, the therapeutic work succeeded in enabling Mark to achieve a fairly well-articulated sense of the pattern. He understood as well how it was related to his mother's efforts to ward off depressive feelings and to the way she used her identification with him in that effort. But it was still very difficult for him to resist the pull of the "shoulds" because he was usually in *conflict*. He could not be sure if he was dealing with a should or with something he really wanted to do. Much energy went into wrestling with these continually unsolveable dilemmas.

In attempting to help Mark go beyond understanding the pattern, and actually begin to break it, I suggested that whenever he had any suspicion that a sense of "should" was even a part of his inclination to do something, he would be best off not doing it. The advice in effect was, "If you're sure you want to do it, do it. But if you're not sure, if you're in conflict, err on the side of resisting the shoulds. If you end up doing nothing, that's okay. You'll be confronting your phobia about becoming a lethargic blob. You'll sense that you can resist a 'should' and not collapse into an inanimate heap. And if you do feel a strong spontaneous desire, then go ahead. In fact, this is the only way we can *make room for* those kinds of desires, the only way you can begin to get clear about what that feels like."

He was asked, however, not to follow this rule just yet when it came to *consequential* things (such as important job matters or issues central to his relationship with his girl friend). Moreover, I addressed quite explicitly that he would encounter some very difficult discriminations. It would be unclear *both* whether he really wanted to do something or was just following a "should" *and* whether whatever it was was important. The basic message was that such dilemmas were part of living and that he should focus his energies in the beginning on the easy ones. In that way he could gradually build a new sense of agency into his life and become clearer about what it actually felt like to want something.

ARE ACTIVE METHODS SUPERFICIAL OR MANIPULATIVE?

Some therapists are hesitant to include methods such as role playing, rehearsal, and graded real life tasks for fear that their use will compromise the depth of the therapy and of the change that can be achieved. In their view, such methods necessarily imply a superficial concern with surface behavior only. Such an attitude, I believe, is rooted in faulty premises, and places unnecessary constraints on the possibilities for promoting the changes the patient is seeking. Far from consigning the therapy to banality and superficiality, active efforts to help the patient change his ongoing behavior in daily life can actually deepen the impact of the therapeutic work. Explicit attention to and assistance with manifest behavior permits a more thorough and affectively alive integration into the patient's life of the understanding he has gained in the therapy. It thereby reduces substantially the likelihood that the therapy will be limited by sterile intellectualized insights that fall short of producing real change.

Because the patient's inner state and his outer behavior are complexly interlinked, changes in the one yield changes in the other. This linking is powerful and goes in both directions; but because it is less than a one-to-one correspondence, it is usually not sufficient to approach change only from one of the two directions. Multifaceted intervention, including both work on the patient's inner states and fantasies and work on his overt patterns of interaction with others, is likely to yield greater change in *each* than efforts that address only one.

In the therapeutic approach described in this book, attention to the manifest patterns of interaction, although crucially important, is clearly only a part of the work's focus. The meaning to the patient of the various actions he might undertake (and, importantly, of the therapist's participating with him in this way); the subjective feeling tone associated with it; and the underlying assumptions and fantasies and less consciously articulated experiences that lie behind (and are in turn maintained by) the manifest patterns—all are within the purview of the therapeutic focus described here.

Overt behavior and intrapsychic processes are not really separate realms. They are most fully understood in relation to each other and in terms of the complex feedback loops that link and maintain them. As I have described in the early chapters of this book, pursuit of one pole of the dialectic of action and insight deepens rather than diminishes our appreciation of and ability to work with the other pole.[6]

Use of the methods alluded to in this chapter furthers and deepens the process of exploration at *all* stages of the therapy, assuring that it will be more fully experiential. But it may be particularly important in the later stages of the work, when the processes of working through are especially emphasized. There is little that can more powerfully amplify and consolidate the experiential dimension of what the patient has learned in the sessions than his trying out his insights in daily life. And there are few better ways of promoting one's genuine experiencing of the hidden dimensions of one's subjectivity than to establish new modes of interacting with others.

A FINAL NOTE ON RESISTANCE

Throughout this book, I have stressed the importance of communicating our understanding to the patient in ways that do not needlessly generate resistance. For some readers, this aim itself may seem problematic. Especially for psychoanalytically oriented therapists, the analysis of resistance is at the very center of therapeutic focus. Indeed, it might be said with some justification that the primary way in which contemporary psychoanalytic practice differs from the methods used by Freud and other early analysts lies in the increasing sophistication with which the task of identifying and analyzing resistances is undertaken. It would seem, from this perspective, that any effort to sidestep or avoid resistance will be counterproductive; only if the resistances are able to be fully addressed will truly deep and lasting change be promoted.

[6]See also Wachtel (1977, 1987), Wachtel and Wachtel (1986), and Wachtel and McKinney (1992).

In considering this issue, it is useful at the outset to remind ourselves that resistance is not recalcitrance, stubbornness, or a lack of cooperation on the patient's part. It is, rather, a manifestation in the therapeutic relationship of the same anxieties and avoidances that are at the heart of the difficulties the patient comes to therapy to address. In this sense, resistance can never be totally eliminated. Where there is a problem appropriate to bring to therapy, there is inevitably anxiety, and hence resistance.

In the evolution of psychoanalytic practice, it was not long before Freud recognized that the behaviors he had experienced as resistance were not merely an annoyance, to be gotten past or conquered as rapidly as possible, but were of intrinsic theoretical and clinical interest in their own right, psychological phenomena as essential to explore as the tendencies they were designed to ward off. With the development of ego psychology and the clarification of the role of anxiety in generating psychological disorder, understanding of the phenomena labeled as resistance took a further step forward. Increasingly, the aim was not to suppress or overcome the resistances but to *analyze* them, to help the patient see and understand *that* he was resisting, *why* he was resisting, and *what* he was resisting.

Much of the core of this conception of the therapeutic process is sound, but its boundaries and details have become blurred, for reasons having to do with the intersection of semantics and history. The term resistance itself is no longer adequate to capture the phenomena to which it refers. A term that has inherently adversarial overtones has come increasingly to refer to an understanding that is *not* adversarial: the patient does not really *resist* the therapy when he manifests many of the behaviors originally labeled as resistance; rather, that is one more way in which he *participates* in the therapy. The behaviors we have learned to label as resistance are in large measure manifestations of the patient's *conflict* and *anxiety*, and if the patient is to bring those conflicts and anxieties into the therapy room (as he must if he is to benefit from the therapy), then perforce he will also give evidence of "resistance."

Not all resistance, however, is a necessary and (ultimately) productive occurrence in the therapy, nor is all of it generated solely by the dynamics and characteristics the patient initially brings with him. Much of it, we need to understand, is artifactual and iatrogenic. If one tries to minimize resistance by avoiding the topics that can arouse anxiety, the therapy is indeed hampered and rendered superficial. But if resistance is minimized by *approaching* the topic, but doing so *skillfully*, the matter is quite different. The essence of dealing with resistance in the most therapeutically effective manner is to keep clearly in mind that ultimately overcoming resistance in a fashion consistent with the therapeutic effort entails helping the patient to overcome the anxiety that motivates it. And this means confronting the object of anxiety, not avoiding it.

In large measure the therapist's expertise lies in dealing skillfully with the resistance, in finding a way to enable the patient to face those aspects of himself and of his life that are causing his difficulties. But the therapist is best able to accomplish this task if she recognizes that the responsibility for what seem to be adversarial elements in the therapeutic relationship does not lie solely with the patient. The therapist's way of inquiring and of interpreting can at times be equally responsible. It is to this obstacle to therapeutic progress that much of this book is directed. My aim has been to enable the therapist to pursue the tasks of therapeutic work without stepping on her own feet, or on the patient's. With sensitivity both to the patient's vulnerabilities and to the ways in which our own communications can contribute to increasing or diminishing those vulnerabilities, we are in a position to use what we have learned to make a lasting contribution to the patient's well-being.

Postscript
Therapeutic Communication with Couples

Ellen F. Wachtel, Ph.D.

The principles of therapeutic communication described in this book are as applicable to work with couples as they are to work with individuals. In certain respects, they can be applied almost without modification, as the foundation for basic clinical effectiveness. In other ways, they must be modified slightly to be applied to the somewhat different context of couples therapy. In this postscript, I spell out both how these principles apply to couples work and how they are modified in such work. Although I will refer to specific chapters or principles from the book in numerous places, my intent is as well to convey more generally how pervasive these principles are in effective work with troubled couples. I hope it will be evident to the reader how much of what is described here, even when not explicitly referring back to the book, is rooted in the same basic principles.

In order to provide a context for this discussion, I will also need to convey something of my overall approach to couples therapy. There are, of course, many different schools and theories of couples therapy, with both divergence and overlap. In the work described here, both psychodynamic and systems principles feature prominently, but both are given a particular shape by their being integrated with each other (see Wachtel & Wachtel, 1986) and by my commitment, consonant with the main themes of this book, to finding and building on the strengths that people bring in and not just seeing what is wrong.

One key difference between individual and couples therapy—which on the one hand requires certain modifications of the principles described in this book, and on the other makes them even more cru-cial—is that in couples therapy whatever one has to say to one person is overheard by a second; indeed, by a second with whom the first may be in conflict. As a consequence, helping couples to really listen to one another and to change habitual patterns of interaction can feel like a balancing act not dissimilar to that of the high-wire walker's. The skill of the couples therapist consists very largely in maintaining a sense of balance; not tilting to one side or the other too much without making rapid and deft corrections and treading with a determined yet light step so that she remains on firm footing with each member of the couple.

Since couples therapy involves talking to each partner in the pre-sence of the other, concern for *how* statements are made and not just *what* is said is perhaps even more important than when speaking to a single individual privately. Carefully wording comments so that they will not be experienced as critical or humiliating not only tremendously increases one's effectiveness in reaching the individual spoken to but also provides some insurance against the potential misuse of these com-ments by an angry partner.

Careful wording of comments made to each individual has two other important functions as well. First, the couple often begins to model the therapist's constructive way of broaching sensitive and difficult topics even without the desirability of doing this being explicitly stated. And second, as discussed later in this chapter, concern with the connotative aspects of one's choice of words and therapeutic focus often provides one partner with a more benign perspective on the difficulties of the other.

Careful attention to the language we use when working with cou-ples is helpful in combating the feelings of despair and futility that most couples are experiencing by the time they have decided to seek some professional help. Not only do couples generally feel quite angry and frustrated, but it is not uncommon for them to feel a good deal of *shame* about their relationship—shame because they may have been spinning their wheels for years, unable to go forward, yet unable to call it quits; shame about the "pettiness" of their arguments; shame about the con-stant "tit for tat" in which they engage; shame about the loss of control or venom in their fights; shame that their children have had to witness emotional and sometimes physical abuse; and even shame that they have lived for years as "friends" and have each accepted a marriage of convenience, without love, sex, or passion.

Because of these considerations, therapists working with couples must take great care that their comments do not inadvertently create more despair or humiliation. Therapy that uncovers what is wrong, without also attending to what is right, is likely rapidly to unravel the fragile thread of optimism that leads a couple to seek some help. A central underlying tenet of the couples work I will be describing is that change is most likely to come about by building on whatever positive aspects of the relationship once existed and still exist in some form. By training herself to notice strengths as readily as pathology, the couples therapist gives the message that change in time-worn interactions might still be possible. Whatever "good" in the relationship is still there, or even *once* was there, must be nurtured so that it can grow to assume a central position in the couple's relationship.

An essential ingredient to all therapy is hope that something better is possible. By taking every opportunity available to build on whatever kernels of strength still exist, the therapist gives the couple some reason to take the risks involved in changing and attempting to meet one another's needs. One might think of the work as akin to renovating and creating additions to a home while using the supporting beams and preserving as much of the old character as possible. The therapist searches, in what may feel to the couple like nothing more than rubble, for foundation stones and valuable aspects of the relationship in which a new and vital structure can be built.

Attention to the "rubble," however, is important too. If a couple is going to value what the therapist finds to preserve, they must know that she has seen as well where the structure has crumbled and where it may even look hopeless to its inhabitants. Attention to "positives" will only be accepted if each member of the couple knows that the therapist truly understands just how bad it has been between them. Each partner must experience the therapist as having empathy for his or her perspective. Each must know that the extent of his or her feelings of deprivation and anger are understood and that the seriousness of the couple's problems is acknowledged. A focus on "positives" can have a powerful impact when the couple experiences it as in the context of the therapist's *realistic* assessment of their difficulties. Building on variations, focusing on the direction of movement, and attending to conflict and ambivalence are but some of the methods described in this book that with only slight modifications, enable the therapist to focus on positives while at the same time she works on the very real difficulties the couple describes.

As in individual therapy, the couples therapist must find a way to balance the need to affirm and the need to confront. Problems need to be focused on while at the same time respect for the couple, and perhaps even for the "logic" of the interactional pattern that developed between them, needs to be conveyed. Just as the individual's defenses must in a sense be "admired" for the functions they have served, the dysfunctional patterns between people often have a logic to them that it is helpful to acknowledge.

The concept of reframing has long been used by family therapists (often, with a partially paradoxical intent) as a means of simultaneously affirming and challenging the couple's interactional patterns and interpretations of each other's behavior. Little attention has been paid, however, to how to talk to the *individuals* in the couple or family in ways that similarly convey acceptance yet push for change. It is not often acknowledged in the couples therapy literature that although in one sense the *couple* is the patient in couples therapy, probably the majority of comments made in a session are to individuals rather than to the couple collectively.

Individuals in couples therapy are apt to be even more defensive and feel even more threatened than they might otherwise be. After all, in many instances they are being asked to be open in the presence of the very person who has become an adversary.[1] Many of the suggestions in this book, particularly those that deal with the use of attributional comments and attention to conflict, are of great help in reducing the defensiveness of individuals in the context of couples work. Attention to how to frame comments so that defensiveness will be minimized is particularly important when working from within an integrative perspective in which individual psychodynamic issues as well as systemic ones are addressed. Even though the couples therapy I describe is problem focused and stresses the finding of new ways to interact, attention to the preconscious and even unconscious conflicts and wishes of each individual is a crucial component in finding interactional solutions that will really meet each person's needs.[2]

Couples therapists often need to make comments and interpretations that are based on information that is not nearly as complete as in individual therapy. The extreme distress of the couple and the sense of urgency they frequently feel to come to some decision as to the salvageability of the marriage necessitates this. Wording statements so that they will not be perceived as "pronouncements" or "interrogations" is thus of particular importance in couples work. Greater care is also needed because the therapist cannot rely on the trust generated by an exclusive relationship, in which the therapist gives the patient *undivided* attention and concern, to cushion the blow of ineptly made or unintentionally

---

[1]It is important to be clear, however, that not all couples who seek therapy treat each other as adversaries. Some couples convey a good deal of love and respect for one another and are puzzled about what is going wrong between them.

[2]Combining individual and systemic perspectives is important in family work as well as with couples. Not enough attention has been given to the individual conflicts and concerns of symptomatic children when they are seen in family therapy. New methods of working with families that address individual and systemic issues equally are important to develop (Wachtel, 1987, 1990, 1991, 1992).

hurtful interpretations. Moreover, though some couples therapy is long-term and some individual therapy short-term, generally the individual therapist's relationship with the patient is of a longer duration, and this shared history together in itself gives the therapist more leeway for error. Careful wording of comments in the ways described in this book, so that they are experienced as giving permission for new ways of acting rather than as rebukes, is of the utmost importance when time is limited and interventions are made rapidly.

When working with couples, it is important that each partner also feel known as an individual. An openness to changing *in* the relationship is enhanced when each person feels understood and appreciated for who he or she is *apart* from the relationship. Couples therapists are apt to see the darkest and most unattractive sides of their patients.[3] The couple knows that the therapist is getting an impression of each of them that is in some sense based on their worst selves. For this reason, it is important to broaden one's perspective and to have an awareness of how each person acts in *other* aspects of his or her life. One can do this simply by talking to the couple about their lives outside the marriage and also by having them each talk about their families through constructing genograms.[4]

ATTENTION TO "INCIDENTALS": THE NOTICING OF VARIATIONS AND MOVEMENT IN POSITIVE DIRECTIONS

Moment to moment, in every session with a couple, therapists make choices regarding what they will respond to. Which *part* of a statement

---

[3]Therapists who know their patients only from individual meetings often do not see aspects of their behavior that may be activated only when in the presence of the spouse. A great deal of knowledge of the patient's emotional reactions can, of course, be obtained from observation of the patient in the transference; but the individual therapist who has seen her patient alone for months or years, and has experienced the full range of transferential responses, may nonetheless be shocked if accorded the opportunity to observe the patient in direct interaction with his or her spouse. There is often an intensity and irrationality in these interactions that is unmatched by anything that is revealed in the transference.

[4]The genogram, a systematic way of obtaining a three-generational family history, can be utilized in a way that makes it a projective instrument (see Wachtel, 1982). One can get to know a good deal about each person in a relatively short amount of time by spending some portion of the session constructing the genogram of each partner in the presence of the other. One quickly obtains a good deal of information not only about the individual's impressions of family members but also about his idiosyncratic world view and unarticulated ego ideals and longings. We get as well a quick glimpse into the unconscious concerns that are relevant to the marital relationship.

the therapist chooses to focus on, as well as how the therapist's comments are couched, greatly influences whether there will be movement or resistance. Being helpful to couples is often as much a function of what we do *not* do and the paths we do *not* take as it is of the utilization of any particular intervention. Attention to what might seem "incidental" to what the couple, and even most observers, might take as the main message is frequently the most helpful path to follow. In effect, at those times the therapist listens to the background chords instead of the melody and calls attention to aspects of their interaction that they might not otherwise notice. Often it is this shift in focus, from the obvious troubles that are usually in the foreground of attention, to various seemingly unimportant and largely unnoticed aspects of the couple's relationship, that is the starting point for useful new perspectives and reframings.

Building on strengths can be implemented at almost every juncture at which the therapist is called on to comment. Even when the primary focus of the statement is on a problematic pattern or negative feature of the relationship, it is important to attend to and highlight any elements of what is being observed that have a positive quality or potential. One can underline positives while simultaneously discussing the couple's difficulties by carefully attending to *variations* and the *direction of movement*—for example, by saying something such as: *I'm struck by how you are more able today, and have been increasingly able in the past few weeks, to not withdraw when you are feeling angry at each other. You really have been hanging in there more.*

From the first session to the last, the therapist must be constantly aware of reinforcing any movement, slight as it may be, towards the therapeutic goals. Crucial to the effective use of underlining positives is the recognition that both individual and transactional behavior is never static (see Chapter 7). Spouses will vary in how defensive, cooperative, controlling, sensitive, gentle, self-centered, or angry they are with one another, and it is important to comment on these variations, especially on those that are in the direction of what the couple hopes to achieve.

If at all possible, I try, even in a first session, to attend to some "incidental" that may reflect something positive in the relationship. Thus, after hearing a couple describe their difficulties and communicating to them my understanding of how distressed and drained they are by these problems, I will then go on to comment on something I have noticed that the couple probably takes for granted. For instance, with some couples it might be pointed out that although they are clearly quite frustrated with one another, it is interesting that they don't contradict each other very much and seem to agree on what has happened. Or perhaps one might notice that although they are both very angry, they are not condemning or attacking in a deep sort of way. Or perhaps one notices that despite the fact that things have been going very badly for them, they laugh together for a few moments in the session. Even something as simple as their letting each other talk without interruption can be noted, since this is by no means true of all couples.

Of course one might notice more significant (less "incidental") positives, and these of course should be commented on too. The couple may clearly show affection for one another, respect each other as people, have a shared sense of values, have a shared way of looking at the world, or may regard each other as being good parents, to name but a few. Often these strengths (from minor to major ones) have been, prior to the therapist's comments, largely unnoticed. Giving this feedback starts the process of building. Most couples respond extremely positively to the therapist's sharing of such observations as long as these comments are accompanied by clear indications that the difficulties of the couple are also being noticed.

If feedback of this kind is to be effective, it must be genuine, or it will be experienced by the couple as nothing more than patronizing manipulation. When therapists train themselves to notice strengths as much as they do problems, these sorts of statements begin to come naturally and to derive from the overall sense the therapist has of the couple. In general, comments about strengths are taken more seriously when they are supported by details that elaborate the point. It is better for therapists not to be terse in explicating the reasons for the positive observations they are making. For example, a statement such as *I think you are trying hard today to understand your husband's point of view* would have more of an impact if some elaboration were offered. One might add to that statement something like: *The gentle way you are speaking and the kinds of questions you are asking indicate a real willingness to take in what is being said.* Or, rather than saying that the couple seem to have a shared sense of humor, it would be better if one added to that statement the observation that the husband smiles at his wife's droll way of describing unpleasant events.

Attentiveness to small variations and subtle changes can powerfully influence future behavior. For example, if a generally closed and defensive person admits in a session to some unconscious motivation such as "well, maybe I was angrier than I realized" or "I guess what I did was a bit provocative," the therapist should note the candor and openness with which he or she is speaking. This acknowledgment not only is likely in itself to lead to more openness, it also offers the therapist an opportunity to inquire about what makes it difficult at other times to be as open as he or she is being today. Raising the issue at a time when one is saying something positive to the patient is likely to be experienced very differently than if one had tried to discuss the undesirable behavior at the time it was actually taking place (see Chapter 7).

Even when a couple is arguing rather intensely in a session, it is possible to offer certain kinds of positive feedback that can help shape their actions in future arguments. By noting such things as, for instance, that although they are very angry they are doing well in maintaining control, or are not hitting below the belt, or are not engaging in character assassinations, the therapist calls attention to positives that can then become incorporated into future self-definitions and consequent actions.

A related but slightly different type of intervention is that of *positive attribution*. This involves something rather similar to what was described in Chapter 9—noticing the slightest bit of motivation for change and attributing to the couple or the individual the wish to do something differently. Thus, for example, if the wife sighs and says "I *really do* have a bad temper," the therapist might comment that she senses that the wife seems disturbed by this and would like to do something about it. Often the therapist might attribute motivation to the patient of which he or she is not yet cognizant. By articulating a yet inchoate feeling, the therapist in fact helps along and encourages moves in the direction now named. As discussed in Chapter 9, such a comment is appropriate only when there is at least some kernel of truth to it that can be expanded upon. In order for attributions to be effective they must actually resonate with an aspect of the individual's experience. People will adopt attributions about themselves if they resonate with at least some part of conflictual feelings. Attributions that are off the mark are unlikely to do harm but will not be accepted.

RESISTANCE AND ANXIETY

As was described at several points in this book, resistance is not solely a result of characteristics of the patient or of struggles to maintain the status quo. Often it is stimulated as well by the subtly adversarial manner in which the therapist couches her inquiries and interpretations. Marital and family therapists too not infrequently provoke resistance. The family therapy literature is replete with references to couples and families which speak about them in an adversarial manner. Images of "doing battle" and outmaneuvering intransigent systems abound. In recent years a number of marital and family therapists have written critically about this "hierarchical," "acting upon" therapeutic stance (Hoffman, 1988; de Shazer, 1985) and the inevitability of resistance has been questioned (Dell, 1982; Anderson & Stewart, 1983).

Though it is undoubtedly true that people frequently are reluctant to change familiar patterns that have proven to be destructive, they are generally *ambivalent*, not just *negative*, about the prospect of change. The interactional patterns couples develop reflect a complex mix of conscious and unconscious forces that can indeed express each partner's psychodynamic conflicts and defense mechanisms.[5] Though these dynamics are important, they do not *inevitably* lead to resistance. "Benefits" gained by the relationship staying static are only one side of the balance sheet. The negatives that result from these unarticulated and often unconscious "contracts" (Sager, 1978) are strong motivators for change and often far outweigh wishes to hold on to familiar though problematic interactions.

Recognizing that it is anxiety that lies behind resistance is as helpful with couples as it is with individuals. When one member of the couple behaves "hostilely" to the therapist, or acts as though all attempts to make clarifying comments are "oversimplifications," or "corrects" everything that the therapist or partner says, or dismisses directly or indirectly all suggestions for new ways of interacting as useless, it is hard not to feel annoyed and to experience that person as someone who is simply "difficult" and "resistant." Understanding the sources of anxiety that lie behind such obstructionist behavior enables the therapist to couch comments in ways that alleviate some of this anxiety and avoid the power struggles that such behavior often evokes.

A common anxiety, for example, often not quite conscious, is that the therapy will help *a little*—just enough to make the marriage tolerable but not really gratifying. In other words, the uncooperative member of the couple is anxious that if the marriage *improves*, he or she may not have the wherewithal to separate, even though a feeling of dissatisfaction remains. This anxiety, that although certain elements of the relationship might improve the less tangible and concrete dissatisfactions will go unchanged, is frequently not fully conscious or articulated. Often, once the concern about "improvement" is verbalized by the therapist, the patient feels better understood and is able to participate more fully in the work. Put differently, and elaborating on a point made in Chapter 8, in couples therapy too a key challenge is to address the most serious of difficulties while affirming the basic value of (in this case) both the individuals *and* the relationship. A key difference here is that whereas in individual therapy the basic value of the individual is never in question, in couples therapy the therapist should be open to the possi-

---

[5]For a discussion of the many ways in which collusive defense mechanisms can operate, see Wachtel and Wachtel (1986).

bility that the relationship (as opposed to the individuals) *may* be so compromised as to not be worth saving.

As the work proceeds, it is important to continue to make clear that the worry about minor changes covering over major dissatisfactions has not been forgotten or resolved simply because it has been spoken about. Thus, when working on the more easily workable difficulties, the therapist might say something like: *I know that the changes we are discussing right now, though important, do not address the heart of the matter as you experience it. But if you would bear with me, I think dealing with some of these issues might clear the path for working on the knottier concerns.*

JOINING WITH THE RESISTANCE

A related concern seen in couples work is the feeling on the part of the couple that what goes on between them is so complex and subtle that the therapist just won't be able to understand it accurately. The therapist's attempts to convey some understanding of what is being described may be met with constant corrections and qualifications. The individual who says "no, that's not what I mean" is not simply being difficult. He or she may genuinely experience the restatements offered by the therapist as only partially correct. It is helpful in these instances to *invite* the person to correct and elaborate on your statements. Often just admitting to the "resistant/anxious" patient that in fact you do *not* fully understand, and that further clarification on his or her part will be helpful, avoids a power struggle and results in a diminished focus on "inaccuracies." Phrasing one's comments in a way that joins with the resistance aids in preventing a clash of wills. One might say something like: *I know that what you are trying to describe is very complicated and not easy for someone who isn't actually living it to understand, but is it something like this?* or *Fill me in; correct what I'm saying.* This approach conveys respect for the patient's concerns and a willingness to take his anxiety seriously. Generally one will see a noticeable change in the patient's behavior when the therapist responds in this way and thereby conveys an acceptance of the patient rather than simply a wish to interpret or change the behavior.

In couples therapy, each individual is, part of the time, in the difficult position of having to listen to what in his or her mind is often a grossly inaccurate version of a story. Some people can quite easily tolerate the therapist temporarily getting a "misimpression," whereas for others the experience of being misrepresented or unfairly blamed, even momentarily, gets them quite agitated. The experience of being unjustly "blamed" is a highly charged one for these patients. If the therapist listens quietly to the other partner for a few moments, this type of person becomes anxious that the therapist is believing in toto every-thing that is being said. He or she feels an urgent need to object, qualify, or give his or her version of almost every statement made. Often these types of individuals come on like steamrollers and deny any truth to what their mate is saying. They resist the therapist's attempts to keep some order and persistently interrupt when their spouse is speaking. Again, it is important to keep in mind that these people are not just being "difficult." Rather, they are anxious that the therapist will see them as the villain.

There are two approaches that, if used in conjunction with one another, often are quite effective in dealing with this kind of behavior. First of all, it is useful to state *explicitly* that as a specialist in couples therapy you've learned to listen with the deep conviction that there are two sides to every story. Requests that the patient contain himself are thus coupled with assurances that he or she will get a turn and will definitely have a chance to express alternative points of view.[6] The second approach involves not only trying to convey to the patient that you understand his or her perception of the problem (e.g., *I know it's hard for you to hear this being said about you because you really feel you've been very supportive*) but also going further and giving the patient some sense that the personal qualities of which he is most proud have not gone unnoticed despite the "biased" reports of his spouse. One must re-member that the other side of the coin of the patient's need to prove himself innocent is the wish for the therapist to have a more accurate (and of course more complimentary) picture of what he is actually like. When "resistant/insecure" individuals receive some feedback regard-ing the therapist's observation of specific positive qualities that they possess, they are generally better able to withstand their partner's "blames."[7]

For instance, in one case a very bright, physically powerful and verbally forceful man who objected to everything his wife was saying in regard to his lack of supportiveness, relaxed when the therapist said, "It's clear from the kind of work you do [public service law] that you are

[6]This is just a temporary measure. Later in the work, the therapist tries to get the couple to really *listen* to one another, rather than listening only with a view toward rebuttal.

[7]It is important to note as well that couples therapy can stimulate countertransference feelings in the therapist that she does not generally feel when working with individuals (Wachtel, 1979). Many of the suggestions offered in this book regarding how to address behavior on the part of a patient that the therapist feels annoyed about are directly applicable when similar feelings arise in couples work. The principle of raising the issue when the patient is *not* doing it, and of judiciously employing some externalization so that the patient does not feel blamed, can easily be incorporated into couples therapy.

a person who cares a lot about helping others who might not have all that you have going for you. I can understand why it's so upsetting to you that your wife regards you as domineering." This statement not only let the patient know that the therapist empathized with the difficulty he would have listening, but incorporated reassuring positive feedback as well.

Certain modality-specific characteristics of couples work—in particular the need for greater directiveness on the therapist's part,[8] combined with the fact that this occurs not privately, but in the presence of an often critical spouse—stimulate, more frequently than in individual therapy, reactions to being controlled. For this reason, somewhat exaggerated versions of the constructions described in this book might be required. In the couples context, patients who might not do so in an individual session may qualify or argue with every point made. Dealing with this reaction through interpretation at an early stage of the therapy often heightens the problem, since the therapist's comments may increase feelings of vulnerability and control. Instead, the therapist should begin by adjusting her comments to accommodate to the patient's reaction. By phrasing one's comments in a low-key or even one-down manner, the therapist attempts to bypass the situation-generated resistance.[9] Though surely the individuals' reactions to the therapist are relevant to aspects of the couple's difficulties, interpretations of that sort should be saved until greater trust has developed. Often statements such as *I may be off the mark here but . . .* , *I'm not quite sure how to explain this, but I think . . .* , or *I'm feeling a bit confused . . .* are enough to reassure the patient that he need not fear domination and humiliation in front of his spouse.

If the patient's resistance is still strong, then the next step is for the therapist to admit his powerlessness by preempting the patient's criticism. Such statements as the following go further than the ones above in conveying to the patient that you will not engage in a power struggle: *I probably won't be able to convince you of this . . .* , *I know you won't like what I'm suggesting and of course I have no power to get you to do anything you don't really want to do but. . . .* Highlighting the reality of one's lack of power

---

[8]If couples therapy is to be effective, it is essential that the therapist "conduct" the sessions much more actively than is typical of individual therapy. Giving the couple free rein to use the hour as they will is likely to result in feelings of futility; they reargue old issues and simply "ventilate" in a way not too dissimilar from what they do at home. Most couples are quite relieved when the therapist takes charge.

[9]I have noticed over the years that my youngest and least threatening graduate students often do quite well with just this kind of patient. It is important that they *not try* to be more of an authority than they in fact feel.

often has the quasiparadoxical effect of gaining greater cooperation and of increasing the impact of one's comments.

WORRY ABOUT NEW PATTERNS OF INTERACTION

Often anxiety is generated by the very fact that the therapy has begun to help, and change in the relationship is clearly on the horizon. There is something reassuring about the known and familiar even if the old patterns have been largely unsatisfying. It is this anxiety that is captured by the notion of homeostasis—the tendency of systems to resist change. Even though the couple has actively sought help in trying to find better ways of interacting, one or both may get cold feet when therapy actually begins to have an effect and may fear the unknown prospects change may bring. When this anxiety is at play, resistance is not generally manifested by overt negativism, but rather takes the form of a reversion to old ways of interacting or a failure to put into action some of the suggestions or agreements that have been made in sessions. It is important to remember once again that there is a difference between ambivalence and resistance. Couples *want* to change at least as much as they want things to stay the same. Frequently couples come in very *upset* by the fact that they have reverted to old patterns and all too familiar arguments. Profoundly discouraged by their own backsliding, they may be pessimistic about the effectiveness of therapy. One must be careful not to assume too quickly that this is an indication of deep resistance to change. Doing so gives more weight to the negative side of the ambivalence than is warranted. Generally it is better simply to offer some reassurance that change almost always involves taking two steps forward and one step backwards. As described in Chapter 7, it is extremely helpful to notice the overall *direction* of change and to help the couple see what they have been able to do and not just what remains problematic.

Of course, when there is persistent failure to put into action the suggestions and understandings achieved in sessions regarding a particular issue, the therapist must do more than offer reassurance. Exploration of the worries that lie behind the failure to change is now called for. What are the anxieties that each member of the couple feels? Do the old and predictable roles serve to ward off experiences and aspects of the self that one partner or the other is uncomfortable with? Are they colluding in helping the other defend against the anxiety of acting differently? Using imagery or even dreams to get at unconscious fears can be very helpful.

For instance, one man, when asked to fantasize about what would happen if he gave up being the protector and self-sacrificing member of the family, visualized himself in a hospital bed, alone and abandoned by his wife. As much as he really wanted to change the old pattern of relating, he feared that he would be of no value to his wife if he did so.

FACILITATING REAL LISTENING

Frequently, by the time couples enter therapy, their relationship has become so adversarial that they listen to one another only with the set of defending themselves against presumed attack. Many couples have become, in a loose sense, "paranoid," in that they hear everything the other says as critical and respond in kind. Often the defensiveness is "justified" in that the relationship has so deteriorated that a good deal of the communication that takes place outside the therapy office is of an accusatory nature.

The initial goal of couples therapy with such couples is to break this cycle of blame and counterattack, in which the listening partner "listens" only with the set of formulating a rebuttal. It is easy to tell when a person is listening in this way. Sometimes they may interrupt to interject corrections, but even when waiting patiently there is a look in the eyes that says: "No! No! No! It was *this* way!" or "That's *not* true; you're *distorting*!" or "I can't believe you are saying that!" Even when blame really is being cast, the other spouse, by responding only to that dimension of his partner's communication and doing so with counter-recriminations, may contribute to the dead-end adversarial cycle.[10]

Helping the couple learn to actually listen to one another rather than debate and rebut is the initial focus of the work. Thus, the central dilemma of therapy, calling attention to something that needs to be "corrected" without being accusatory, is at play in the very first session with most couples. I find it best to interrupt their adversarial discussion as early as possible in the process with a statement that explains that this mode of communication, though quite normal and understandable when couples have been having a difficult time, is, *as they themselves know*, unproductive (see discussion of attribution of knowledge in Chapter 9). I often say that part of my job as a couples therapist is to help them to try to listen and talk with each other in a different way. By explicitly

---

[10]In my experience, it seems easier initially to break this cycle by working on the "blamed" partner's response rather than starting off with getting the "blaming" partner to speak differently. In time, less blaming statements will become natural and authentic. As the therapy makes clear the cyclical nature of the couple's difficulties, the couple generally spontaneously adopts the therapist's facilitative mode of addressing difficulties.

stating that this is my job, I share responsibility for change and further normalize and reduce any sense of blame.

In keeping with the premise that it is far more effective to build on positives than just to point out negatives, I then tell the couple *how* they can begin to break out of this adversarial mode. I ask them each to listen to what the other is saying with the mental set of looking for *anything* that is said with which they can agree. After just a few moments, I will remind the listener again to try to find *anything* that he or she thinks is basically right in what is being said and to try to see if it is possible to see anything of what is being said from the spouse's point of view. By reminding and instructing them before much of an adversarial discussion has taken place, I am trying to prevent having to "criticize" and instead provide some guidance upon which they might be able to build.

Throughout the work, I continue to give some reminders of how I'd like them to listen, and I express empathy for the fact that this is not at all easy to do. If someone is having a hard time doing this, or rejects my request as impossible or foolish, I will see if they can at least agree to *think* about what the spouse is saying and not respond immediately. If this too is rejected or just doesn't seem possible to do, I regard this as "resistance" that emanates from anxiety and take instead one or several of the tacks described above.

The other tack I take that helps break the cycle of bitter mutual recriminations is (consistent with some of the principles I have already outlined) to respond first to any movements in the right direction and to variations in how the couple is communicating and listening, and only later to the more problematic features of how they are communicating. Thus, I might choose to preface a discussion of the content of what is being stated by saying something like: *Before I ask you to respond to what your husband just said, I just want to mention how struck I am by my sense that you were really listening very openly; I could tell by your expression that you weren't formulating a rebuttal.* This not only positively reinforces and shapes the desired mind set but also, as discussed in Chapter 9, imparts a "suggestion" that may in fact lead to a more productive response.

When couples are accustomed to arguing rather than talking, they often ignore or don't even notice moments when they have actually reached an agreement. One person may continue therefore to argue for something even *after* the partner has already assented to what is being requested. The therapist can encourage real listening by halting a discussion at the point where some agreement actually has been reached—by, for example saying something like: *Wait a minute. Before you go on, I have a feeling that you both didn't quite notice that you've been talking about this in a way that actually already has resulted in some agreement being reached.* By saying something like this, the therapist underlines the unnoticed accomplishment and prevents the "undoing" that is so characteristic of discussions that go on too long. This in turn enables the couple to continue in a more positive mood and increases the chance that they will have a further meeting of the mind.

HELPING THE COUPLE CHANGE THE QUALITY OF THEIR ARGUMENTS

Often couples seek therapy because of the frequent escalation at home of minor disagreements into long and bitter arguments. Helping couples shorten the length, breadth, depth, and impact of arguments is one of the goals that determine choices at therapeutic junctures. Unraveling the content of their arguments may be considerably less important than figuring out how in the future they can prevent something minor from mushrooming into a major upset.

Escalation of relatively insignificant differences into intense arguments, of course, often reflects underlying difficulties and bitterness that may subside spontaneously when the more significant issues between the couple are addressed in the therapy. But though therapists often assume that when the reason for maladaptive behavior no longer exists new and more productive behavior will emerge automatically,[11] frequently couples have gotten into power struggles so habitually they do not really know how to behave differently even if they want to. Concrete advice offered in a "normalizing" respectful manner is generally welcomed.

One might say something such as: *There are specific things one can do to avoid arguments or put to rest disagreements even when no resolution has been reached, but many couples have never been taught them. A lot of this is the kind of thing that grandmothers used to impart.*[12] This type of statement, by normalizing the difficulty, not only minimizes any feelings of foolishness in having to be taught the obvious, but also can be seen as another

---

[11] In the family therapy field this assumption is reflected in what I call the "trickle down" approach to children's symptoms; it is often assumed erroneously that when the marital or family interaction changes the child's symptoms will spontaneously disappear (see Wachtel, 1987, 1990, 1991).

[12] The behaviors I am talking about are things that include: keep to the current point and don't bring up old history; speak about behavior, not character; talk in terms of one's own wishes and needs rather than what is right and wrong; and so forth. Many couples respond well to jokingly offering them "grandma tips" such as *You generally catch more flies with honey than you do with vinegar* or *Never accuse her of being just like her mother.*

version of the "externalization in the service of therapy" described in Chapter 6.

When a couple reports on a bad argument they had in the past week, I try to be alert to any steps in the right direction or any variation in the way they argued that can be reinforced despite the "relapse." Thus, in response to a couple saying something like "On Friday night we had a terrible argument, and although we did a lot of things together the rest of the weekend, the atmosphere was kind of cool," the therapist, in order to build on any movement, can defer asking about the content of the argument and instead ask what each of them did to enable them to do things together the next day, even if coolly, without rehashing the previous night's battle.[13] The answer to this question is likely to involve the articulation of ego strengths that have been taken for granted, such as self-control, desire to make things better, or the acceptance of differences. Neither the argument nor the fact that they stayed cool for two days is the initial point of intervention chosen at this choice point, since once again a key guideline for choices is to start, whenever possible, with the underlining of strengths.

Even when discussing the actual content of the argument, the therapist continues to look vigilantly for movement in the right direction. For instance, the therapist might preface her comments about the content of the argument with mentioning almost as an aside that although there was something that needs to be worked out that led to an argument, it seems that the argument was a little different from in the past; it seemed more confined to the topic at hand and did not become one in which old hurts and other related issues were dredged up.

CHANGING RIGID CONCEPTIONS OF SELF AND OTHER

Couples often describe themselves as polar opposites. They are locked into one-dimensional, rigidly defined roles in which each is seen, so to speak, as possessing only half of what a full human being requires. Not uncommonly, although they may disagree on almost everything else, neither partner protests when his or her spouse describes "traits" by saying, "I'm emotional and he's the logical one" or "I'm good with people, and my wife is much more of a loner." These generalizations, though they undoubtedly contain an element of truth, are not the whole truth. Such broad characterizations deny the complexity of people and

---

[13]Compare this example to the case of Jill in Chapter 7.

the fact that all people have subtle facets to their personalities and times when they behave "uncharacteristically."

The couple's shared view that "this is the way I am," or "this is the way he is" (and that not much can be done about it) can be a major obstacle to change, locking people into maintaining roles that they may wish to shed. The therapist can increase the couple's flexibility regarding how they see themselves and each other by vigilantly attending to variations and exceptions to expected behavior. Noticing "uncharacteristic" behavior is the best antidote to rigid entrenched positions and conveys to the couple the notion that there are clearly untapped potentials in each of them that a changed relationship can help them actualize. For example, if the nonemotional person says anything even mildly involving the expression of feelings, the therapist could say: *I know you say you are not emotional, but before we discuss what you are saying, I just want to point out that to me, what you just said really seemed to come from the heart—and to me that's emotional.* [Turning to the wife]—*Did you notice that? Does he sometimes talk that way?* It is also important to notice and comment on things the *partner* may be doing that facilitate this kind of openness. One might say, *I noticed that you seemed very responsive to what your husband had been saying earlier on in the session, and I guess that helped him in turn to be less guarded.* These types of comments not only notice variations but use reframing in various ways. First of all, the therapist is providing a new definition of "emotional" in that anything said sincerely is "from the heart" and thus emotional. Second, whether an individual is "emotional" or "unemotional" is implicitly discussed not as an individual characteristic per se but rather as something the couple *elicits* in one another. These "incidental" or "by the way" type comments are over time extremely effective in helping individuals change their self-perceptions as well as their experience of their partner.

ADDRESSING "UNSOLVABLE" PROBLEMS

Couples often describe a difficulty in their marriage in terms that are so broad, general and momentous that they feel a certain futility about ever overcoming these difficulties: "I think my wife is afraid of intimacy; she doesn't have any close friends and hardly ever sees her family." "I'm not sure if there was ever really anything there." "My husband has a 'split personality'; he just suddenly blows up over nothing" "A big problem in our relationship is that we have very different interests; we just don't like the same things." "We have different sex drives; I'm much more interested in sex than he is." Such statements present issues that can seem unresolvable.

It is best, if possible, to defer discussion of these issues for some time. When some progress has been made on more "resolvable" issues, these big differences often don't loom as large as they did earlier. Also, it is very important that when these issues *are* discussed the couple feels confident that the therapist really knows them well, both as a couple and individually. Feeling known is an essential element in the trust that is necessary if reframings and interpretations offered by the therapist are to be taken seriously and not dismissed as glib manipulations.

When the time does come to wrestle with the larger issues, the therapist can use the method of addressing "incidentals" as a source of facilitative "mini-reframings." I call these "mini-reframings" because they do not attempt to cast the whole relationship in a different light, but rather they simply involve a slightly off-centered reaction to something that has been said. By responding with what might seem at first almost to be a nonsequitur, or off-the-point comment, the therapist shifts the discussion to pathways that lead to options rather than closed doors.

For example, in response to the first statement described above—"I think my wife is afraid of intimacy; she has no close friends and hardly ever sees her family"—one might say, *I am struck by how even though you are angry and upset about this, and want something more from her, you can see it's that she's afraid of intimacy, not that she doesn't want to be intimate with* you. Such a response casts the problem in a way that more readily leads to exploration rather than rejection, blame, and impasse. This response doesn't immediately deal with the content of the concern but instead underlines something that neither of them may have focussed on—the lack of personalizing the intimacy problem.

As discussed in Chapters 9 and 10, reframings and attributions often have elements of suggestion that if accepted, can be helpful in opening up new ways of responding. For instance, if the husband accepts the suggestion that he is no longer "personalizing" the problem, the therapist might then ask if he can guess or understand the nature of his wife's anxiety. Or the wife might be asked not to dismiss her husband's characterization immediately but instead to think about whether there is any truth to what he is saying. Or she might be asked to see if she could understand why he might feel that she has trouble with intimacy.

It is important to note that not every individual comment can be reframed in this way. To do so would be glib and disruptive of dialogue. Often it is only after considerable straightforward discussion of an "unresolvable" problem that the therapist can respond to it from an angle that really resonates and thus opens up new pathways to resolution. For instance, with a couple who despair of the fact that they share no interests, a variety of interpretive reframing may emerge that recasts the problem from one of a stubborn closed-mindedness with regard to each other's interests to something less accusatory and potentially more solvable.

When the therapist listens to the problem with the set of looking for facilitative constructions, she is likely to find interpretations which, though they may not be *the* meaning or *only* truth, do provide a useful new perspective with which to engage the couple. For instance, to name but a few of the possible reframings for this particular problem of lack of mutual interests, one might see in this interaction a fear of losing one's identity by merging too much with the other, a valuing of intensity of interests with a corresponding dislike of doing things that are not deeply meaningful, or an issue of loyalty or authenticity to one's true identity. New interpretations in turn lead to new behavioral solutions, which work because, as described earlier, they address underlying psychodynamic issues and idiosyncratic concerns.

A CAVEAT REGARDING THE LIMITATIONS OF THIS APPROACH

The reader should keep in mind that the focus on positives does not mean being "pollyannaish." The examples offered in this chapter take place in the context of a therapy that continually helps the couple articulate their concerns and complaints. If this aspect of the work is not attended to, then no amount of attention to strengths is likely to be effective. A delicate balance must be maintained, in which the therapist listens simultaneously to both negatives and positives.

There are also occasions of course when the negatives in a relationship are so strong and have gone on for so long that it is virtually impossible to build on strengths. The approach described above has been almost surprisingly powerful, but of course it is limited by the assets and resources the couple possess.

When all is said and done, any psychotherapeutic approach is only as good as the therapist applying it. Psychotherapy is not an exact science. It requires sensitivity to nuances that cannot be completely spelled out and a readiness to acknowledge that, whatever one's theoretical orientation, it is but a very provisional map of a vast and still largely unexplored territory. I believe that the principles of therapeutic communication described in this book should be extremely helpful to the practicing therapist and are likely to improve one's effectiveness with a wide range of cases. They are by no means a substitute for the personal qualities that mark the excellent therapist. But in the hands of a therapist who manifests those qualities, they can suggest new ways of being helpful and provide a much needed additional tool for this most demanding kind of work.

REFERENCES

Anderson, C., & Stewart, S. (1983). *Mastering resistance*. New York: Guilford Press.

Bowen, M. (1978). *Family therapy in clinical practice*. New York: Jason Aronson.

Dell, P. (1982). Beyond homeostasis: Toward a concept of coherence. *Family Process, 21*, 27–42.

de Shazer, S. (1985). *Keys to solutions in brief therapy*. New York: Norton.

Hoffman, L. (1988). An interview with Lynn Hoffman, *The Family Therapy Networker, September–October*, 56–58.

Sager, C. (1978). *Marriage contracts and couples therapy*. New York: Harper & Row.

Wachtel, E. F. (1979). Learning family therapy: The dilemmas of an individual therapist. *Journal of Contemporary Psychotherapy, 10*, 122–135.

Wachtel, E. F. (1982). The family psyche over three generations: The genogram revisited. *Journal of Marital and Family Therapy, 8*, 335–343.

Wachtel, E. F. (1987). Family systems and the individual child. *Journal of Marital and Family Therapy, 13*, 15–25.

Wachtel, E. F. (1990). The child as an individual: A resource for systemic change. *Journal of Strategic and Systemic Therapies, 9*, 50–59.

Wachtel, E. F. (1991). Breaking a taboo of family therapy: Working with the individual child. *The Family Therapy Networker, July–August*, 46.

Wachtel, E. F. (1992). An integrative approach to working with troubled children and their families. *Journal of Psychotherapy Integration, 2*, 207–224.

Wachtel, E. F., & Wachtel, P. L. (1986). *Family dynamics in individual psychotherapy: A guide to clinical strategies*. New York: Guilford Press.

References

Alexander, F. (1961). *The scope of psychoanalysis*. New York: Basic Books.

Alexander, F. (1963). *Fundamentals of psychoanalysis*. New York: Norton.

Alexander, F., & French, T. (1946). *Psychoanalytic therapy*. New York: Ronald Press. (Reprinted by University of Nebraska Press, 1974.)

Apfelbaum, B. (1966). On ego psychology: A critique of the structural approach to psychoanalytic theory. *International Journal of Psycho-Analysis, 47,* 451–475.

Apfelbaum, B., & Gill, M. M. (1989). Ego analysis and the relativity of defense: Technical implications of the structural theory. *Journal of the American Psychoanalytic Association, 37,* 1071–1096.

Arkowitz, H., & Messer, S. M. (1984). *Psychoanalytic therapy and behavior therapy: Is integration possible?* New York: Plenum.

Aron, L. (1991). Working through the past—working toward the future. *Contemporary Psychoanalysis, 27,* 81–109.

Ascher, L. M. (1989). Paradoxical intention: Its clarification and emergence as a conventional behavioral procedure. *The Behavior Therapist, 12,* 23–28.

Bandura, A. (1969). *Principles of behavior modification*. New York: Holt, Rinehart & Winston.

Bandura, A. (1977). *Social learning theory*. Englewood Cliffs, NJ: Prentice-Hall.

Basescu, S. (1990). Show and tell: Reflections on the analyst's self-disclosure. In G. Stricker & M. Fisher (Eds.), *Self-disclosure in the therapeutic relationship* (pp. 47–59). New York: Plenum.

Bateson, G. (1972). *Steps to an ecology of mind*. New York: Random House.

Bateson, G. (1979). *Mind and nature*. New York: Dutton.

Berger, P., & Luckmann, T. (1966). *The social construction of reality*. Garden City, NY: Doubleday.

Bergin, A. E., & Garfield, S. L. (1986). *Handbook of psychotherapy and behavior change*. New York: Wiley.

Bowlby, J. (1969). *Attachment*. New York: Basic Books.

Burke, W. F., & Tansey, M. J. (1991). Countertransference disclosure and models of therapeutic action. *Contemporary Psychoanalysis, 27,* 351–384.

Butler, G., Cullington, A., Munby, M., Amies, P., & Gelder, M. (1984). Exposure and anxiety management in the treatment of social phobia. *Journal of Consulting and Clinical Psychology, 52,* 642–650.

Chambless, D., & Goldstein, A. J. (1980). Agoraphobia. In A. J. Goldstein & E. B. Foa (Eds.), *Handbook of behavioral interventions* (pp. 322–415). New York: Wiley.

Chapman, A. H. (1978). *The treatment techniques of Harry Stack Sullivan.* New York: Brunner/Mazel.

Coleman, M. L., (1956). Externalization of the toxic introject. *Psychoanalytic Review, 43,* 235–242.

Coleman, M. L., & Nelson, B. (1957). Paradigmatic psychotherapy in borderline treatment. *Psychoanalysis, 5,* 28–44.

Dollard, J., & Miller, N. (1950). *Personality and psychotherapy.* New York: McGraw-Hill.

Ellenberger, H. (1970). *The discovery of the unconscious.* New York: Basic Books.

Emmelkamp, P. M. G. (1982). *Phobic and obsessive–compulsive disorders: Theory, research and practice.* New York: Plenum.

Erikson, E. H. (1963). *Childhood and society* (2nd ed.). New York: Norton.

Fay, A. (1978). *Making things better by making them worse.* New York: Hawthorne.

Feather, B. W., & Rhoads, J. M. (1972). Psychodynamic behavior therapy: II: Clinical aspects. *Archives of General Psychiatry, 26,* 503–511.

Fenichel, O. (1941). *Problems of psychoanalytic technique.* New York: Psychoanalytic Quarterly.

Fiedler, F. E. (1950a). The concept of the ideal therapeutic relationship. *Journal of Consulting Psychology, 14,* 239–245.

Fiedler, F. E. (1950b). Comparisons of therapeutic relationships in psychoanalytic, nondirective, and Adlerian therapy. *Journal of Consulting Psychology, 14,* 436–445.

Flavell, J. (1963). *The developmental psychology of Jean Piaget.* Princeton, NJ: Van Nostrand.

Fogarty, T. F. (1979). The distancer and the pursuer. *The Family, 7,* 11–16.

Frank, J. D. (1973). *Persuasion and healing.* Baltimore: Johns Hopkins University Press.

Frank, J. D. (1982). Therapeutic components shared by all psychotherapies. In J. H. Harvey & M. M. Parks (Eds.), *Psychotherapy research and behavior change* (pp. 5–37). Washington, DC: American Psychological Association.

Frank, K. A. (1990). Action techniques in psychoanalysis. *Contemporary Psychoanalysis, 26,* 732–756.

Frank, K. A. (1992). Combining action techniques with psychoanalytic therapy. *International Review of Psycho-Analysis, 19,* 57–79.

Frankl, V. (1960). *Man's search for meaning: An introduction to logotherapy.* Boston: Beacon Press.

Freud, A. (1936). *The ego and the mechanisms of defense.* New York: International Universities Press.

Freud, S. (1904). On psychotherapy. *Collected Papers,* Vol. 1 (pp. 249–264). New York: Basic Books, 1959.

Freud, S. (1910). The future prospects of psycho-analytic therapy. *Collected Papers,* Vol. 2 (pp. 285–297). New York: Basic Books, 1959.

Freud, S. (1912). Recommendations for physicians on the psychoanalytic method of treatment. *Collected Papers*, Vol. 2 (pp. 323–333). New York: Basic Books, 1959.

Freud, S. (1914). On the history of the psycho-analytic movement. *Collected Papers*, Vol. 1 (pp. 287–359). New York: Basic Books, 1959.

Freud, S. (1916). *A general introduction to psychoanalysis*. Garden City, NY: Garden City Publishing, 1943.

Freud, S. (1919). Turnings in the ways of psycho-analytic therapy. *Collected Papers*, Vol. 2 (pp. 392–402). New York: Basic Books, 1959.

Freud, S. (1920). Beyond the pleasure principle. *Standard Edition*, Vol. 18 (pp. 3–64). London: Hogarth Press, 1959.

Freud, S. (1922). Psycho-analysis. *Collected Papers*, Vol. 5 (pp. 107–130). New York: Basic Books, 1959.

Freud, S. (1926). Inhibitions, symptoms, and anxiety. *Standard Edition*, Vol. 20 (pp. 87–172). London: Hogarth Press, 1959.

Freud, S. (1938). Constructions in analysis. *Collected Papers*, Vol. 5 (pp. 249–264). New York: Basic Books, 1959.

Freud, S. (1940). *An outline of psychoanalysis*. New York: Norton, 1949.

Gergen, K. (1985). The social constructionist movement in modern psychology. *American Psychologist, 40*, 266–275.

Gill, M. M. (1951). Ego psychology and psychotherapy. *Psychoanalytic Quarterly, 20*, 62–71.

Gill, M. M. (1954). Psychoanalysis and exploratory psychotherapy. *Journal of the American Psychoanalytic Association, 2*, 771–797.

Gill, M. M. (1979). The analysis of the transference. *Journal of the American Psychoanalytic Association, 27* (Supplement), 263–288.

Gill, M. M. (1982). *Analysis of transference*. New York: International Universities Press.

Gill, M. M. (1983). The interpersonal paradigm and the degree of the therapist's involvement. *Contemporary Psychoanalysis, 19*, 200–237.

Gill, M. M. (1984). Psychoanalysis and psychotherapy: A revision. *International Review of Psycho-Analysis, 11*, 161–179.

Goldfried, M. R., & Davison, G. C. (1976). *Clinical behavior therapy*. New York: Holt, Rinehart & Winston.

Greenberg, J., & Mitchell, S. (1983). *Object relations in psychoanalysis*. Cambridge: Harvard University Press.

Greenson, R. R. (1965). The working alliance and the transference neurosis. *Psychoanalytic Quarterly, 34*, 155–181.

Greenson, R. R. (1967). *The technique and practice of psychoanalysis*. New York: International Universities Press.

Harre, R. (Ed.). (1986). *The social construction of emotions*. Oxford: Basil Blackwell.

Harvey, J. H., & Parks, M. M. (Eds.). (1982). *Psychotherapy research and behavior change*. Washington, DC: American Psychological Association.

Havens, L. (1986). *Making contact: Uses of language in psychotherapy*. Cambridge: Harvard University Press.

Heller, T., Sosna, M., & Wellbery, D. (Eds.). (1986). *Reconstructing individualism:*

Autonomy, individuality, and the self in Western thought. Stanford, CA: Stanford University Press.

Hoffman, I. Z. (1983). The patient as interpreter of the analyst's experience. *Contemporary Psychoanalysis, 19*, 389–422.

Hoffman, I. Z. (1991). Toward a social-constructivist view of the psychoanalytic situation. *Psychoanalytic Dialogues, 1*, 74–105.

Hoffman, L. (1981). *Foundations of family therapy*. New York: Basic Books.

Horney, K. (1945). *Our inner conflicts*. New York: Norton.

Horney, K. (1950). *Neurosis and human growth*. New York: Norton.

Jacobson, N. S. (1989). The therapist–client relationship in cognitive behavior therapy: Implications for treating depression. *Journal of Cognitive Psychotherapy, 3*, 85–96.

Kantrowitz, J. L. (1983). The role of the patient–analyst "match" in the outcome of psychoanalysis. In *The Annual of Psychoanalysis*, Vol. 14 (pp. 273–297). Madison, CT: International Universities Press.

Kernberg, O. F. (1976). *Object relations theory and clinical psychoanalysis*. New York: Jason Aronson.

Kernberg, O. F. (1977). Contrasting approaches to the psychotherapy of borderline conditions. In J. F. Masterson (Ed.), *New perspectives on psychotherapy of the borderline adult* (pp. 77–104). New York: Brunner/Mazel.

Knight, R. P. (1954). Evaluation of psychotherapeutic techniques. In R. P. Knight & C. R. Friedman (Eds.), *Psychoanalytic psychiatry and psychology* (pp. 65–76). New York: International Universities Press.

Kohut, H. (1971). *The analysis of the self*. New York: International Universities Press.

Kohut, H. (1977). *The restoration of the self*. New York: International Universities Press.

Kohut, H. (1979). The two analyses of Mr. Z. *International Journal of Psycho-Analysis, 60*, 3–27.

Kohut, H. (1984). *How does analysis cure?* Chicago: University of Chicago Press.

Kohut, H. (1985). *Self psychology and the humanities*. New York: Norton.

Laing, R. D. (1960). *The divided self*. London: Tavistock Publications.

Laing, R. D. (1969). *The politics of the family*. New York: Pantheon.

Lambert, M. J. (Ed.). (1983). *Psychotherapy and patient relationships*. Homewood, IL: Dorsey Press.

Lambert, M. J., Shapiro, D. A., & Bergin, A. E. (1986). The effectiveness of psychotherapy. In J. C. Norcross (Ed.), *Handbook of eclectic psychotherapy* (pp. 436–461). New York: Brunner/Mazel.

Langs, R. (1973). The patient's view of the therapist: Reality or fantasy? *International Journal of Psychoanalytic Psychotherapy, 2*, 411–431.

Langs, R., & Stone, L. (1980). *The therapeutic experience and its setting: A clinical dialogue*. New York: Jason Aronson.

Liebowitz, M. R., Stone, M. H., & Turkat, I. D. (1986). Treatment of personality disorders. In A. J. Frances & R. E. Hales (Eds.), *Psychiatry update: American Psychiatric Association annual review*, Vol. 5 (pp. 356–393). Washington DC: American Psychiatric Association.

Linehan, M. M. (1987). Dialectical behavior therapy for borderline personality disorder. *Bulletin of the Menninger Clinic, 51*, 261–276.

Linehan, M. M., & Wagner, A. W. (1990). Dialectical behavior therapy: A feminist–behavioral treatment of borderline personality disorder. *The Behavior Therapist, January* 9–14.

Loewenstein, R. (1956). Some remarks on the role of speech in psycho-analytic technique. *International Journal of Psycho-Analysis, 37*, 460–468.

Lomas, P. (1987). *The limits of interpretation*. London: Penguin.

London, P. (1964). *The modes and morals of psychotherapy*. New York: Holt, Rinehart, & Winston.

Lukes, S. (1973). *Individualism*. New York: Harper & Row.

Lux, K. (1990). *Adam Smith's mistake: How a moral philosopher invented economics and ended morality*. Boston: Shambhala.

Marks, I. M. (1989). *Fears, phobias, and rituals: The nature of anxiety and panic disorders*. New York: Oxford University Press.

Maslow, A. H. (1962). *Toward a psychology of being*. Princeton: Van Nostrand.

Meichenbaum, D. (1977). *Cognitive–behavior modification: An integrative approach*. New York: Plenum.

Messer, S. B., Sass, L. A., & Woolfolk, R. L. (1988). *Hermeneutics and psychological theory: Interpretive perspectives on personality, psychotherapy, and psychopathology*. New Brunswick, NJ: Rutgers University Press.

Mischel, W. (1973). Toward a cognitive social learning reconceptualization of personality. *Psychological Review, 80*, 252–283.

Mitchell, S. (1988). *Relational concepts in psychoanalysis*. Cambridge: Harvard University Press.

Nelson, M. C. (1962). Effect of paradigmatic techniques on the psychic economy of borderline patients. *Psychiatry, 25*, 119–134.

Orne, M. T. (1972). Can a hypnotized subject be compelled to carry out otherwise unacceptable behavior? *Internation Journal of Clinical and Experimental Hypnosis, 20*, 101–117.

Orne, M. T., & Evans, F. J. (1965). Social control in the psychological experiment: Anti-social behavior and hypnosis. *Journal of Personality and Social Psychology, 1*, 189–200.

Poland, W. (1986). The analyst's words. *Psychoanalytic Quarterly, 55*, 244–272.

Polanyi, M. (1958). *Personal knowledge: Towards a post-critical philosophy*. Chicago: University of Chicago Press.

Polanyi, M. (1966). *The Tacit Dimension*. New York: Doubleday.

Rabinow, P., & Sullivan, W. M. (1979). *Interpretive social science*. Berkeley: University of California Press.

Racker, H. (1968). *Transference and countertransference*. New York: International Universities Press.

Reich, W. (1949). *Character analysis*. New York: Noonday Press.

Reppen, J. (1982). Merton Gill: An interview. *Psychoanalytic Review, 69*, 167–190.

Rice, L. N. (1983). The relationship in client-centered therapy. In M. J. Lambert (Ed.), *A guide to psychotherapy and patient relationships*. Homewood, IL: Dow Jones-Irwin.

Rieff, P. (1966). *The triumph of the therapeutic: Uses of faith after Freud*. New York: Harper & Row.

Rockland, L. H. (1989). *Supportive therapy: A psychodynamic approach*. New York: Basic Books.

Rogers, C. R. (1942). *Counseling and psychotherapy: Newer concepts in practice*. Boston: Houghton Mifflin.

Rogers, C. R. (1951). *Client-centered therapy: Its current practice, implications, and theory*. Boston: Houghton Mifflin.

Rogers, C. R. (1959). A theory of therapy, personality, and interpersonal relationships as developed in the client-centered framework. In S. Koch (Ed.), *Psychology: A study of a science*, Vol. 3 (pp. 184–256). New York: McGraw-Hill.

Rogers, C. R. (1961). *On becoming a person*. Boston: Houghton Mifflin.

Rorty, R. (1979). *Philosophy and the mirror of nature*. Princeton: Princeton University Press.

Safran, J. D., & Segal, Z. V. (1991). *Interpersonal process in cognitive therapy*. New York: Basic Books.

Sandler, J., & Rosenblatt, B. (1962). The concept of the representational world. *Psychoanalytic Study of the Child, 17*, 128–145.

Schafer, R. (1976). *A new language for psychoanalysis*. New Haven: Yale University Press.

Schafer, R. (1978). *Language and insight*. New Haven: Yale University Press.

Schafer, R. (1981). *Narrative actions in psychoanalysis*. Worcester, MA: Clark University Press.

Schafer, R. (1983). *The analytic attitude*. New York: Basic Books.

Schimek, J. G. (1975). The interpretations of the past: Childhood trauma, psychic reality, and historical truth. *Journal of the American Psychoanalytic Association, 23*, 835–865.

Schlesinger, H. J. (1969). Diagnosis and prescription for psychotherapy. *Bulletin of the Menninger Clinic, 33*, 269–278.

Schneider, P. (1991). The analyst's questions to the patient: Implicit aims and functions. *Contemporary Psychoanalysis, 27*, 552–573.

Schotte, D. E., Ascher, L. M., & Cools, J. (1989). The use of paradoxical intention in behavior therapy. In L. M. Ascher (Ed.), *Therapeutic paradox*. New York: Guilford Press.

Schwartz, B. (1986). *The battle for human nature: Science, morality, and modern life*. New York: Norton.

Searles, H. F. (1965). *Collected papers on schizophrenia and related subjects*. New York: International Universities Press.

Seligman, M. E. P. (1975). *Helplessness*. San Francisco: W. H. Freeman.

Selvini Palazzoli, M., Cecchin, G., Prata, G., & Boscolo, L. (1978). *Paradox and counterparadox*. New York: Jason Aronson.

Shapiro, D. (1965). *Neurotic styles*. New York: Basic Books.

Shapiro, D. (1981). *Autonomy and rigid character*. New York: Basic Books.

Shapiro, D. (1989). *Psychotherapy of neurotic character*. New York: Basic Books.

Shawver, L. (1983). Harnessing the power of interpretive language. *Psychotherapy: Theory, Research and Practice, 20*, 3–11.

Singer, E. (1968) The reluctance to interpret. In E. Hammer (Ed.), *Uses of interpretation in treatment* (pp. 364–371). New York: Grune & Stratton.

Spence, D. P. (1982). *Narrative truth and historical truth: Meaning and interpretation in psychoanalysis*. New York: Norton.

Spence, D. P. (1987). *The Freudian metaphor: Toward a paradigm change in psychoanalysis*. New York: Norton.

Stein, M. H. (1979). Review of H. Kohut, "The Restoration of the Self." *Journal of the American Psychoanalytic Association, 27,* 665–680.

Stone, L. (1961). *The psychoanalytic situation*. New York: International Universities Press.

Sullivan, H. S. (1947). *Conceptions of modern psychiatry*. New York: Norton.

Sullivan, H. S. (1953). *The interpersonal theory of psychiatry*. New York: Norton.

Sullivan, H. S. (1954). *The psychiatric interview*. New York: Norton.

Swenson, C. R. (1989). Kernberg and Linehan: Two approaches to the borderline patient. *Journal of Personality Disorders, 3,* 26–35.

Tansey, M. J., & Burke, W. F. (1989). *Understanding countertransference: From projective identification to empathy*. Hillsdale, NJ: Analytic Press.

Tenzer, A. (1984). Piaget and psychoanalyis, II: The problem of working through. *Contemporary Psychoanalysis, 20,* 421–436.

Truax, C. B. (1966). Reinforcement and nonreinforcement in Rogerian psychotherapy. *Journal of Abnormal Psychology, 71,* 1–9.

Wachtel, E. F., & Wachtel, P. L. (1986). *Family dynamics in individual psychotherapy*. New York: Guilford Press.

Wachtel, P. L. (1977). *Psychoanalysis and behavior therapy*. New York: Basic Books.

Wachtel, P. L.(1981). Transference, schema, and assimilation: The relevance of Piaget to the psychoanalytic theory of transference. In *The annual of psychoanalysis*, Vol. 8 (pp. 59–76). New York: International Universities Press.

Wachtel, P. L.(1982). Vicious circles: The self and the rhetoric of emerging and unfolding. *Contemporary Psychoanalysis, 18,* 273–295.

Wachtel, P. L. (1985). Integrative psychodynamic therapy. In S. Lynn & J. Garske (Eds.), *Contemporary psychotherapies* (pp. 287–289). Columbus, OH: Charles E. Merrill.

Wachtel, P. L. (1987). *Action and insight*. New York: Guilford Press.

Wachtel, P. L. (1989). *The poverty of affluence: A psychological portrait of the American way of life*. Philadelphia: New Society Publishers.

Wachtel, P. L. (1991a). The role of "accomplices" in preventing and facilitating change. In R. C. Curtis & G. Stricker (Eds.), *How people change* (pp. 21–28). New York: Plenum.

Wachtel, P. L. (1991b). From eclecticism to synthesis: Toward a more seamless psychotherapeutic integration. *Journal of Psychotherapy Integration, 1,* 43–54.

Wachtel, P. L., & McKinney, M. (1992). Cyclical psychodynamics and integrative psychodynamic therapy. In J. Norcross & M. R. Goldfried (Eds.), *Handbook of integrative psychotherapy* (pp. 335–370). New York: Basic Books.

Waelder, R. (1960). *Basic theory of psychoanalysis*. New York: International Universities Press.

Wallerstein, R. S. (1986). *Forty-two lives in treatment: A study of psychoanalysis and psychotherapy*. New York: Guilford Press.

Wallerstein, R. S. (1988). Psychoanalysis and psychotherapy: Relative roles reconsidered. *The Annual of Psychoanalysis, 16*, 129–151.

Wallerstein, R. S. (1989a). The psychotherapy research project of the Menninger Foundation: An overview. *Journal of Consulting and Clinical Psychology, 57*, 195–205.

Wallerstein, R. S. (1989b). Psychoanalysis and psychotherapy: An historical perspective. *International Journal of Psycho-Analysis, 70*, 563–591.

Watzlawick, P., Weakland, J., & Fisch, R. (1974). *Change: Principles of problem formation and problem resolution*. New York: Norton.

Weeks, G. R., & L'Abate, L. (1982). *Paradoxical psychotherapy: Theory and practice with individuals, couples and families*. New York: Brunner/Mazel.

Weiss, J. (1971). The emergence of new themes: A contribution to the psychoanalytic theory of transference. *International Journal of Psycho-Analysis, 52*, 459–467.

Weiss, J., & Sampson, H. (1986). *The psychoanalytic process*. New York: Guilford Press.

Werman, D. A. (1984). *The practice of supportive psychotherapy*. New York: Brunner/Mazel.

Whitehead, A. N., & Russell, B. (1910–1913). *Principia mathematica*. Cambridge: Cambridge University Press.

Whorf, B. L. (1956). *Language, thought, and reality*. Cambridge, MA: MIT Press.

Whyte, L. L. (1960). *The unconscious before Freud*. New York: Basic Books.

Wile, D. B. (1981). *Couples therapy: A nontraditional approach*. New York: Wiley.

Wile, D. B. (1982). *Kohut, Kernberg, and accusatory interpretations*. Paper presented at the symposium "Do we have to harm clients to help them?" 1982 American Psychological Association Convention, Washington, DC.

Wile, D. B. (1984). Kohut, Kernberg, and accusatory interpretations. *Psychotherapy, 21*, 353–364.

Wile, D. B. (1985). Psychotherapy by precedent: Unexamined legacies from pre-1920 psychoanalysis. *Psychotherapy, 22*, 793–802.

Zeanah, C. H., Anders, T. F., Seifer, R., & Stern, D. N. (1989). Implications of research on infant development for psychodynamic theory and practice. *Journal of the American Academy of Child and Adolescent Psychiatry, 28*, 657–668.

Zetzel, E. R. (1956). Current concepts of transference. *International Journal of Psycho-Analysis, 37*, 369–376.

Index